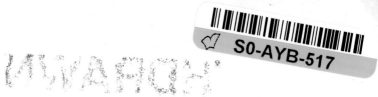

The Gift of Healing Herbs

Also by Robin Rose Bennett

Healing Magic: A Green Witch Guidebook to Conscious Living

The Gift of Healing Herbs

Plant Medicines and Home Remedies for a Vibrantly Healthy Life

Green Treasures from Mother Earth

ROBIN ROSE BENNETT

Foreword by Rosemary Gladstar

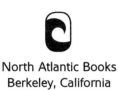

North Atlantic Books
Berkeley, California

Published by
North Atlantic Books   Cover art courtesy of Matthew Wood
P.O. Box 12327   Illustrations by Karen Flood, www.karenflood.com
Berkeley, California 94712   Cover and book design by Suzanne Albertson

Printed in the United States of America

The Gift of Healing Herbs: Plant Medicines and Home Remedies for a Vibrantly Healthy Life is sponsored by the Society for the Study of Native Arts and Sciences, a nonprofit educational corporation whose goals are to develop an educational and cross-cultural perspective linking various scientific, social, and artistic fields; to nurture a holistic view of arts, sciences, humanities, and healing; and to publish and distribute literature on the relationship of mind, body, and nature.

MEDICAL DISCLAIMER: The following information is intended for general information purposes only. Individuals should always see their health care provider before administering any suggestions made in this book. Any application of the material set forth in the following pages is at the reader's discretion and is his or her sole responsibility.

North Atlantic Books' publications are available through most bookstores. For further information, visit our website at www.northatlanticbooks.com or call 800-733-3000.

Library of Congress Cataloging-in-Publication Data
Bennett, Robin Rose.
The gift of healing herbs : plant medicines and home remedies for a vibrantly healthy life / Robin Rose Bennett.
      pages cm
   Includes bibliographical references and index.
   Summary: "Guides and inspires readers to explore herbal remedies and home recipes for health and encourages readers to discover the personal, symbolic story that lies underneath manifestations of illness"—Provided by publisher.
   ISBN 978-1-58394-762-3
1. Herbs—Therapeutic use. 2. Health. 3. Self-care, Health. I. Title. RM666.
   H33B46 2014
   615.3'21—dc23   2013037861

1 2 3 4 5 6 7 8 9 UNITED 19 18 17 16 15 14
Printed on recycled paper

For Estherelke Keyawis Kaplan (June 18, 1940–July 7, 2009),
my sister who loved Earth and the herbs so much. May we harvest
together again one day, singing our songs.

• • • • • • • • •

I am writing this book to give back, to pass along what methods, skills, understanding, and wisdom have been gifted to me in the realms of healing your body with herbs and healing your soul by re-connecting with the Earth and realigning with your true Self.

This green path slowly but surely returned me to a natural yet heretofore elusive state of joy and delight at being alive in a body on this beautiful planet Earth. That is too good to keep to myself, and thus, this book is my sharing of what has filled me up, overflowing, because it isn't mine—it's ours. My prayer and blessing for each reader is this: May you live in joy, feel vibrantly well with the help of healing plants, and freely share your unique gifts with the rest of us for your own happiness and the benefit of all beings. I am dedicated to every child on Earth having a life to smile about. Adults need to wake up for this to happen. So, let's wake up! Our children are waiting.

CONTENTS

PART I. *What Is Healing?*

PART II. *The Herbs and Your Body Systems*

PART III. *Everything Is Medicine*

PART IV. *Additional Remedies, Tips, and Thoughts on Healing*

LIST OF RECIPES

FOREWORD BY
ROSEMARY GLADSTAR

You hold in your hands a treasure, a book of green wisdom that delves deeply into the heart and soul of herbalism and retrieves an abundance of emerald jewels for us to savor. I have the good fortune to know Robin; we dance in the same herbal circles and play in the same green meadows. A true wise woman, deeply compassionate and heartfully giving, Robin Rose brings a joyful spirit and an open heart to all she does. So it's not surprising that her books on herbal healing (this is her second in what we hope will be a series) are so heartful, wisdom-filled, and imbued with spirit. I read them as much for spiritual insights as I do for herbal information; both are so richly interwoven, embedded together, wedded like body and soul.

Robin's own life was transformed by plants. In her late twenties she went through a period of great physical exhaustion and discovered she had severe anemia. While using herbs to bring her body back into balance, she also discovered a joyful awakening of her spirit: "Plants transformed my health and my life, and enriched my spiritual practice by connecting me deeply with Earth." It is this soulful or spirited side of healing that she is most attuned to, and shares so enthusiastically, so gratefully, in all she does. As you read *The Gift of Healing Herbs*, expect to journey deep into the soulful healing of the plant world.

Herbal healing is far more than just a physical system affecting our physical bodies, and the pages of *The Gift of Healing Herbs* contain far more than the simple directives found in most herb books—what herb to take for what illness, proper dosages, and safety issues. While this information is, of course, shared—there are very thorough instructions for using all of the herbs and herbal recipes—Robin goes beyond the sharing of simple recipes and erudite information about herbs. She invites us to look at healing as a soulful journey, and plants as spiritual teachers: "Soulful healing asks that while you are healing your body you look for the meaning ... as it relates to your whole being." And with simple and clear direction, she offers us techniques and gifts to do this—how to relate more deeply to the plants, how to seek their medicine gifts, how to offer them gifts in return....

And how to listen to our bodies. "Bodies don't lie," she admonishes. "They tell the truth, no matter how uncomfortable or inconvenient that truth may be." And she goes on to instruct us how to listen to and love our bodies, because, when all is said and done, "Love is what heals."

But—lest you think you'll find only wise adages and spiritual passages in Robin's book—let me assure you, in the tradition of the best of those well-written herb books, *The Gift of Healing Herbs* is filled with the practical as well. There is a full compendium of herbs, all of which Robin has worked with personally and knows well, so the writing is in-depth and thorough. There are excellent herbal recipes and remedies, and instructions for treating a variety of common health issues. There are suggested dosages and safety issues. In other words, one finds the practical advice one needs to put this information to good use. But it's how Robin shares that's so unique.

She teaches through stories. If there's a case to be made, or a teaching to offer, there's a story to tell. It's the way I learn best, and the way many people learn best—and this book is rich with story. In page after page, Robin presents heartful sharings of her own healing journey and the healing journeys of those she's worked with in her herbal practice and met through her classes. We not only learn about red clover, yarrow, motherwort, and a host of other common medicinal herbs, we actually hear real cases of how these plants have helped various individuals that Robin has personally assisted. Each person is unique, so the formulas vary and change. There's no standard "this remedy for that illness"; instead, Robin wisely attends to each person as an individual on his or her personal healing journey: "I have found that if I tend to a person's illness, rather than to a person, I treat that person as if they *are* their illness."

As I read, I kept discovering gemstones: "Healing, like life, doesn't often progress in a straight line. It spirals." Working with individuals with chronic conditions, Robin, like most compassionate healers, has learned that healing isn't always an end goal—that often the journey is the healing process.

Robin presents a practical and useful book, but the teachings are profound—and delightful as well. Imagine for a moment a little girl running joyfully towards her parents, a huge smile on her face, as she presents a single dandelion blossom. A wise child then, a wise woman now, Robin offers years of experience that she's gleaned from working soulfully with plants and people, and offers it to us so gracefully in this book, *The Gift of Healing Herbs*.

Rosemary Gladstar, author of *Herbal Healing for Women* and *The Family Herbal*, founder of the California School of Herbal Studies and United Plant Savers

PREFACE

Journal entry, New York City, 1991 What is it about plants? What is it about feeling the Earth under your feet or under your fingernails, about seeing the wild plants and grasses pop up through the cracks in the sidewalks or lining the city streets? I can't fully explain how it happens, but I know that plants help people remember how to be happy, how to feel our natural joy. I see it in eyes that begin to shine during an afternoon's medicinal plant walk in any of the city parks. Saying hello to this plant and that, discovering their virtues, uncovering our own. Plants love us. They help us reclaim our health and our whole selves. Plants are healers.

I WAS NOT BROUGHT UP TO KNOW THE EARTH in intimate detail. No one I can remember from my childhood ever suggested that the land I lived on and was surrounded by contained anything important to me. My sense of kinship was connected to my house, my bedroom (my one almost personal space), my family, and my friends. I had no conscious sense of connection to the wild; the closest I came was that I deeply loved the trees in our small suburban backyard.

Recently I was guiding a walk focused on identifying and learning about wild medicinal plants in the woods near my home in New Jersey. My friend Marian was there. We've known each other since we were three years old and our families lived a few doors down from each other. When I introduced everyone to a sassafras tree, Marian excitedly announced that there had been a sassafras tree in my backyard when we were growing up. I told her that I didn't remember any sassafras tree there. Surely she must be mistaken. But would I have known if it had been there? It's not a tall and impressive-looking tree, and since no one at home would have taken me outside and pointed out the wonder of three different-shaped leaves on a single tree, or titillated my senses by giving me a leaf to rub and smell for the unforgettable root beer-like fragrance, I could easily have missed the inconspicuous sassafras tree. I have since learned that this tree is gifted at turning itself invisible—but that's another story for another time!

I sit now and try to remember whether there really was a sassafras tree growing behind the house in which I grew up. These days I love sassafras so much it amazes me to think I might have grown up with one right in my own small backyard. I gather sassafras leaves for tea every summer and fall, and dig some roots, too.

But I don't remember this tree at all because I didn't know her, though I clearly remember a tall oak tree I was especially fond of, a young maple tree out front, and an old weeping willow tree out back that I dearly loved. Despite my tearful protests, the willow was eventually chopped down to make room for a patio. I enjoyed the patio, but have never forgotten the lovely willow.

It is only over the past twenty-five years of my life that I've become aware of the gift of healing herbs, Earth's green treasures—her medicinal and nourishing herbs, plants, and trees. For the first twenty-five years of my life, I was not conscious of the plants at all. I knew, certainly, that trees and plants and wildflowers were beautiful, but not much more.

When I was first heading upstate from my home in New York City to study herbal medicine at the Wise Woman Center in Saugerties, New York, my father told me he could understand my wanting to learn about herbal medicine (a progressive attitude in 1985), but he didn't quite understand why I needed to go and live in the country and learn about *plants*. I tried to answer him but didn't do a very good job. I knew it was important, but I didn't know why—or if I did, I couldn't articulate it, I was that disconnected. Even though I knew it intellectually, I didn't really, truly understand that the herbs I could buy in jars and bottles were plants, and that there were things I needed to learn about and from plants! I did know it though, in my gut and in my bones.

The most telling compliment I receive upon teaching an herbal medicine class is, "You're helping me remember something I feel like I've always known." It was the compliment I gave to my first plant-medicine teachers, and exactly how I still feel anytime I learn the truth about something fundamental.

The book is divided into four main sections, followed by a resource list.

The first section explores the spiritual nature of health and illness, and offers detailed directions and practical guidelines for making every form of herbal preparation mentioned, from infusions to steam baths to smoke blends.

The second section delves into the plants, our body's systems, and the relationship of each body system to the primal elements of Earth, Air, Fire, and Water.

The third section invites us to realize that "everything is medicine," as we celebrate the abundance of healing herbs found in our kitchens' spice racks and pantries.

The fourth section provides the "how-to's" of herbal aid for wounds and bruises, additional remedies, recipes, and tips for home and travel, and concludes with some thought-provoking "Ideas about Healing."

NOTE TO THE READER

A CAVEAT/CONFESSION ABOUT MY OWN recipes throughout this book:

I never make anything the same way twice, whether it's dinner or medicine, so I'm trying my best to give you recipes with actual quantities (and names!); but the truth is that I don't make these blends exactly the same way over and over again. So start with the recipes the way they are written, and as you get more and more familiar with the herbs you can apply your own intuition and artistry to the blends and proportions, and add or subtract your own touches.

I also highly recommend using simples, or one herb at a time. This is an excellent way to get to feel and know the effects of the herbs in your own body. My best recipes are created when I physically have my hands on the herbs. If you like exactness, when you get a recipe exactly how you want it, write it down. I admit I wish I'd been writing mine down throughout the years. This book would have taken a lot less time to write!

A general tip is that for best results when you are making medicine, it is important to focus and be totally attentive to what you are doing. Imagine that you were sitting with one of the greatest healers in the world. You wouldn't be talking on the phone or watching television while you sat with them, would you? No, you'd be listening. So listen while you make medicine. Or chant or sing. This opens other channels of receptivity to wisdom.

Finally, the term "traditional medicine" is often used incorrectly, misapplied to modern (conventional, allopathic, Western) medicine. Throughout *The Gift of Healing Herbs* I refer to herbal healing and other ancient systems accurately, as "traditional medicine."

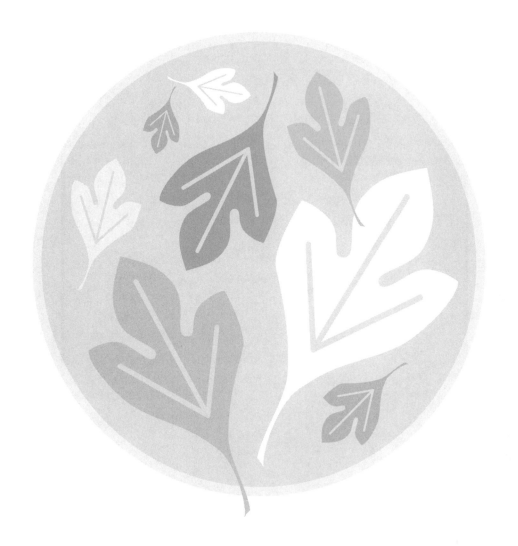

PART I

What Is Healing?

Here's a "Greet the New Day" ritual that I do each morning to get my day off to a lovely start. Ideally, stand outside and face each of the directions as you chant to the elements, or turn slowly in a circle before you begin, or walk around a medicine wheel if you have one handy. The elements are what we are made of, and all around Earth they provide a universal framework for our place within and as a part of nature. This chant can be said indoors too, of course, but at least open a window.

Simple "Greet the New Day" Ritual

A spoken-word Earth chant

Good morning, day!
Dearest Earth, Air, Fire, and Water
I am *Robin, Gaia's Daughter.

Below, Above, and the Center—
Mother Nature you're my mentor.

From below
And from above,
Infuse my heart
And soul with love.

Pure joy fills me
Through and through
When I walk in
Harmony with you.

*Fill in your own name if you want to say this spoken chant to your own new day. If you're male, after you greet the elements, change the next line to, "I greet the new day that's begun; I am _____, Gaia's son!" Or make up your own rhyme—or don't worry about rhyming at all. It's your sincerity that matters.

What Is Soulful Healing?

*Listening to the Voice of the Soul
within the Body's Symptoms*

Soulful healing asks, while you are healing your body with herbs from Earth, that you look for the meaning in what is happening within your body as it relates to your whole being. This is not a whiny or despairing "Why is this happening to me?" or a one-size-fits-all New Age generalization that you and you alone created your reality. The questions are: "What is the deeper teaching in this experience?"; "What is here for me?"; and "How can I make this experience an ally for my growth and transformation?"

Patterns form invisibly and then descend into form. Life is a web of meaningful patterns. It takes an active, open curiosity and passion to arrive clearly at your truth. And it must be *your* truth for it to have any import for you. When you are willing to "go there" the most magical healings happen. Miracles happen every day, but they often require the courage to look inward.

It can be hard work to release limiting patterns of belief that you find—beliefs that have a part in keeping you ill. Bodies always tell the truth. "I'm fine, but I have a headache." I feel fine, but my stomach is upset." Fine? Really? I don't think so. Being in a body, it is as if you were born with a fierce and loving teacher who is within you and yet also well-known for helping prevent or relieve pain and swelling in the joints. This wild, native medicinal plant is an indigenous "weed" that grows from Maine to Florida and as far west as Texas. It is best-loved and most often used in the American South, where "poke salat" made from the leaves is a traditional food. This dish needs to be prepared carefully, before any red appears in the stalks, and even then must be cooked in two or three changes of water for it to be safe and healthy to eat. Both roots and berries are considered medicinal but should be used with caution and only taken with guidance.

· · · · ● · · · ·

One additional point I'd like to make here is that when we read herbal books, there are long lists of "anti" herbs—antibacterial, antiviral, antiparasitic, antimicrobial, antifungal, and so on. I use these terms, too, as in anti-inflammatory and antidepressant. But I wonder—where are all the "pro" herbs? Can't we re-name some of these terms? How about pro-circulatory, pro-respiratory, pro-digestive, spirit-lifting, etc?

I think affirming what the herbs can help us with is more in keeping with the energy and spirit of herbal medicine! So I will be inserting affirming names of categories for the healing properties of herbs wherever possible throughout *The Gift of Healing Herbs.*

Healing is a journey. Mark Twain said, "A real journey is one where, halfway through, you wish you were home." Healing can surely be like that, whether you are challenged by chronic asthma, stuck in bed with a migraine headache, or dealing with an illness like multiple sclerosis. Here is where it becomes so important to remember that evolutionary intelligence is at work in your body's natural orientation and impulse to heal. The body is brilliantly designed for and always oriented toward healing. I can't count the number of times I've seen and heard about people who got better though they had conditions they were told *absolutely could not improve.*

I'm not saying that physical healing *always* takes place, but true healers approach the mystery of healing with humility and the knowledge that *nothing is impossible.* I have always felt this to be true, and when I heard Oaxacan midwife/herbalist, Doña Enriqueta Contreras utter these exact words not long ago I got "truth bumps" everywhere. (Seneca Elder Twylah Nitsch taught me that what we call "goose bumps" are actually "truth bumps." Yes!) To put it in the affirmative, *anything is possible.*

Bodies always tell the truth. They give us hints of how to listen for it, and to recognize it when we hear or see it. I keep a fortune from a cookie on my writing table, which says, "Impossible is a word found only in the dictionary of fools." Amen.

I suggest that this journey toward personal insight be undertaken with as much kindness, compassion, and humor as you can muster, because it is difficult. Soulful healing takes courage. However, it is always liberating and can even be fun. Reconnecting with the patterns of meaning in your own healing journey will inevitably, ultimately, increase your joy in being alive. This approach helps you to heal your soul while you heal your body, and that healing allows you to reconnect with and reintegrate your whole self.

Like other pivotal events in our lives that cause us to stop, physical illness calls us to remember our purpose here, to remember what matters to us and what (often simple) things bring us joy. Visionary astrologer Caroline Casey said, "Shock transforms the circle of habit into the spiral of growth." Illness can be that transformative shock if we allow it to be, whether the illness is a "well-timed" common cold ("well-timed" meaning disruptive, coming at a "bad" time) or the now all-too-common cancer, or anything else.

For years I kept a letter to the editor of *The Sun* magazine up on my refrigerator. A woman wrote that a man she knew was diagnosed with a terminal illness and given no hope of recovery. He had always wanted to live a simple life, living on a small boat, sailing around with few possessions to tend to. So he decided it was now or never. He sold what he owned, went to Florida, bought a small sailboat, and finally began living the life he'd always wanted. Some time later his doctor called with great news. He'd been misdiagnosed; not only was he not dying of the disease but he didn't even have it. His x-rays had gotten mixed up with someone else's. The writer concluded with, "I often think of that guy, sailing around in his little boat, enjoying his life, all because he believed he was going to die one day."

can do—she offers her help to let the light of love shine through your body as she aids you on your healing journey.

There are many more physical, chemical, clinical details that could have been added to these briefest of plant biographies, but this was the information I chose to provide my friend with. I came up with this idea of introducing him to each plant in this way because he had never responded well to herbal recipes or simples no matter how appropriate they were; or, rather, he'd respond beautifully for one or two days, and then they would stop helping him. This was the first time that herbs had helped him on a long-term basis. I think this was because they had become spiritual allies rather than mere physical substances. He'd always felt more at home in the realm of spirit.

Jim took two droppers of the blend in boiled water or tea, three times daily, for about nine months. He also planted a hawthorn tree, which he grew to love as he tended it. He felt that the herbs helped him greatly in his remarkable recovery process, which also included supportive friends and family, physical therapy, acupuncture, sound-healing work, counseling, and his own relentless determination to regain his full well-being, especially his mobility and speech. He used the herbal tincture blend until he intuitively felt that it was time to stop.

The stroke had damaged the part of his brain connected with swallowing, so he sometimes struggled with a feeling of choking. He continued to have weakness in that area, and with breathing in general. This had been an ongoing vulnerability most of his life, and was exacerbated by the fact that he currently lived at an altitude over 12,000 feet.

About a year passed before he called and asked me to help him address this symptom too with herbs. I made some hyssop and elderberry syrup and sent it to him. He liked it so much that he decided to continue taking it, so I taught him how to make it for himself. The syrup recipe is below.

I also suggested mullein; I had introduced him to the mullein plants in his area when I last visited. He began to take mullein flower tincture internally, and to massage mullein flower oil on his throat. He went outside and communed with the wild mullein plants nearby. These herbs became great herbal allies for him.

Jim recovered nearly full functioning in his movement and speech. His medical team had prophesied that this level of recovery was highly unlikely, though possible, and if it did happen, that it would take far longer than it actually took him.

ELDERBERRY-HYSSOP SYRUP

1 cup dried hyssop leaves and flowers

½ cup dried elder berries

4 tablespoons local honey per cup taken, or to taste

Put the herbs in a half-gallon jar. Cover them with boiling water, and steep for 8–12 hours. Decant the herbs, squeeze them out, and compost them. Put the infusion into an open saucepan and decoct it over the lowest possible heat, slowly steaming off half the liquid. When the liquid is at half-volume, take the pot off the heat and add honey.

Take this syrup straight, by the tablespoon, or stir it into water, tea, or infusion. Use three times daily, or more as needed, to help with bronchial irritation and inflammation, to facilitate productive coughing, and to strengthen the respiratory and immune systems.

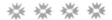

The perfect approach for one person could be another person's total turn-off, or simply a foreign language that doesn't compute because it seems incomprehensible. Yes, we're all the same, and yes, we're all different. It's so important to honor your uniqueness, to learn what works best for you regarding what helps you to heal.

When you begin to know who you truly are, how precious you truly are, you return to a sense of interconnection and oneness with the web of life, with no fear of losing yourself. You recognize that this web includes a place for each of us and all our relations, and you are likely to feel your heart fill with gratitude for the generous plant people, the green healers who ask for so little and offer us so much.

Some Spiritual Herbal Allies

Herbs can be taken in a variety of creative ways when calling on them as spiritual allies. The following herbs can be imbibed as teas and infusions, bathed in, used as flower essences or anointing oils, taken as tinctures, or put into a medicine bag that you wear. You could also put freshly harvested branches, leaves, stalks, and/or flowers in a vase on your altar or bedside table to share in their essence and presence while you meditate or sleep and dream with them.

Cedar, Grandmother (*Thuja* species) is for divine alignment, for creating sacred space both inside and outside the body, for healing from trauma (especially sexual and/or violent trauma), and even for invisibility when needed.

Elder (*Sambucus nigra* and other species). Guide through the chaos of transformation; helps you connect with the wisdom of your ancestors.

Flowing Cherry (*Prunus* species). Commonly called "weeping cherry," this tree tells me she is flowing, not weeping. She helps release habits of sadness—the places within you where, when they are triggered, you automatically and habitually get stuck in sadness and despair.

Ginkgo (*Ginkgo biloba*) is for journeying into the past or future, developing the gift of prophecy, retrieving ancient wisdom, rebirthing yourself, astral traveling, recalling past lives, and for clear mental focus.

Hawthorn (*Crataegus* species). Traditionally known as a magical tree, long held sacred by the fairies, hawthorn is helpful for claiming the physical body as sacred space, for marrying sexuality with spirituality, and for learning to have healthy boundaries without defensiveness. She supports the ability to stand one's ground and to claim one's space, and strengthens the ability to say no while keeping the heart light, free, and open.

Kwanzan Cherry *(Prunus serulata)*. The flowers from this familiar cultivated Japanese tree share and evoke the energy and spirit of pure joy.

Lavender (*Lavandula* species*)* helps bring ease, forgiveness, and sweetness, helping you make peace with any bitterness that's been held and directed toward yourself, circumstances, or other people.

Linden (*Tilia* species). Dance into other dimensions and other worlds; protective, comforting, and magical guide through times of grief.

Mugwort, aka Cronewort *(Artemisia vulgaris)*. The Anglo-Saxons called this plant "eldest of worts"; she opens the third eye for insight, wisdom, and perception of the dimension of beauty, helps with night-dream recall, and reawakens dreams of the heart.

Mullein *(Verbascum thapsus)* helps you open to the present moment, stand up for yourself, embrace male and female within, and see far and wide for a broader overview of your own situation.

Oak (*Quercus* species) is a sacred tree to people in many cultures. Traditionally, Druids met in oak groves, and contemporary Native American teachers from South and Central America also consider oak to be the "chief standing person." Oak's Celtic name, *duir*, means "door." Any part of oak can be helpful in crossing through the doorway of conventional time and space into the liminal space between the worlds to access spiritual guidance.

Rose (*Rosa* species) opens the heart to forgiveness of self and others, and to boundless self-love, expands one's point of view to see others' perspectives with more compassion and understanding, and stimulates the open-heartedness that helps open the mind.

White pine *(Pinus strobus)*. Tree of peace; helps relieve the tendency toward martyrdom and perfectionism; supports flexibility and self-esteem.

Wild carrot *(Daucus carota)*. A shape-shifting ally helpful for learning the art of shape-shifting, flowing with change, healing sexual confusion, supporting creativity, and learning to focus intention, while developing playfulness and exuberance; it opens the third eye and crown chakras, and increases awareness of energy and oneness.

Any plant or tree, anywhere, that ever calls to you in that way.

Herbal Preparations

The following are detailed descriptions of a variety of ways I've found effective for preparing herbal medicines for internal and external use, and are the methods I use most often.

Every herbalist has her or his own favorite methods, just as every cook has her own style in the kitchen. No one's method is "wrong." I love to do things in ways I find aesthetically pleasing or downright beautiful, and I'm open to learning new things and trying out new suggestions. When I discover a better way to do something, I adapt. I want to be as healthy as possible, so I always seek the best yet easiest ways to prepare and use my herbal medicines. I have other things I need, want, and like to do in my life, just as you do.

Helpful Tips and Reminders

Please note that all tea, infusion and decoction recipes are made using *dried* herbs unless otherwise specified.

Most tinctures, vinegars, honeys, and oils are made with *fresh* herbs unless otherwise specified.

Herbs that are burned for their smoke are always used *dried.*

Herbs used in crafting pillows or bags are always used *dried.*

For topical applications: A compress is when the herbal material is wrapped inside a cloth and the cloth is applied to the body. A poultice is when the herbal material is touching the body directly. A fomentation is when a cloth is dipped into an herbal tea or infusion and is then applied to the body. All of these topical preparations can be made from dried herbs with boiling water poured over them, or fresh herbs mashed or chewed, though some herbs or applications will prefer one over the other. When this is the case it is noted in the specific recipe. A tip about making any fresh plant-leaf poultice: If you have no access to boiling water and it isn't a plant you can easily or palatably chew up to soften, rub the plant briskly between your palms to help open the plant's cell walls and release its medicinal properties before applying it.

Honey preparations don't need to be refrigerated.

Another preparation that doesn't need to be refrigerated is a tincture. A tincture is a preparation where the herb is steeped in alcohol to extract its medicinal qualities.

Please only buy vodka or brandy in glass bottles. Otherwise, as the plastic breaks down, it will leach into the vodka or brandy that is the menstruum for your tincture, and you don't want that in your medicine. "Menstruum" is the term used in herbal medicine for any liquid solvent used to extract the medicinal properties from your herbs.

When infusing herbs in alcohol, vinegar, or oil, keep them in a cool, dark place away from heat sources, moisture, and direct sunlight. When a recipe calls for "decanting," pour the liquid off the herbs and then squeeze out the herbs to get the last drops of healing substance from them. Carefully pour the liquid off and squeeze out the spent plant material, to get every precious bit of liquid medicine out of it. You can do this in your hands, or wring it out fully in a piece of muslin or cheesecloth. Don't just press down into a metal or bamboo strainer because you will not get much out of the herbs that way, and you are likely to break the strainer. And be careful to get the liquid into your jar!

All water-based preparations need to be refrigerated. All the other preparations should *not* be refrigerated (except for optional refrigeration of honey balls).

To avoid mold and spoilage, *do not* wash fresh plant material that is going to be made into an infused oil, with the possible exception of roots.

If freshly dug roots are washed, chop them and let them dry completely before pouring oil over them, or they will mold. If possible, harvest them when it's not muddy, and simply dry-brush them clean. Personally, I don't wash plants that I am making into medicine, as this causes them to lose medicinal chemicals, oils, vitamins, and more as soon as the water is added to them. I make a practice of picking my medicine plants as carefully as possible so that they are clean.

When you harvest and make preparations, be aware that everything you are thinking, feeling, and talking about becomes part of your medicine. Gathering and making medicine is a simple process, but it is also a sacred act. Be mindful. Be open-hearted. Your medicines will reflect this and be stronger for it. I like to sing when I gather and make medicine, so the medicine has music in it, too. Create a sense of sacred space when you craft medicine, and when you decant it.

Harvesting

Teaching harvesting is something that is best done hands-on, out in the lawn, field, or forest, or by the seashore, and so is beyond the scope of this book. Some things need to be shown and seen, in person. However, I will include some general practical and philosophical information about wild harvesting here—and strongly encourage you to go outside and meet the plants. They are eager to meet you!

Herbalists love to guide people on weed walks. Find someone in your area who is knowledgeable, and take a walk together. It's fun and empowering to learn what is growing around you.

Harvesting food and medicine from the wild, even if the wild is your backyard, offers endless teachings on mindfulness. Foraging wild plants for food and medicine invites you to be in the present moment, aware of what is going on in front of, underneath, and all around you. You must watch for insects, soil conditions, animals, birds, and of course for specific details that let you know you are gathering the correct plant. It is important that you learn if there are plants that are illegal to harvest in your region, or if certain plants are deemed at risk or endangered. United

Plant Savers (see Resources, page 511) is a great organization for such information. Most but not all of the plants in *The Gift of Healing Herbs* are common, abundant weeds, making them far less likely to be on such lists.

Always be mindful of how much of a plant you are taking. When in doubt, be conservative, as in conservation-minded. How much to take will depend on the plant being gathered, and how much there is of it in the area. If plants are endangered or sparse, please leave them. Generally, take no more than ten to fifteen percent of one type of plant from a given area. This will allow the plant community to continue to grow and thrive. If a plant is considered invasive—dandelion, for example—and thus possibly subject to herbicides and other such reactionary measures, then gather it freely! In public lands like parks, you can call the parks department to check if they have done any spraying recently. And while you're calling, voice your objections to such dangerous practices!

One of the great gifts that harvesting provides is the opportunity to slow down. I remember a student on a summer weed walk in Central Park saying, "You shouldn't call these weed *walks*, you should call these weed *sits*. We never go more than a few steps before you spot another plant to talk about, and then we sit down again!"

I apologized for "false advertising," and she protested, "Oh no, I love it. I am usually never this slow, calm, and focused. It's great!"

Still, we can make mistakes. After all, we're human. So I want to tell you that when you gather plants there are at least four times for you to fully observe what you are harvesting for medicine:

1. upon observing the plants, before gathering them;
2. while gathering the plants;
3. while hanging the herbs up to dry; and
4. when taking the herbs down to use them or put them away.

First, check the plants, and make certain that you've correctly identified them. Carefully check that they aren't infested with bugs or cocoons, that they are devoid of obvious fungal infections, and that they are vibrantly healthy.

Increasing your observational skills is vitally important. It awakens your awareness of and respect for other forms of life, and opens your eyes and all your senses so that you can take in and embrace life more fully. As you practice, this helps you yourself become more fully alive.

I enjoy using harvesting as a form of moving meditation and mindfulness practice. For example, when I'm harvesting a tree's leaves and one leaf falls to the ground, I won't pick another leaf until I've located the one that fell, and picked it up. On the purely practical level, I know the leaf will nourish the ground and doesn't need me to pick it up, but it is a way of showing my respect for what the tree is freely gifting to me. These are free classes on mindfulness, led by an ever-changing roster of master teachers. Their only fee for these teachings is my full attention and appreciation, and since these continue to serve me in every area of my life, the benefits far outweigh the cost.

I always offer a "give-away" when I'm harvesting plants for medicine. It's respectful to give a gift to the grandmother plant. Choose the plant that looks the oldest, largest, and/or healthiest, and ask for her permission to harvest from her family, and for her blessing on your harvest. This reminds you that you are receiving something of worth. The reality is that anything you have to offer was given to you by the Earth in the first place, wasn't it? So the gift is symbolic—but the request isn't. After you ask, listen. If you get the feeling you shouldn't harvest the plant you came there to gather, listen to that feeling, and don't do it.

I encourage anyone who is going out to wildcraft (harvest wild plants from the land) to create a give-away bag or bundle filled with one or more herbs you love. Tobacco is a traditional give-away of many indigenous peoples because it's used in sacred ceremonies, and therefore highly valued. I like to include herbs that I use in ceremony and highly value, such as rose, lavender, white sage, or artemisia in my give-away bundles. I've had students who've given away gifts of substances they hold in high esteem ranging from chocolate-chip cookies to bagel chips! Small crystals can be given, or water can be shared. You can offer a hair from your head, or a song, or your silence. It doesn't always have to be an object, as long as it is meaningful and valuable to you.

I've had—and I'm sure will continue to have—many opportunities to practice forgiving and accepting myself when I mess up, for example, by bringing home a harvest bag full of bugs. Fortunately, I've found that the plants themselves are quite forgiving and accepting. I am happy to spend my life being guided by them, and learning how to be present in the moment, the precious *now* that is all there truly is.

Basic Supplies for Your Herbal Kitchen

If you simply plan to make teas, infusions, and decoctions, you'll need:

Ingredients
Dried herbs

Water

Tools
Several wide-mouthed quart and half-gallon glass jars with good lids

Stainless-steel, coated-enamel, or glass saucepans and soup pots with lids

Small and large fine-mesh strainers

Optional Tools
Wide-mouth funnel (helpful for pouring boiling water into infusion jars)

Kitchen scissors

Cheesecloth (unbleached)

Wooden chopsticks—handy for many things including poking down your medicines and taking vertical measurements when you're steaming off liquid to make a decoction (see below).

BASIC-PLUS SUPPLIES FOR YOUR HERBAL KITCHEN
If you also want to make your own syrups, infused oils, ointments, tinctures, honeys, elixirs, and more, then you'll need the following.

green all year. The larch tree, also known as tamarack *(Larix laricina)*, wouldn't be used for a fresh winter infusion because that conifer drops its needles in the fall, when the deciduous trees shed their leaves.

I use a minimum of one cup of fresh herbs, well cut-up, for each quart of infusion, and then steep it to taste, depending on the herb. With the exception of the evergreens and black birch twigs, when I make infusions with fresh herbs such as mints and lemon balm fresh from the summer garden, it is more for general tonifying and tasty beverage teas than for medicinal brews.

AMOUNT OF STEEPING TIME

The timing of steeping infusions can be tricky; it can enhance or actually ruin your medicine. Too little steeping can leave your medicine weak, tasteless and, at worst, ineffective. Too much time can make a good infusion turn sour, or cause oils in it to turn rancid. When you're taking herbs internally, you want their properties extracted into your water or chosen menstruum—hence the long steeping times. Some helpful guidelines are given below. Still, I find there is no substitute for experience and learning optimal preparations plant-by-plant. There are always exceptions to the rules, much as in cooking.

General Guidelines for Steeping Times

Flowers: Steep 1–2 hours (though some can't steep this long, while others stand up to longer steeping—see list below)

Leaves and stalks: Steep about 8 hours

Roots and barks: Steep at least 8 hours

As you can see, steeping time varies! When plants are rich in the volatile oils that make them aromatic, it's important not to over-steep them. On the other hand, some hard berries and most fresh evergreens do best when steeped for a very long time.

Some specific exceptions are:

- Calendula blossoms: 30–60 minutes
- Chamomile: 5 minutes
- Evergreen needles: 8–24 hours

- Ginger root: 1–2 hours
- Goldenrod: 20 minutes
- Hawthorn berries, elder berries and rose hips: 8–12 (up to 24) hours
- Jasmine: 3 minutes
- Lavender: 20 minutes
- Linden flowers: 8 hours
- Mushrooms: at least 24 hours
- Red clover flowers: 8 hours
- Rooibos: 3–6 minutes
- Rose: 75 minutes
- Rosemary: 15–20 minutes
- Garden sage: 1 hour
- Most seeds: 15–20 minutes
- Yarrow flowers: 1 hour (can be brewed longer)

Simple Meditative Infusion Ritual

While your herbs are steeping,
Gently twirl your jar back and forth, back and forth,
Inviting magical energy to enter into your infusion.
Watch the plants dance and swirl as you twirl the jar.
Let their beauty and flowing movements in the water
beckon you to daydream....

DECANTING INFUSIONS

When your infusion has steeped for its full length of time, set a strainer on top of a pot of an appropriate size for the volume of liquid in the herbs. Line the strainer with a piece of unbleached cheesecloth, if you like. Pour off the liquid through the strainer into the pot.

Squeeze the herbs thoroughly, either with your hands or by wringing the herbs in the cheesecloth, until you can't get any more liquid out. Compost the plant material. You can refrigerate your infusion for later use, or heat it up in a saucepan on the stove and pour the infusion into a stainless-steel or glass-lined thermos (no plastic, please) for drinking throughout the day. When you refrigerate your infusion, it can last anywhere from several days to weeks, depending on the herb.

Don't use a microwave oven to reheat your herbal infusion, unless that's the only way you'll use your herbs at all. Microwaves scramble the molecules of anything that is heated in them, and then your body doesn't assimilate the medicine or food as well. If you don't have time to decant your infusion when it's ready, put it in the refrigerator with the herbs in it, and decant it when you get a chance. If you want to just pour off some infusion to drink before straining it, you can do that, and then strain the rest when you can.

There are some herbs that will spoil if they sit too long. A general tip is that aromatic flowers like chamomile, lavender, and roses can't sit too long without going off.

Simple Teas

Generally speaking, tea is made as an enjoyable beverage rather than as a medicine. Simple teas are made by steeping a small amount of herbs—about one teaspoon per cup—for a short time, from five to fifteen minutes. And though some simple teas are indeed medicinal, I use the term "tea" to refer more to an herbal beverage than an herbal medicine. A simple tea can be made using any herb—fresh or dry, loose or in a tea bag. As with infusions, though, there are exceptions. For example, if I steep chamomile tea for five minutes, it is already medicinal, and the same is true with jasmine. But these are the exceptions and not the rule. If I steep stinging nettle or red raspberry for five minutes, I'll have a nice beverage tea, but won't get the range of benefits these herbs will offer as a full-strength infusion.

DOSAGE

When you are well, drink one or two cups of an infusion daily for nourishment (vitamins, minerals, and chlorophyll) and enjoyment. Specific infusions can be chosen as seasonal tonics, as medicine for an organ or body system that may need extra help, or for maintenance of health after a condition has improved.

When ill, drink two to four cups a day of infusions, either making them individually or filling a thermos to sip throughout the day. Drink more if desired, but generally no less than two cups daily, at least five days a week, for best results.

Decoctions

I enjoy making decoctions. Begin by making and decanting an herbal infusion. The pot of decanted infusion is put on the stove, uncovered, on the lowest possible heat. Slowly steam off half the liquid. How long this takes depends on how much liquid you start with; the larger the volume you're steaming off, the longer it will take.

This preparation requires you to be reasonably close at hand and attentive so you don't steam off all the liquid, lose your medicine, and burn your pot as the final insult-to-injury.

In the winter I put an open decoction pot on the woodstove to steam off the liquid at a nice, slow pace. A chopstick is a handy tool for medicine-making; in this instance I simply scratch a little mark in the stick to denote the height of the liquid when I begin. I then check periodically, and when it's halfway down the chopstick, I know that my simple decoction is done. This method makes your infusion twice as strong each time the liquid is halved.

If I halve it again, it will be four times stronger, and so on. This method is great for bitter brews that you want to be able to take in smaller quantities, such as for children or those who don't want to or can't drink as much infusion as they need for effective healing.

A decoction, being a water-based preparation, needs to be refrigerated. How long it will last depends primarily on what herb was decocted. For example, a pine needle decoction might last for six months, whereas a dandelion root decoction might last for only a month. Look at it, and smell it. If it has fermented and gone "off," you'll know it is no longer good, the same as if your milk has soured. A decoction can be used as is, preserved with the alcohol of your choice (about a tablespoon of alcohol for every four ounces of decoction), or it can become the base for syrup.

Syrups

A decoction can easily be turned into syrup by adding a sweetener. That's really all there is to it, though syrup often also contains alcohol. My favorite sweetener is honey because it's medicinal as well as delicious. It also helps preserve the syrup.

White sugar is traditional, but I never use that in my medicinal syrups. Other options include raw sugar, sugar cane, vegetable glycerin, maple syrup, agave (highly processed, so I don't recommend it) and, for iron-tonic syrups, blackstrap molasses.

Alcohol preserves syrup better than a sweetener alone. When the decoction is complete, take it off the heat and stir in your sweetener. I don't like my syrups overly sweet, so I use approximately one tablespoon of honey per cup of syrup. (Many traditional recipes call for equal parts of decoction and sugar by weight; I find this undrinkable!)

I generally add about one ounce of alcohol for each cup of syrup. Brandy will add an anti-spasmodic quality to your syrup. It works especially nicely if you're making the syrup for spasmodic coughs, or the muscle cramps that can often accompany them—it's like an old-fashioned hot toddy with an herbal twist. Speaking of herbal twists, I also like to use an herbal brandy tincture as the preserving alcohol, so that the additional medicinal qualities of whatever herb I've tinctured in brandy are added to my syrup.

I keep my syrups refrigerated, and find that they last for about three months without alcohol, and six months to a year with alcohol, though these timeframes vary.

DOSAGE

Take decoctions and syrups by the tablespoon. For a preventative or tonic medicine, take one or two tablespoons daily. For an acute situation, such as a cough that comes with a cold, you might take a tablespoon every few hours, up to about eight tablespoons or so, as needed.

Herbal Baths

Baths are a great way to take your medicine. They are one of my favorite ways to use herbs for physical and spiritual healing. Skin is the largest organ of assimilation and elimination, so even though soaking in an herbal bath is external medicine, it affects you through-and-through and is a natural, pleasurable way to practice herbal self-care. Immersing yourself in herbal-infused water in your bathtub encourages you to relax and take time just for you.

A sponge bath is good when you can't get into a tub. It can be done over the whole body, or targeted to specific areas. A sitz bath is where you sit in a basinful of herbal infusion with the liquid to just above your hips. This encourages circulation in the pelvic area, and can be useful for healing problems in that area of the body. Hand and foot baths are taken to benefit hands or feet, of course, but can also be used as an avenue to circulate herbs to wherever they're needed. A foot bath is a practical way to give healing herbs when a person can't eat or hold anything down, such as in diarrhea or vomiting from flu, or when someone is too weak to ingest much at all.

When taking a full-body bath, I suggest adding a half-gallon of full-strength infusion to your bath water, and soaking in it for a minimum of twenty minutes. Another way to prepare an herbal bath, if you don't have time to steep an infusion, is to bring herb(s) to a boil in a half-gallon or more of water, and then simmer them for perhaps an hour.

Sitz, sponge, hand, and foot baths generally require about one quart of infusion—half the amount of herbs as for the full body. No matter what kind of bath you're preparing, pour the liquid through a fine strainer into your bathtub (or bowl for your hands, or bucket for your feet), and enjoy.

then fill the jar the rest of the way with your chosen menstruum—vodka, brandy, or other alcohol.

Please note that there are different schools of thought regarding what proof of alcohol is "right" to use for medicine-making. I know herbalists who say that nothing less than ninety-five percent alcohol (that's 190-proof) makes good medicine. This spirit can be used as is, or diluted with water to achieve a lower proof but, again, that is not the simpler's method that I advocate for home remedies. There are some traditional herbalists who teach that anything stronger than wine hurts the spirit of the plant. The first group says their way is scientifically verifiable by measuring extracted constituents. The other group says the strong alcohol smothers the spirit of the plant rather than bringing it out.

Which is the truth? I can't speak to alcohol proofs, but I do know from my own experience that the love and respect you put into growing and gathering the plants and making the medicine is the strongest "proof" of all, and will create healing medicines no matter what alcohol is used. I believe that tinctures should taste as much like the plant as possible. When the alcohol is too weak or too strong, you taste the alcohol more than the herb.

I like to use 100-proof vodka because it is half alcohol and half water, and therefore will extract both water-soluble and alcohol-soluble constituents of the plants. I also like using brandy to tincture certain herbs. A basic tenet of the wise-woman approach to healing is to use what is accessible and abundant, and to use the best-quality medicine and other ingredients that you can afford. Vodka and brandy are generally accessible, so make your medicine, bless it, and give thanks for it. It will be fine medicine for healing, filled with the power of your love.

MAKING SINGLE- OR MULTIPLE-HERB TINCTURES

I usually, but not as an absolute rule, make single-herb tinctures, and continue to suggest this approach to budding and experienced medicine makers alike. On the practical side, this gives you a better opportunity to get to really know the herb you're using—its taste, texture, character, and effects. It also gives you the greatest flexibility in adjusting dosages.

Spiritually or energetically, I have the feeling that when the herbal preparation is itself whole and complete, its presence in the tincture blend you craft with other herbs will be more powerful, just as, when you mix herbs together into a tea or infusion, they are first simply themselves. I liken it to two whole people coming together to share themselves, rather than two people who feel incomplete trying to complete themselves through each other. It's healthier for two people to join together as two wholes rather than two halves trying to become whole; the two help each other grow, and become greater than the sum of their individual parts.

I apply this thinking to most of my plant tinctures: The plant has its own integrity before it's tinctured into a long-term relationship with the menstruum. But I can understand why some people like to move them into relationship with other plants more quickly by tincturing the fresh herbs together. If you are strongly attracted to making multiple-herb tinctures, I suggest you work with the plants individually first; but there are no absolutes in herbalism. Total consistency would represent a lack of imagination!

DECANTING TINCTURES

Let tinctures sit for at least six weeks before using them. It's not necessary to shake them if you've torn or cut up the fresh plant material well, but you may choose to shake or twirl them from time to time, or sing to them, or hold them in silence, to help infuse them with your intentions and healing love and energy. If you have used dried herbs to make tincture, then I do recommend shaking them.

I like to turn my bottles upside-down and right-side-up, over and over again in a swinging motion like a seat on a Ferris wheel. Tinctures can sit with herbs in them almost indefinitely without evaporating or spoiling, but I like to decant my tinctures the same year I make them unless a preparation whispers or sings to me to leave it longer.

For decanting, get a beaker, measuring cup, or other pitcher large enough to hold the contents of your tincture bottle. It should ideally have a pour spout and a wide enough opening to work with easily, but if that's not available, a clean jar or bowl will work fine. Carefully pour all of the herbal liquid into the clean pitcher through a piece of cheesecloth on a strainer or sieve, or directly through a fine-mesh strainer. You may find it easier to set your strainer inside a funnel. After pouring, squeeze out the plant material to capture the strongest part of the medicine you've just made.

Either bring together the corners of the cheesecloth and wring out the herbs over the pitcher or, if you didn't use a cloth, pick up the herbs and squeeze them out over the strainer. Be careful in both cases not to take more than you can handle; you want the liquid to go into your pitcher rather than over the sides. When you've squeezed out every drop that you possibly can, pour the herbal tincture back into the original jar—it's pre-labeled! Or pour it into a new jar for use or storage.

Compost the plant material; this final give-away to the Earth completes the making of your medicine. If you live in a city apartment, save the spent plants you've tinctured (in herbalism this is called the "marc") to bring to a park or place under a tree or bush on the street, where they can decompose and feed the soil that feeds the plants and trees.

DOSAGES

One dropper of herbal tincture equals approximately twenty-five to thirty drops. Five to six droppers equals approximately one teaspoon. Tincture dosages are often given as "1 dropper in water or tea" per cup, but this can vary widely depending on the plant, and also on the herbalist and the situation. Some herbalists use tiny dosages, and some use very large amounts. I find that what I suggest depends on whom I am helping, and have no qualms about going low or high in my dosing, as needed. I tend to go high when I am helping someone with extreme pain.

Consider whether you tend to be highly sensitive to substances, or are average in sensitivity, or require twice as much of anything to achieve a desired result. For example, perhaps you drink a half glass of wine to the same effect that your friends and companions get from a bottle, or perhaps your dentist has told you that you take twice the amount of Novocain anyone else needs before your mouth gets numb.

Use common sense, get guidance when you can, and remember that you can always increase the amount if you feel you are not using enough, or decrease the amount if you discover you don't need as much as you thought.

This is one of the great things about using gentle, potent herbs, especially for acute conditions. If you take five drops of motherwort *(Leonurus cardiaca)* tincture for anxiety or menstrual cramps and it doesn't help you in ten or fifteen minutes, you'll know it, and you can increase your dosage. If you take five more drops and it still doesn't help, you can take more until you get relief. One person may find five drops miraculous, and someone else may find a whole teaspoon is the perfect dosage for them. But on average, one full dropper of tincture is a good place to start. Dosage suggestions are given in all medicinal tincture recipes.

Glycerites

Glycerites are not as strong as alcohol tinctures and don't extract all the medicinal properties as well, but this sweet, syrupy preparation can still be a wonderful choice for people averse to using alcohol (but still desiring the convenience of a tincture), and for children. I find that fresh flowers such as chamomile, linden, lavender, and rose are especially lovely to prepare as glycerites.

I make fresh-flower glycerites by filling a jar of any size with the flowers and then covering them with vegetable glycerin. These are decanted the same way that alcohol tinctures are. I make dried-flower glycerites by filling the jar about half-full of flowers, covering them with a 60/40 mix of water and vegetable glycerin, and stirring or shaking the preparation well.

I like to include glycerites as simples or in recipes when I'm working with someone who is addressing a fierce sweet tooth or sugar addiction. I also often include glycerites in recipes for helping someone with low spirits, as their sweetness tends to be uplifting. Glycerites can be used in food, too, drizzled over fruit, over ice cream, yogurt, pancakes, etc. They can also be used as sweeteners in herbal cough syrups.

Herbal Vinegars

The process for making infused herbal vinegar is simple; it basically follows the same instructions as those given for making tinctures. After harvesting or buying the fresh herb, tear or chop it up finely and place the plant material into a clean glass jar. Fill it to the top with the herbs. Then pour apple cider vinegar over the plants, filling your jar to the tippy-top. I use raw, unfiltered apple cider vinegar even though it's a little pricier than the pasteurized vinegar in the supermarket, but use whatever kind you have available, or the best you can afford.

Use a chopstick or small branch to push down the plants and poke holes throughout the plant material, to make sure the herbs are thoroughly saturated in the vinegar. Top the jar up with vinegar several times over the next five minutes to make sure it is as full as possible, then screw the lid tightly closed. One difference between a tincture and infused vinegar is that with vinegar you need to close your jar with a plastic lid, or a cork or glass stopper, because a metal lid can rust closed from the acidic vinegar. If you only have a metal lid, line it with plastic wrap, wax paper or—my favorite—unbleached parchment paper. Again, shake the jar if you like. Say a prayer, or sing a song. Give thanks for the good medicine that's coming.

Vinegar that has had herbs infusing in it for six weeks or more is no longer just a flavored culinary item. Vinegar is a valuable food medicine that excels at extracting vitamins and minerals from whatever herbs are infusing in it. Vinegars offer you nourishing medicines that can be incorporated into everyday usage as food to nourish your bones, muscles, hair, skin, nerves, and digestion.

Some herbal vinegars can be enhanced by adding honey and/or molasses into the jar while they're steeping. There are recipes for some of those preparations (sometimes called "oxymels") in Part III, Everything is Medicine.

DOSAGE

Vinegar preparations can be substituted for tinctures when necessary. Vinegar, however, doesn't extract all the alcohol-soluble constituents of herbs, so I replace each dropper of alcohol tincture with one or two tea-spoons of infused vinegar. But my primary usage of vinegars is in and as food, providing preventative medicine and good nourishment. Herbal vinegars can also be used in the bath by adding approximately a half cup of vinegar per bath.

Herbal Oils and Ointments

Cut or tear up fresh plant material that you've gathered (or purchased) on a dry day. Do not wash it. Fill a glass jar neither loosely nor jam-packed, within a half-inch or so of the top. Cover the herbs with olive oil. Poke through with your chopstick to release as many gas bubbles as possible, and to make sure all the plant material is thoroughly saturated with oil. As the plant material absorbs the oil and lowers the level of it in your jar, top up the oil several times. Cap and label the jar in the same way as for tinctures and vinegars. I often place my label on the lid rather than the jar itself, so that when I top up the jar with more oil, I don't risk smearing my label and having to re-do it.

Set the oil on a saucer out of direct sunlight. It will often seep out over the sides while it's infusing, as more gas is released from the plant. For the first week or two, top up the medicine with oil as needed, and continue to poke all herbal material under the oil to discourage mold. It is essential to keep the oil filled to the top, so there is no air space there in which mold could grow. Wait four to six weeks before decant-ing, but not much longer—herbal oils should be decanted as promptly as possible.

The moister the plant, the trickier it is to keep the preparation from molding. Some particularly moist plants are violet leaf, comfrey leaf, and dandelion blossoms, and their oil recipes offer some trouble-shooting tips. Another tip is to make sure that your jar and lid are completely dry.

After decanting your preparation, let the oil sit for about twenty-four hours, and then pour it off one more time, carefully leaving behind the water layer that sits on the bottom. That tiny bit of watery oil will not keep, but it is good for immediate use. Store the remainder in a clean, dry glass jar in a cool, dry place.

HERBAL OINTMENT

After you've decanted infused oil, whether immediately or weeks or months later, you can turn it into an herbal ointment. Gently heat the oil and stir in grated beeswax, then let it cool. Use anywhere from one teaspoon to one tablespoon of beeswax to an ounce of decanted herbal oil to achieve the desired firmness; some people like their ointments gooey, and others like them rather solid. The more beeswax, the more solid.

Stir the beeswax into the oil over a low flame. As soon as the beeswax has completely melted and there are no little pieces of wax left in the saucepan, pour the mixture into a jar and cap it. It will be ready to use in fifteen to thirty minutes, depending on how big a container you're using, and on the ambient temperature. If you don't like the texture at that point, scoop it out of the jar, re-melt it, and add either more oil or more beeswax. Remember to use a wide enough jar to get your finger into even when it's almost empty.

Poultices, Compresses, and Fomentations

These preparations are worth getting to know well enough to be comfortable with using them. They are useful for many applications including relaxation, dissolving growths, relieving pain, healing skin rashes, wounds, and bruises, healing infections, knitting broken bones, easing the itch of mosquito bites, drawing out foreign objects, and more.

When you are using herbs externally, as in poultices and compresses, you want the medicinal properties to stay in the herbs—hence the short steeping times detailed below. Generally speaking, the more frequently the herbs are applied with these methods, the more effective they will be. The length of time to leave the herbs on will vary depending on the herb and the situation. A general guideline is approximately twenty minutes per application, but that can vary in either direction.

POULTICES

To make a poultice: Pour just enough boiling water over fresh or dried leaves to completely moisten them, and let them sit for five to ten minutes. Or bring the water and herbs to a boil, and then turn the water off and let them sit for five to ten minutes. Removed the softened leaves from the water, and lay them over the area of the body that is in need of healing. Some herbs can simply be chewed or rubbed briskly between your hands to soften them, and then applied immediately. A poultice can be left alone, secured with a band-aid; or a cloth can be wrapped around it to keep it in place.

COMPRESSES

To make a compress: Open up the herbs in the same way as for a poultice, then wrap the softened leaves, flowers, and/or roots in a soft, porous cloth like cheesecloth or thin cotton before applying the plant material to the body, rather than applying herbs directly to skin. This comes in handy for open gashes and lacerations, where you don't want herbs to get into and irritate the wound. A compress can also be appropriate for scratchy herbs that you don't want against your skin, or any area of the body that's extra-sensitive, like the eyelids, or places where poultices would fall off otherwise.

FOMENTATIONS

To make a fomentation: Steep the herbs in boiled water for a longer time than for poultices and compresses. Then dip a soft cloth into this tea, wring it out, and put the wet cloth over the area of the body that you are healing. This step can be used in-between the others, or as an easier way to apply herbal medicine externally. It is easy and effective, but not as strong as using the herbs themselves.

HERBAL SPRAYS

Herbal sprays are usually used externally. Start by making an herbal tea or infusion. After decanting it, put the liquid into a small plastic or glass spray bottle that can be easily carried and used for a variety of purposes.

You might use your herbal spray as a bug repellent, as an antiseptic, to cool you off, to calm you down, or to lift your spirits. Store any excess tea or infusion in the refrigerator, where it will keep longer.

Another popular way to make an herbal spray is to put water inside a spray bottle and add a few drops of essential oil. Shake the bottle gently before spraying it on your skin. This form doesn't need to be refrigerated, and you can add water to the same bottle a few times before you need to refresh the essential oil in it.

Please note that essential oils are not the same as infused oils. Essential oils are highly concentrated substances. Making them requires an enormous amount of plant material, and they are expensive to purchase. Only tiny amounts of these oils are needed for the desired medicinal effect. I suggest using them sparingly, and always diluting them in water or infused oil. Essential oils are made from plants, but they have been turned into manufactured products, and no matter how lovely they smell, they are far from their original, earthy form and need to be used with sensible cautions.

Herbal sprays can also be used internally, especially for sore throats and/or infections in the throat. An example of an effective herbal throat spray is one made with propolis. Propolis is a sticky, resinous substance collected by bees from flower buds and used to maintain the health of their hives. Add a few drops of propolis tincture into the water in a spray bottle to create an anti-microbial spray that can be directly applied into the throat.

HERBAL SMOKE

Smoke, whether from one plant or more, has always been a part of traditional medicine. It is used ceremonially and in prayer, whether it is frankincense and myrrh in a church or sage in a moon lodge. Smoke is considered a sacred substance because it is in-between form and formlessness, or matter and spirit; the smoke is the bridge between them. It carries our prayers and blessings. Smoke can be wafted around a person's body for spiritual healing, or used to clear an area of stale energy. Medicinally, herbal smoke can be used to dilate the bronchia to make breathing easier, and is thus useful for specific acute situations. It can be gently blown into an ear for help with ear pain. I often include a smoke blend when someone is releasing a tobacco habit. Herbs must be dried to be able to light them. White sage is well-known, but many other herbs can be used as smoke, some of which are included in *The Gift of Healing Herbs*. (See my earlier book, *Healing Magic: A Green Witch Guidebook to Conscious Living* for more suggestions).

PILLOWS AND MEDICINE BAGS

You don't always need to ingest or imbibe herbs; sometimes you can wear them, lie on them, or sit with them to receive their gifts. This is especially true for spiritual healing, but can impact practical matters, too. An herbal pillow can help bring a better night's sleep and dispel nightmares. An amulet or medicine bag that contains an herb whose energy benefits you can be worn or carried to give you more confidence, calm you, or make you feel safer. It is also fun to create beautiful things with the dried plants, and they can make thoughtful, personal gifts to share with someone you love.

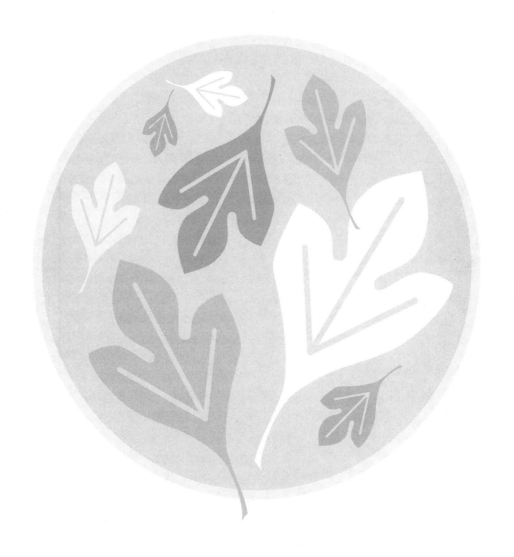

PART II

The Herbs and Your Body Systems

Nourishing Health, Preventing Ailments, and Rebuilding Vitality

Our biography becomes our biology.
—Caroline Myss, medical intuitive and international
teacher of energy medicine

E very system of the body is interdependent with every other system.
In truth, there is no separating them, any more than you can separate
your body and psyche. Here we will look at some of the workings of the
body systems discussed later, and explore how to apply herbal medicine
for optimum nourishment and healing, and some of the common challenges connected with each system, especially relative to your whole being,
physical and emotional health, and spiritual evolution.

I say that bodies tell your true stories. I have seen that bodies always
speak to you in the language of love—yes, *always*. They never communicate punishment or disapproval through illness or injury. Your body asks
you to pay kind attention to yourself, and to bring self-awareness and
love where love seems lacking. When necessary and beneficial, you can
transform your biography/biology with focused attention and by choosing
the herbs and healing practices that are right for you, and by doing those
practices consistently and with conscious intent.

In this section we'll also explore the connections between your body's
systems and the primary elements: Air/breathing and circulating movement, spaciousness and inter-being; Fire/digesting and assimilating life

with passion and joy; Water/flowing nourishment, releasing wastes freely, boundaries and boundlessness; and Earth/stillness and stability, focused movement.

These connections are not specifically correlated with ancient, established systems such as India's Ayurvedic medicine or Traditional Chinese Five Element theory. They are offered rather as an intuitive, metaphoric foundation for connecting your personal healing with the healing of the Earth and all forms of life upon her.

A special note on the element Water: There is no life without water, at least not on Planet Earth. Just as the Earth herself is mostly composed of water, so are we. Water is an intrinsic part of each of our body systems' optimal functioning, as well as a fundamental expression of who and what we are as evolving human beings with bodies that are far more fluid than solid, and that contain far more space than substance.

6

The Cardiovascular System

Herbs and more for health, acute illnesses, and chronic challenges of the cardiovascular system; how to nourish veins, arteries, heart and kidneys for good circulation, healthy blood pressure and a healthy and strong heart.

The circulatory system, powered by the grapefruit-sized muscular organ we call the heart, is connected to the element Fire, and needs warmth, stimuli, and movement to be healthy. Like fire, the heart and the blood it ceaselessly pumps around our bodies are never still.

This system and its health, acute illnesses, and chronic challenges often offers us teachings around joy and gratitude, playfulness or over-seriousness. Holding grudges, a lack of willingness to forgive, and withholding of love for self and others are all challenges that can impede the successful workings of this fantastically exuberant system. These challenges can cause us to "harden" our hearts, which can lead to hardening of the arteries, or arteriosclerosis.

In Traditional Chinese Medicine (TCM) the heart is associated with the nervous system and with Spirit. It is vitally connected to our sense of joy. Joy is beneficial to the heart, and a healthy heart is beneficial to our joy. Grounded joy is not manic nor in need of jumping up and down and talking and laughing loudly. It can be expressed as wild rejoicing, but natural joy stems from peace within; it is peaceful and present, vital, and accepting of what is, even as it naturally tends toward increasing joy for all.

The heart is a powerful, muscular organ. It is kept so busy providing blood to every cell in our bodies, and continuously bringing the blood back to itself and then to the lungs to be oxygenated, that we have an additional, separate circulatory system for it; the coronary circulation system exists solely to feed the heart muscle itself! The heart is designed to give and receive continuously, which is as apt a metaphor as you could want for the heart of being human.

· · · ● · · ·

Some of my favorite cardiovascular-system herbal allies are: hawthorn berries and flowers, rosemary, linden, grape leaves, nettles, seaweeds, parsley, yarrow, violet, and ginkgo biloba.

The first herb I think of in connection with the health of our dear hearts is the sacred hawthorn tree, beloved of the mischievous faeries and all who believe that a life devoid of magic is not really worth living.

Hawthorn (*Crataegus* species)

Grandmother hawthorn sounds like a snake
When wind moves through her leaves,
Making them shake.
They rustle and hiss
As they touch one another—
Sounds like a snake may be Grandma's lover!

But sly humor and magic isn't all there is to hawthorn, not by a long shot. Hawthorn strengthens and protects the heart and cardiovascular system, as well as the coronary circulation. Her leaves, flowers, and fruits contain chemicals that increase the blood flow to the heart muscle. Hawthorn increases the ease of circulation by toning the arteries as it strengthens and soothes the heart, and is considered specific for angina pectoris and functional heart disease. She is a member of the rose family and, like rose, is a direct tonic to the heart, arteries, nerves, blood, and intestines.

Hawthorn is rich in a variety of bio-flavonoids including the anti-inflammatory quercetin. The flowers of hawthorn are sweet and musky, while the fruits are sour and astringent. All parts are high in vitamin C, and are nourishing, calming, and restorative. Hawthorn infusion or tincture relieves a feeling of oppression in the chest and can help with fatigue and difficulty breathing. Hawthorn can normalize blood pressure and reduce fluid congestion around the heart. For that last purpose, combine it with mullein leaf. Hawthorn is used for palpitations, and for that purpose combines well with motherwort.

Hawthorn is an essentially safe plant medicine. Eating or drinking an infusion or tincture made from her fruits is akin to eating apples (another member of the rose family). Hawthorn provides nourishment to the blood, strengthens the blood vessels in the digestive system, and increases digestive enzymes as well, increasing the efficiency and ease with which fats and proteins are digested.

I love hawthorn and have found many delightful ways to ingest this healing plant. Hawthorn berries and flower infusions are one of my "regulars"—the herbs I turn to again and again as a source of iron, antioxidants, and optimal nourishment for veins, arteries, and heart. It is also a vital medicine for the spiritual heart.

Herbalists vary in the dosages they suggest, and generally speaking dosages need to be adjusted to the person using the herb. I typically suggest starting with 1 dropper of tincture several times daily, or 2–4 cups of infusion on its own or blended with other plant medicines. Here's a great recipe:

HEALTHY HEART BLEND—VARIATION I

½ cup dried hawthorn berries

½ cup dried hawthorn flowers and leaves

½ cup dried linden blossoms

½ cup dried nettle leaves and stalks

Mix these herbs together into a half-gallon jar and pour boiling water over them, to the top. Cap it tightly and let it steep for about 12 hours. Drink 1–4 cups daily.

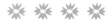

This infusion is useful for an ailing cardiovascular system, or to help maintain a healthy one. This blend of herbs will provide medicinal benefits for the heart muscle itself, while each of the herbs improves circulation and helps the lungs. Linden flowers are soothing and anti-inflammatory, and both she and hawthorn are specific for normalizing blood pressure. Nettle aids hawthorn in protecting the integrity of the veins and arteries, and sees to the health of the supportive, hard-working kidneys. This infusion does all this and more, and tastes absolutely superb.

If you are healthy, you can use this blend or rotate the individual herbs into your life periodically. If you are engaged in healing your heart or blood pressure, drink a minimum of two cups daily, at least five days a week. If you are taking heart medication, I'm sure you are having your health monitored. If you have a physician who supports your use of herbs, food, and other traditional approaches to healing, so much the better. Depending on how long you have been ill and how long you've been taking pharmaceuticals, after using these herbs regularly, individually or blended together, you may need to have your prescriptions reduced and re-evaluated.

HEALTHY HEART BLEND—VARIATION II

½ cup dried hawthorn berries

½ cup dried hawthorn flowers and leaves

½ cup dried linden blossoms

½ cup dried violet leaves and stalks (and flowers, optional)

Substitute violet for the stinging nettles when there is a need to moisten tissue, ease heart pain, or soothe the nerves. I generally use sweet blue violet, *Viola odorata,* but would happily use whatever species is local. Another species of violet, common pansy *(Viola tricolor)* is nicknamed "heart's ease" for a reason—it is beneficial to the heart, building strength and reducing pain.

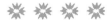

According to pioneering herbalist Juliette de Bairacli Levy, violet tea is sweetened with honey and taken by the wineglass every four hours for heart pain and to reduce blood pressure.

She also writes of the beautiful calendula blossom as a tonic treatment for the heart, veins, and arteries. This bright yellow or orange flower induces joy merely by looking at it. Best gathered in the sunshine, calendula, like nettles, is sometimes seen as an herbal "cure-all." Here it is useful for stimulating the circulation and reducing varicosities in the veins, thus making the heart's job easier.

Esteemed twelfth-century herbalist St. Hildegard of Bingen wrote about the tonic effects of parsley on the cardiovascular system. A recipe for parsley wine that's been passed down is:

PARSLEY TONIC WINE

12 sprigs fresh parsley

1 quart white or red wine

2 tablespoons white-wine vinegar

9 ounces honey

Put all the ingredients except the honey together into a soup pot. Boil for 10 minutes, and then add honey.

Strain and pour into bottles. Take 1 tablespoon 3 times a day.
Red wine contains resveratrol, a chemical compound that is of benefit to the heart—but use whichever kind of wine you like best. Both white and red wines are perfectly good for tonic preparations; I prefer red. Some versions of the recipe call for the vinegar, and some don't. You can make infused fresh parsley vinegar (see page 53), and use that in the tonic wine if you like. You can also use a heart-healing infused honey (see page 45) made with linden, rose, or holy basil, making it even more healing and tasty. If you can afford raw honey, I'd highly recommend that.

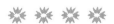

The first herbal medicine I ever gave to my dad was hawthorn berry-infused brandy when he was having angina attacks. I put a quart of homemade hawthorn berry brandy tincture in a pretty glass bottle with a cork, and asked him to put it on his nightstand and take a big swig from it every night before he went to bed. His eyes lit up. "That's my medicine? I can do that!" And hawthorn has continued to be one of his primary healing allies as he has continued to support his cardiovascular system with herbs for the past couple of decades—during which he has thankfully been free of angina attacks.

HAWTHORN BERRY BRANDY

Fresh hawthorn berries

Unflavored brandy

Cut up or mash well a batch of fresh-picked hawthorn berries from any wild species of hawthorn tree, seeds and all. Do watch out for little worms! Of course, discard any berries that have worms. Fill the jar with the berries, and then cover them with the brandy of your choice. I use any commonly available oak-aged brandy. Wait a minimum of 6 weeks before decanting for use.

This is simply a fresh-herb tincture using brandy as the menstruum. You could leave the berries in there for years, and your brandy tincture would still be fine. If you use dried hawthorn berries, fill the jar about 25% with the dried berries and then fill all the way with brandy, and leave for 6 months–1 year before decanting for use.

This fabulous medicine is easy to make, though cutting up fresh hawthorn berries is time-consuming. Use everything—the seeds will get squeezed out with the rest of the plant material when you decant the tincture.

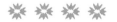

Years later, my father called me because he'd started having terrible headaches and lightheadedness. Upon examination, his doctor agreed with my long-distance assessment that he was overmedicated for his high blood pressure, and took him off one of the drugs. His pressure and symptoms worsened, and he called me again after it had continued for several days.

The health of the kidneys is directly connected to regulating blood pressure. Simple parsley tea, so tonifying to the kidneys, can help bring down high blood pressure quickly. I asked him to go to his spice rack and get some parsley. Having visited recently, I knew the quality wasn't the greatest; it was not organic, and not too fresh, but it was the best that was immediately available. I had him make parsley tea to drink and, adapting a tip from Maria Treban for him, I suggested he give himself a sage bath using a washcloth saturated in regular garden sage tea, rubbing it over his head and chest. Mineral-rich sage can be used as a restorative herb after a stroke, or in this case as a preventative measure. His blood pressure was nearly normalized by the next morning, and the doctor pronounced it perfect the following day.

He drank a cup of parsley tea daily, and has been feeling much better since then. After his pressure was fine for a good while, he stopped drinking the parsley regularly and only uses it occasionally when he feels the need. He has gotten to know his own body so much better by using the plant medicines. I bless these herbs, and feel such gratitude for their gifts! And I plan to make him the parsley wine because he is a fan of red wine, and I know that's a sure way to get him to consume more parsley!

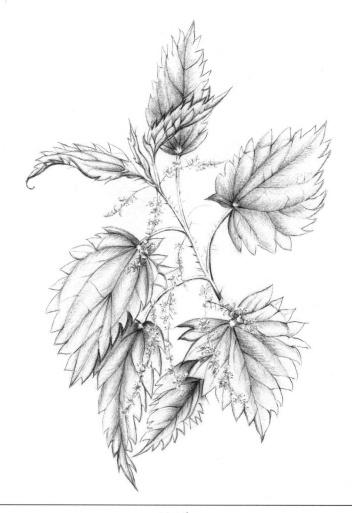

Nettles

Nettles (*Urtica dioica* and other species)

Body: builds blood, strengthens adrenals, kidneys, and lungs; elasticizes veins and arteries; supports immune strength and recovery from allergies and debilitating chronic conditions.

Mind: sharpens focus.

Heart: opens the heart to fierce love.

Soul: supports self-respect on the deepest level.

Stinging Nettles

Nettles has her way with us—
Demands respect
And asks for trust.

When we brush by
She burns and stings,
"Persevere" is what nettle sings.

Use this plant internally
She helps tone veins
And arteries.

She builds our strength,
Kidneys and lungs,
And helps us heal whatever comes.

Her minerals that nourish
Blood, nerve, and bone
Help us flourish.

Green stamina
For you and me,
Charged with herb electricity!

Nettle has abundant seeds
And vitamins
to meet our needs.

Fuels adrenals for energy
And strong,
potent immunity.

Drink your nettles quite a lot

Or eat them cooked

In your soup pot.

You will be glad!

I tell you true,

'Cause nettles are so good for you.

One of the most amazing herbs on Planet Earth has to be the common weed called stinging nettles. I use nettles regularly. It is like having herbal health insurance! Nettle is almost a panacea, with healing benefits for nearly every major body system—lymph, glandular, respiratory, skin, urinary, and cardiovascular. In the cardiovascular system its tonic and rejuvenating effects on the veins and arteries, along with its healing properties for the kidneys, make it a great herb to know.

One story about stinging nettles that's made an indelible impression on me is the one told in the book *Song of the Seven Herbs* by Walking Night Bear and Stan Padilla. It seems that originally wild nettles, now covered in stinging formic acid and other phytochemicals, looked completely different than the weedy green plant we know today. Nettle was a magically attractive plant, so obviously full of rich blessings that people and even animals took undue advantage of her, harvesting too much without gratitude or respect. She was bright and shining to look at—the color of gleaming gold (and we know how some people act around gold).

Finally nettles called out to Creator for help, concerned for her own life and well-being. Creator thought and thought, and finally turned nettles into her current form for her own protection, hiding her riches under scruffier, simpler green skin and irritant exudations. Nettles still gets to give her gifts to the people, animals, and land, and so fulfill her purpose on Earth, but people can't simply come and take from her without gratitude and respect anymore. The story ends with the sentiment that now only those with the eyes to see are able to see nettles' true "heart of gold."

What a powerhouse! Nettle is a supremely chlorophyll-rich plant that generously proffers her dark-green healing virtues to everyone. High in mineral nutrients such as calcium and silica to support bones and joints, lungs and connective tissue, as well as vitamins A, C, E, and notably K, which helps prevent hemorrhage, nettle offers optimum nourishment. Nettle helps those moving through long-term illness and/or recuperating afterward. She contains highly assimilable iron and protein that offer daily sustenance and strength when someone feels weak and exhausted. Nettle helps the body fight a variety of infections by tonifying the lymph, lungs, and blood circulation. Nettle helps restore kidney essence and function, and re-energizes depleted adrenal glands.

She rebuilds healthy hair from the shaft up, and helps in the creation of healthy boundaries too. She has a way of helping the body and psyche set so many different things right when they've gone wrong that I have to acknowledge it can sound unbelievable as you listen to a wise woman talking about nettles. But the truth is that, although it's not a magic bullet or cure-all plant, nettles is certainly a "cures-much" plant, and turns up in many healing stories in this book. Recipes containing nettles are found throughout, and here are two delicious, nutritious, and medicinal infusion recipes that use the combination of red, green, and yellow herbs that I particularly favor.

GREAT WAY TO START THE DAY
INFUSION—VARIATION I

¾ cup dried stinging nettles

½ cup dried hawthorn berries

¾ cup dried sassafras leaves

Mix the herbs together in a half-gallon jar. Pour boiling water over them, and cap tightly. Leave out to steep on your counter overnight, or 8–12 hours. In the morning, squeeze out the plant material as fully as you can, and compost the herbs. Store the infusion in the refrigerator and heat on the stove to drink.

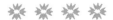

This is a magnificent tea to wake up to after it's steeped overnight. Even after you've decanted it, the tastes and chemical constituents keep blending and settling, and the infusion gets even better as it becomes more fully what it is. The hawthorn and sassafras leaves both add a spirit-enlivening, joyous quality to the nettles' zing and power. Drinking this invites your blood and lymph fluid to flow and circulate freely, with both nettles and hawthorn toning the veins and elasticizing the arteries all the way down to the tiniest blood vessels—the capillaries, a mere hair-width thick or less. Bioflavonoid-rich hawthorn strengthens your heart and general immunity, and the moistening, demulcent qualities of sassafras leaf also help offset any dryness from astringent, tissue-toning nettles. The taste too is sweet and rich—simply fantastic!

GREAT WAY TO START THE DAY INFUSION—VARIATION II

1 cup dried stinging nettles

½ cup dried red clover

½ cup dried oatstraw

Mix the dried herbs together in a half-gallon jar. Pour boiling water over them, and cap tightly. Leave out to steep on your counter overnight. Squeeze out the plant material completely, and compost the herbs. Store the decanted infusion in the refrigerator and reheat gently on the stove to drink. You can put this in a stainless-steel thermos and drink it all day.

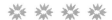

This version is a great blend, too. It is a bit more calming and less uplifting than Variation I. Each plant in this blend is a nutritional powerhouse on its own! The oats and red clover add lightness and grace to the brew. Red clover brings a substantial amount of usable protein to the mix, and oats stabilizes blood sugar and aids digestion. There is an abundance of vitamins, minerals, trace minerals, and amino acids in this recipe. Either of these infusions, with a good hearty breakfast (much more than an apple a day!) is a great way to start a day.

Nettle is like green mother's milk and the salty ocean of life. She imparts a green so rich it turns red inside us and becomes blood itself.

And in fact, chlorophyll and red blood cells have a nearly identical molecular structure; the only difference is that chlorophyll contains magnesium where hemoglobin has iron. Nettles can help build rich, healthy blood.

It's never too late in your life to start drinking or eating stinging nettle. It restores the integrity of the walls of veins and arteries, and thus helps circulation beautifully. One of my apprentices had years and years of leg pain, but has had none for the past several years thanks to her regular ingestion of nettles infusions. (She's also integrating more stretching into her life. Herbs can't do everything!)

I most often think of nettle leaves and stalks as an everyday healer that I use frequently to build and maintain superb vitality. If nettle is too drying for someone (through its astringency as an excellent diuretic) I will mix it with a demulcent herb appropriate to the person and their needs—perhaps linden, mallow, or violet. As long as there is no contraindication for the use of honey (as in diabetes, for example) I might also mix it with naturally moisturizing honey.

Rosemary *(Rosmarinus officinalis)*

Rosemary is not only a delicious aromatic herb, but it is also an esteemed and currently underused tonic for the cardiovascular system, increasing circulation and benefitting the heart itself with calcium, manganese, and magnesium. I like to prepare it as a simple tea with fresh or dried rosemary.

ROSEMARY TEA

1 tablespoon fresh rosemary leaves (or 1 teaspoon if dried)

Pour one cup of boiled water over the fresh or dried rosemary leaves and steep for about 15 minutes.

Rosemary can also be used as a tincture. A cup of tea a day or 25–30 drops of tincture per cup of hot water is a lovely way to take care of your heart—and since rosemary is for remembrance, do remember to try some!

Grapes *(Vitis vinifera)*

When the Vikings arrived on the shores of North America, they called it "the land of the wild grapes." Grapes and grape leaves, vines and tendrils (*Vitis vinifera* and other species) are another underutilized herbal remedy. They are delicious and of great benefit. Many species of grape are useful; one detail for identification purposes is that all of the species of grape have spiral tendrils.

I love grape leaves, vines and tendrils, both internally and topically for enhancing circulation of blood and improving the health of the blood vessels. Grapevines help the circulatory system with their array of antioxidant bioflavonoids. Grape tea or tincture is pain-relieving, anti-inflammatory and helpful with leg pain and varicosities, including hemorrhoids. Fresh leaf poultices applied directly to the veins are beneficial for shrinking swollen veins, as are applications of grape leaf vinegar and even grape tincture diluted with the distilled witch hazel you can buy in the drugstore.

For a fun way to take your grape medicine, here is an elixir I made as an experiment, which turned out to be divine:

CHAMPAGNE GRAPE ELIXIR

1 cup fresh Champagne (Corinth) grapes

1 cup 100-proof vodka

2 cups wildflower honey

Gently mash the grapes. Mix them in with the honey and vodka in a wide mouth glass jar. Adjust the proportions to suit your taste and to fill the jar to the top, and then wait six weeks. It's fantastic for your circulation, and tastes absurdly good.

You could make this with any type of red or purple grape you love.

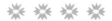

Grape leaf-infused vinegar is another excellent way to use this medicine, both externally on the skin over swollen veins and broken capillaries and internally—it's delicious in food, on salads, cooked greens, in sauces, etc.—or you can add a tablespoon to water and simply drink it. It can also be mixed with an equal amount of honey for helping heal inflamed joints.

GRAPE LEAF VINEGAR

Fresh grape leaves, vines and tendrils

Apple cider vinegar

Chop up the fresh plant material well and fill a wide-mouthed jar of any size with it. Pour apple cider vinegar over the herbs, filling the jar to the top. Wait a few minutes and top the jar up one or more times, to get the preparation as full to the brim as possible, and then cap the jar with a plastic lid, a cork, or a metal lid lined with waxed or unbleached parchment paper (to prevent the metal lid from rusting closed).

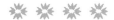

The main mission of our tiniest blood vessels, our capillaries, is to be a bridge between our veins and arteries, so they need to be permeable. Capillaries are so thin that they are fragile and break easily as we age, especially because most of us spend too much time sitting in chairs or with our legs crossed. Grape, used internally and/or externally, will strengthen the elasticity of those hair-thin capillaries and reduce breakage.

My dad had varicose veins for a long time and his legs would tire, but years later when he began to have so much pain at night that it was keeping him from sleeping, and even sometimes waking him up, he found a renowned doctor who performed surgery on one leg, and planned to do the other. They needed to wait several months for his healing, however, before the second surgery.

We added grape leaf into his herbal-care practices, and after several months the surgeon agreed with my dad's assessment that he no longer needed the surgery. It's been over ten years now. Grape, used internally and externally, helps tissue where the blood is leaking out of the vessels, causing purplish blotches on the skin, and also helps heal badly discolored purple, black, and yellow bruises.

GRAPE LEAF OIL

Fresh grape leaves, vines, and tendrils

Olive oil

Chop up the fresh plant material very well and fill a wide-mouthed jar of any size with it. Pour olive oil over the herbs, filling the jar to the top. Wait a few minutes and top the jar up one or more times to get the preparation as full to the brim as possible, and then cap the jar.

    The well-chopped plant parts can be heated on the stove in the oil; let them steep over several days, turning the flame on and off, under a watchful eye. After steeping for 1–2 days, bottle the oil with the herbs still in it, and let it stand even as you start to use it. When the leaves start to stick up out of the oil, decant it, squeezing the leaves well.

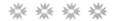

Other Herbs for Cardiovascular Support

Yarrow flowers, stalks and leaves *(Achillea millefolium)* are anti-inflammatory and pain-relieving, and can be useful in cardiovascular recipes, especially where there is high blood pressure, because of the tonic influence this astringent herb exerts on the blood vessels and circulation. It dilates the peripheral vessels even as it tones them. Herbalist David Hoffman suggests combining yarrow with two of my other favorites, hawthorn and linden, for high blood pressure. He also suggests combining it with European mistletoe *(Viscum album),* which I have yet to try—but he is in agreement here with Austrian herbalist Maria Treban. She has written several best-selling herbal books, and her information is nearly all based on direct, personal experience. I have found that her reference books are particularly helpful, and return to them again and again.

    Maria Treban sings the praises of yarrow for the circulatory system as well as for nudging sluggish kidneys to work better, and for relieving vascular spasms. She also sings the praises of European mistletoe for both high or low blood pressure and other circulatory problems. Mistletoe berries are poisonous, so only the leaves and twigs are used, and she helpfully informs us that they must be harvested in March, April, October, November, or early December to be worthwhile medicinally.

Yarrow is warming, drying, and also one of my favorite wound-healing herbs. It's best-known for its usefulness for colds and fever. Yarrow is also classically used externally in a sitz bath, or as an infused oil to help shrink hemorrhoids, the varicose veins that form just inside or outside the anus, often in response to the pressure of constipation or pregnancy. Internal use of yarrow tincture or tea is useful in strengthening the veins, and as an anti-spasmodic to relax the smooth muscles of the digestive tract. If the bitterness of yarrow, with its rich complement of aromatic, volatile oils, is too intense for you, mix in a little honey.

Ginkgo biloba, also known by the lovely name "Maidenhair tree," is a bit thinning to the blood, and can be found in many heart recipes as well. The leaves are rich in a variety of flavonoids. These antioxidant compounds protect the heart muscle and blood vessels, and help reduce the effects of free radicals, while the terpenoids in the leaves encourage increased circulation by dilating the blood vessels. Ginkgo improves peripheral circulation and circulation in the head and respiratory system, and can positively influence the nervous system's synergistic working with the heart.

The yellow autumn ginkgo leaves, prepared as an infusion or simple tincture, are mild and not prone to creating side effects caused by stronger preparations. To summarize, ginkgo helps reduce inflammation in blood vessels, tones the arteries, and reduces platelet clumping. It has also been used successfully for irregular heartbeat, but my personal experience is that hawthorn and motherwort excel at regulating heart rhythms, so I've never tried ginkgo for this.

Further exploration of physical, emotional, and spiritual heart-healing herbs such as linden, rose and lavender, and simple practices such as ritual baths, will continue in the Nervous System section. (See Healing Herbs for Heartache, Heartbreak, Grief, and Shock, page 216.)

The Digestive System

Herbs and more for health, acute illnesses, and chronic challenges of the digestive system; nourishing herbs for the health of the gastro-intestinal tract; herbs to strengthen, relax, tone and/or stimulate the digestive tract and organs, to improve absorption, assimilation and elimination of food and relief from indigestion, constipation, diarrhea, and other digestive woes.

This brilliantly designed system snaking through the center of your body is a tube that starts at the opening of the mouth and ends at the anus. The tube is an organ in itself, and protects the rest of your insides from being exposed to the digestive juices and bacteria that dissolve the food you eat into a form of cellular nourishment that your body can use to survive and thrive.

In between these two openings, among the veins and arteries, nerves, blood, and lymph, you have the throat, esophagus, stomach, small and large intestines, rectum and anus, and the associated organs—the appendix, pancreas, liver, and gall bladder. Many of these vital parts and organs are critical not only for digestion but for healthy immune, endocrine, and nerve functioning.

The processes of digestion—eating food, breaking it down in order to assimilate nutrients that circulate and feed your body, and the elimination of any unusable portions—are chemical and muscular. Given good nourishment, the body will secrete enzymes, acids, and other digestive juices to break down the carbohydrates, fats, proteins, etc. in food into usable forms. Muscular contractions called peristalsis help the food you swallow to move all the way through this tube in a smaller and smaller form, extracting nutrients all along the way, until only the unusable part remains to be evacuated.

Chewing your food begins the muscular part of physically breaking it down to prepare it for the next chemical step, when enzymes in your saliva continue breaking it down. Even before that, your sense of smell stimulates specific digestive juices to begin flowing—the exact juices that will be needed to digest the particular substance you're about to eat. Brilliant!

Chewed food moves down the throat into the esophagus and arrives at the stomach in seconds, aided by rhythmic, physical contractions. In the stomach, digestive enzymes and acid turn the food into a creamy soup called chyme. Rolling muscular waves churn the food every twenty seconds or so, mixing it all together and continuing to prepare the nutrients to enter the circulation at a cellular level.

That process happens mostly in the small intestine, aided by juices from the pancreas and liver. The liver is the heavy-hitter of this system, with hundreds of known functions to perform. In addition to producing bile to break down fat, the liver provides one of the most important filter systems for detoxification of the body. Nutrients that are absorbed all along the journey through the digestive tract are transported to the liver by the hepatic portal system for further filtering, and then sent out for distribution all around the body.

There are mucous membranes throughout the digestive system and, contrary to some popular diets and philosophies, mucus—nourished by slimy, slippery foods and herbs like okra and slippery elm bark—is not only a good thing, it's essential for your health. The mucosal tissues lining the stomach protect it from hydrochloric and other acids produced in the stomach. If the stomach lining or intestinal mucosal tissues get dry or abraded, it leads to a cascade of other problems such as heartburn, difficulty digesting, constipation, ulceration, bleeding, and more.

Mucous membranes are at their best when they are smooth and glistening with moisture, like healthy skin on the inside of your mouth. This kind of tissue is protective, and helps things slide along. Each part of the system is designed perfectly to perform specific chemical and/or mechanical jobs and ensure that you end up well-nourished.

It's now understood that the appendix, the pouch at the entrance to the large intestine that was once thought useless, is not only part of the lymphatic system but helps repopulate the gut flora. Healthy bacteria are needed throughout the gastrointestinal tract, and especially in the colon; these bacteria are essential for fermentation and the final stages of assimilating nourishment from our food. The large intestine absorbs any excess water, as well as some minerals and vitamins. This is followed by the elimination, through a bowel movement, of the insoluble fiber and other wastes the body can't digest and use.

Our contemporary obsession with antibacterial cleansers in soaps, sponges, and detergents is wreaking havoc with our normal profusion of bacteria. Scientists tell us that we have over 100 trillion microbes living in and on our bodies, which is many times more than the number of human cells that make up our bodies! Destroying bacterial populations en masse is also affecting the natural processes of life feeding life on land and in the water. The potential harm to all growing things on Earth is considerable. Meanwhile, in the human body, when gut flora is lacking, whether through antibacterial products, overuse of antibiotics, poor diet, or over-cleansing the digestive system with enemas and colonics, restoring that flora isn't optional for healing—it's crucial.

To start with, the quality of foods and liquids you ingest and imbibe is important, as is your mental and emotional state before, during and after you consume food. The gastrointestinal tract is like the town hall of your body, its central meeting place. There is a lot going on in there, all the time. The gastrointestinal tract is replete with nervous, endocrine, and lymph-system cells. Since they all meet there, problems in any one of those systems can impede and block healthy digestion. This also means that digestive challenges can be approached through tending appropriately to each of these other systems as well.

The digestive system is connected with the element Fire, digesting and assimilating life with passion and joy. Digestive fire (called *agni* in Ayurveda, the ancient system of healing that originated in India), is required for you to be able to alchemically transform food into a form that you can use for your nourishment. The digestive system gives you the ability to assimilate and digest food (life) and then let go the waste products you can't use—experiences that no longer serve you, or wounds you've finished mining for their "gold," that is, their spiritual nourishment for your growth and evolution.

This system's health, acute illnesses, and chronic challenges often offer you teachings and challenges about accepting, assimilating, and ultimately releasing past experiences that have affected you, especially on an emotional level. Consider that any opening into the body creates an energetic and physical interface—where what is inside you meets the world outside you—and this system is open at both ends.

There is an entire nervous system in the gut called the enteric nervous system. When you are growing inside your mother's womb, it splits off from the central nervous system to create a separate system that contains even more neurons (nerve cells) than your spinal cord. Your emotional well-being and the health of your nervous system have a profound impact on your digestive health. In this context, the idea of "having butterflies in your stomach" takes on a clearer significance. Similarly, honoring your "gut feelings" and "trusting your gut" also take on a more meaningful resonance. With this in mind, you can see that challenges within the gastrointestinal system can also revolve around how much you believe, or don't believe, in your own inner guidance, your "gut instincts."

We can help ourselves with herbal medicines when things go awry. Even better, we can use herbs for optimum nourishment and to prevent problems from occurring in the first place.

. . . .

Some of my favorite digestive-system allies are: slippery elm powder, dandelion root, burdock root, marshmallow leaf, flower and root, red clover blossoms, angelica root, ginger root, yarrow leaf and flower, mugwort leaf and stalk, sweet and bitter orange peels, plantain leaves and seeds, chickweed leaves, stalks and flowers, yellow dock root, rosemary, garlic, chamomile flowers, comfrey leaf, cinnamon, and oat straw.

Let's start with a great, all-around soothing recipe that helps to keep the digestive tract moist, and keeps everything moving through it smoothly and freely.

DIGESTIVE AID HONEY BALLS–VARIATION I
(for diarrhea or constipation)

Slippery elm powder

Honey

Mix these together into a nice paste consistency. Roll up into cherry-sized balls, or into one large ball from which you can take 1 or 2 1-teaspoon-size doses (or take 1–2 small balls) a day.

This recipe is great for healing the stomach or intestinal lining thanks to mucilage-rich slippery elm. Slippery elm is an amazing herb because it's helpful if you have loose stools and a tendency to diarrhea, but also if your mucous membranes aren't lubricated enough to deal with the fiber that needs to pass through the colon, resulting in constipation.

Slippery elm is just that—slippery, gooey, and slimy—and that is the quality it brings into your body. Slippery elm doesn't tone the tissue or increase peristalsis, but it does reduce inflammation. It lubricates, coats and soothes inflamed tissue, and in that way helps ease pain and restore healthy bowel movements.

Maintaining Digestive Health

A lot of herbal information for the digestive system is coming up in the section titled "Everything is Medicine" (page 381). As mentioned there, the first things I generally turn to for help in preventing or easing simple digestive distress are whole-milk yogurt (cow, sheep, or goat, store-bought or homemade) and slippery elm powder (*Ulmas fulva* or other species).

Adding 1 teaspoon–1 tablespoon of slippery elm to a half-cup of yogurt works quickly in many situations to relieve gastric distress.

Adding cooked apples, and/or cinnamon, ginger, and turmeric powder, warms the blend. Other possibilities include seeds that help with gas, such as cumin, cardamom, and/or fennel. If you are having trouble digesting, I recommend grinding the seeds, or making simple tea with them. I consume some slippery elm and yogurt most every day.

Flax seeds are helpful for providing mucilage, essential fatty acids, and lignans to benefit the digestive, immune, and sexual-reproductive systems. If you want to use powdered flax seeds, it is important to freshly grind them before use, as the oils in these seeds turn rancid quickly. I suggest keeping flax in the refrigerator, whole or pre-ground. The brown or golden variety can be used daily—about one tablespoon per serving—to help prevent or resolve constipation. Flax seeds can be added into yogurt or hot cereal, or sprinkled on salads and into other grain dishes such as into quinoa, rice, or amaranth. I consume flax seeds almost every day.

DIGESTIVE AID HONEY BALLS–VARIATION II
(for restoring integrity to the gut lining and
increasing circulation and peristalsis)

¼ cup powdered calendula blossom

¼ cup powdered plantain leaf

¼ cup slippery elm powder

¼ cup cinnamon powder

¼ cup turmeric powder

⅝ cup rose honey (to start; increase as needed)

Mix these together into a nice paste consistency. Roll up into balls, or into one large ball, and take 1 or 2 1-teaspoon-size doses a day.

This recipe can be useful where there is poor assimilation of nutrients, bloating after eating, and/or constipation with resultant hemorrhoids. It helps repair damage to the tissue of the gastrointestinal system, whether from straining to have bowel movements, poor diet, not enough liquid, unrecognized food allergies or intolerances, or certain illnesses. The underlying causes need to be sought out and treated as well.

These honey balls are strong but wonderful-tasting, and can be broken up and added into oatmeal or yogurt, along with fruits and seeds, for an easy way to take your medicine. The plantain and calendula both provide tissue-healing for the stomach and gut linings. The plantain leaf is mildly moistening, yet also astringent. Plantain leaves also encourage peristalsis, relieve pain, and are tissue-healing inside and out.

Calendula is used as a vulnerary, healing any abrasions in the digestive tract and helping to rebuild healthy tissue. Cinnamon is warming and stokes the digestive fire, and it stimulates circulation in the blood vessels that are abundant in the gastrointestinal tract. Turmeric is a bitter anti-inflammatory that helps protect and heal the liver. Any honey can be used, but rose honey tastes delicious and has an affinity for the digestive system; it is astringent and toning to the intestines, and helps cool down an overheated liver. The honey can also help counter the drying quality of the turmeric powder.

* * * * * * * * *

Following are some other herbs specifically beneficial to the gastrointestinal system.

Angelica *(Angelica archangelica)* root is a warming digestive bitter that can be used as a tincture before meals to stimulate the production of digestive acids and therefore more efficient digestion. The difference between using angelica and dandelion root before a meal to stimulate digestive juices (see: dandelion below) is that dandelion is cooling and beneficial to the liver and lymph while angelica is quite warming and antibacterial in the digestive tract. The choice of which to use could be a combination of which plant is available to you and which better matches your constitution and needs. When I am going to take a plant regularly, or suggest a plant to be taken regularly (as opposed to a one-time, in-the-moment use for an acute situation) I always try to use plants that touch on a number of concerns rather than just one symptom or condition.

Burdock is an overall aid to the gastrointestinal system, helping normalize bowel movements and stimulate them as necessary. Burdock root strengthens the liver and gall bladder and moistens the mucous membranes of the intestines. Burdock root can be taken in any number of ways for this purpose; it can be eaten raw or cooked, dried and prepared as an infusion, consumed as infused vinegar, or taken as an alcohol tincture in water. (See the Burdock section, page 110.)

Chamomile (*Matricaria* species) is deservedly famous as a relaxing, antibacterial, gut-healing tea. I use it as a simple, and find it underrated as an antispasmodic. It seems so gentle that its potency may seem imperceptible, but it is helpful for cramps and spasms in the belly—even intense ones, sometimes called gripes. I have worked with people who are allergic to chamomile, so I suggest starting slowly to make sure it agrees with you. Most people do just fine with it, but some find it makes their eyes itch and/or nose run, as if they were having a hay-fever or pollen attack. These symptoms subside as soon as the chamomile is removed.

Chickweed (*Stellaria media* and other species) is a nourishing plant that is delicious to eat as well as highly medicinal. I've had great success using it for people with rectal bleeding with no known cause, or sometimes where there was a cause, such as when a colonoscopy damaged tissue, causing bleeding. Chickweed can used for hemorrhoids, too, taken orally as a tincture and applied topically as infused oil. It is soothing and cooling, and helpful when mixed with more astringent, tissue-tightening plantain, yarrow, or witch hazel. Chickweed is good as a tincture, as it extracts well into alcohol. Eat fresh chickweed leaves, stalks, and flowers in season to benefit from an abundance of minerals and to enjoy the sweet taste as the cooling, moistening juices soothe inflammation in the gut. Chickweed helps to emulsify fats, so is also a useful ally for releasing excess pounds.

Cinnamon makes a delicious tea that is helpful for nausea or indigestion. Perhaps you made the mistake of having what you thought would be a friendly political debate over dinner, which didn't turn out that well. If your stomach is still doing flip-flops and your digestive acids are working overtime, it's time for some cinnamon tea. Any species can be used for this purpose—*Cinnamomum cassia* or the so-called "true" cinnamon, *Cinnamomum verum* (formerly *zeylanicum*). I use about six bruised cinnamon sticks per quart of boiled water, steeped for about an hour.

Comfrey leaf is, to me, invaluable for specific purposes such as healing gut tissue. I write about the warnings concerning internal use of comfrey in the chapter on the musculoskeletal system. So please do your own research and draw your own conclusions. I'll repeat my mother's oft-heard advice, too: "When in doubt, don't."

Dandelion is an all-around supporter of healthy digestion. The root in particular helps the liver to do its many jobs involved in breaking down and assimilating food, stimulating healthy bile production and helping the liver and lymph work together to detoxify metabolic wastes. The root can be eaten in moderate quantities and/or used as tincture or infusion. This plant is gently aperient (slightly laxative), and will let you know if you are using too much of it!

Dandelion also supports the health of the pancreas, helping to balance blood sugars and stimulate the release of pancreatic enzymes to help absorption and assimilation of food. Dandelion root is rich in inulin (a sugar molecule that is called "nature's insulin"), which supports healthy bacteria in the small and large intestines.

Taking dandelion root tincture (about 25–30 drops in water) just before or after a heavy meal (15–30 minutes in either direction), will help stimulate digestive juices such as hydrochloric acid and strengthen the digestive fire. At the same time, dandelion cools down any area of the system that may be overheating.

Every part of dandelion except the yellow flower petals is bitter, arguably the most important flavor for the digestive health, and often the missing link in many Western diets. Dandelion greens make great nourishing bitters in salads, and hold up well when sautéed, steamed or boiled. If you include the green parts of the flowers (the sepals and bracts behind the petals) then the flowers are bitter, too. Bitters stimulate the production of digestive juices such as bile, leading to a digestive system in good working order.

In terms of nourishment, dandelion root is a great tonic to take in rhythmic waves of 2–6 weeks at a time, or seasonally, rather than daily, whereas the leaves and flowers are good eaten or drunk as tea, or used as vinegars, any time at all. (If dandelion root is being used to heal liver disease or some other chronic problem, it may be used for longer periods of time; it's simply not my practice to do so when using it as a tonic for general digestive-system health.)

Dandelion flower infused oil is sweet-smelling, and very nice to massage around your whole belly to bring relaxation and pain relief when there is cramping, indigestion or bellyache.

Ginger is a great warming root that raises the fire of the digestive system. This tropical plant is most useful for easing cramps, indigestion, and nausea. I like to use fresh ginger as an infusion, steeped for about an hour; I also infuse it in honey or glycerin for a sweet yet hot gingery treat that aids assimilation and counters nausea and inflammation.

Marshmallow (*Althaea* spp.) leaves, roots, and flowers are sweet, carbohydrate-rich, and somewhat akin to slippery elm bark in their effects in the body. Marshmallow is very mucilaginous, and is a perennial plant that can easily be grown in a garden, whereas elm tree populations have declined due to Dutch elm disease, so marshmallow provides another option. Marshmallow infusion, made from any part of the plant, can be helpful for soothing damaged tissue and moistening a dry digestive tract. In this case, make sure you are drinking enough water and other fluids.

Marshmallow is best prepared by soaking 1 cup of dry root per quart in cold water overnight, then heating the liquid gently *after* squeezing out the roots. This preserves and brings out the medicinal properties of the roots, whereas high temperatures can damage them, making the medicine less effective. I prepare the leaves and flowers together as a regular infusion, covering them with boiling water and letting them sit, steeping, overnight.

Motherwort *(Leonurus cardiaca)* is a bitter mint-family plant. This tincture is my remedy of choice for constipation brought on by nervousness or traveling (having difficulty moving one's bowels in new and unfamiliar locations is not an uncommon challenge).

Mugwort/cronewort is an aromatic bitter that stimulates the flow of bile from the liver and tones and strengthens the liver as well. I often use the leaves in cooking, or use the infused vinegar in meals. One or two tablespoons of the infused vinegar can be taken in water to aid digestion, and can be used successfully to forestall a hangover if you have overindulged in alcohol.

Oat straw makes a fine infusion to nourish digestion and balance blood sugar, with the sole warning that this infusion might not be for you if you have gluten allergies. Some people who find gluten irritating but are not allergic to it can drink oat straw without any problems. Oat straw is a great boon, as it is soothing and moistening to the digestive tract; although it doesn't provide the fiber of oatmeal, it nourishes the nervous system in the gut as well as its tissue, and can be helpful as a nourishing tonic to build and maintain the overall health as well as specific challenges of the digestive system.

Orange (*Citrus* species) peels from both sweet and bitter oranges make good digestive bitters, with bitter orange being more intensely bitter, naturally! I tincture the peels, and also dry them for tasty teas. Orange peels taste great added into other infusions too.

Plantain leaves nourish, tone, and heal the digestive system with a combination of astringency, soothing demulcent action, and fiber. Our wild plantains are a close relative to psyllium, and the seeds provide a bulk laxative that, when mixed with water, brings a gel-like bulky moisture into the intestines, improving elimination. If you use the leaves in food, infusions, vinegars, or even as tincture, plantain will slowly but surely improve the tone of the intestinal tissue and peristaltic contractions, reducing the need for the more laxative seeds or for synthetic laxatives and enemas. The seeds make a tasty addition to salads with a texture akin to sunflower seeds and their own unique, nutty taste.

Red clover blossoms make delicious infusions. I value red clover as an alkalinizing plant for the digestion, and find it to be most helpful for someone who suffers with acid indigestion and/or GERD (gastroesophageal reflux disease) and heartburn. As an alterative, it slowly helps turn the situation around. Fresh red clover blossoms can also be eaten freely in salads.

Rosemary tea is an invaluable aid in liver-related digestive distress, stimulating circulation throughout the body including the digestive tract. It has proven helpful in cases of gas, bloating and irritable bowels, and it is one of my favorite teas or tinctures for digestive headaches. Rosemary-infused vinegars and oils used in meals are lovely for gently stimulating a sluggish liver.

Yarrow flowers and leaves can be used as a cooling, aromatic tea, infusion or tincture to help when there is a bacterial infection in the digestive tract. This tea can also be drunk as a simple bitter, to stimulate the liver and aid digestion. It can be helpful to relieve nausea, including nausea from post-nasal drip.

Yellow dock root (*Rumex crispus* and other species) is my go-to plant for healing serious constipation. It is bitter and drying—not suitable for every day use—but can be used for extended periods of time when the need is there. I've used this for single incidents of constipation, but even more so for people who've had difficulty moving their bowels for years. I've also used it successfully for people who were ill and suffering from impacted feces. It facilitates bowel movements, and is classified as an aperient rather than a true laxative. (An aperient opens and relaxes the bowels, and a laxative stimulates them.) Yellow dock restores tone and function to the entire digestive system and is an astringent tonic for the liver and also encourages lymphatic circulation.

HEMORRHOID HEALERS

Herbs to help heal hemorrhoids (also known as piles) appear in various sections of *The Gift of Healing Herbs,* notably in the section on lady's mantle (see page 370) and several places in the section on the cardiovascular system. It's important to know what is causing hemorrhoids, and whether it is situation-specific and acute, as in pregnancy, or whether there is an ongoing, chronic challenge that results in these anal varicosities. Generally speaking, it is important to nourish the veins and vascular circulation, and to make sure that if constipation is causing them the constipation itself is addressed. Constant straining to move one's bowels is a common cause of this problem.

To summarize, the most helpful herbs for use externally as oils or as fresh or dried leaf poultices or sitz baths are: plantain, witch hazel, chickweed, yarrow, lady's mantle, and white oak bark.

Internally, nourish the circulation with abundant greens and dark berries, and for good vascular health drink grape leaf, nettle, rose, plantain, and hawthorn berry infusions, all of which can also be used preventatively or simply as nourishing tonics. You can include herbs like white oak bark or witch hazel as tinctures or infusions, internally and externally, when you need strong astringency to cool down and shrink inflamed hemorrhoids. If hemorrhoids (or, as I like to call them, "assteroids") are bleeding, then yarrow, witch hazel, and/or lady's mantle should be included.

I've had mixed results with it, but one of the most famous herbs for piles is stone root *(Collinsonia canadensis)* a mint-family plant with lovely lemony flowers, one of the few mint plants whose root is tinctured for medicine.

It's important to resolve any issues with constipation, as this can lead to many other problems in addition to hemorrhoids. Slippery, moistening, fiber-rich foods such as seaweeds, and infusions of burdock, dandelion, and yellow dock roots, are most helpful, as well as making sure you are moving your body, whether through walking, dancing, yoga, sports, or whatever pleases you.

Finally, fermented foods are a potent ally for feeding healthy gut bacteria, and important to include in your diet on a daily basis. Yogurt was mentioned earlier. Other important fermented foods that can be included are: kefir (a fermented grain drink), sauerkraut, pickles, beet kvass (fermented beets), miso (soybean paste), tamari, kimchee, and more. You can buy these foods or learn to make your own. Numerous classes, books, and online videos give instructions on fermentation. (See Resources, page 515.)

Now let's take a look at the "other" opening of the digestive system, as it's often left out of discussions regarding the health of this system.

Herbs for the Health of Your Mouth

The focus here is on nourishing healthy tissue in the mouth; preventing and healing gum infections; and preventing and healing bone loss.

When I was eight years old I had a wicked crush on my handsome Armenian dentist. No matter how much I hated the sound of his drill, I always tried to be a perfectly cooperative good girl when I was at his office, because I wanted him to like me too.

One time I had an abscess in and around my back molar. The infection was horribly painful. He told me he was going to give me a shot of novocaine, then open the infected tissue, drain out the pus, and put me on antibiotics. (This is still the standard treatment for a dental abscess.) He clearly was a believer in empowered, informed patients, even if they were only eight years old, but he scared the living daylights out of me. No one saw it coming that day when I got up and ran out of his chair, across the office, and down the stairs to exit the building. I couldn't imagine anyone touching that painful tissue, and my sense of self-preservation had kicked into high gear. I didn't stop running until I was halfway down the block of the broad city avenue, with my mother in hot pursuit. Of course she caught me, and eventually sweet-talked me into going back inside to have the procedure done. Miserable pain and swelling lasted for a long time after the treatment.

For many years before and after this experience, I spent an awful lot of time (and a lot of awful time) opening my mouth for dentists, periodontists, and oral surgeons. I had been going through dental hell almost since I was born. We all have our weak links, our areas of special vulnerability, and this was and is one of mine. I had no idea then, thank goodness, how many more painful dental experiences were in store for me. I suffered infection after infection, with gum disease, bone loss, tooth loss, and more.

By the time I was just sixteen years old I was told by a man considered to be one of the top dental specialists in New York City that I wouldn't have a tooth left in my mouth by the time I was twenty. He told my mother and me that I should have all my teeth pulled out or ground down and capped, as preventative medicine. It would take close to a year of visits and cost a fortune, he said, but in the end he said I'd have a "movie-star smile." I didn't run away that time, but I left there sobbing in fear and dismay.

That day, I decided there had to be a better way. There had to be options I didn't know about, answers that would help me heal myself. So I began the search that led me to herbal medicine, and thanks to herbal medicine my mouth is now healthier than it has been in my whole life. In fact, when I first started seeing my current dentist about ten years ago he began preparing me for pulling all the teeth he "knew" would have to come out as well as for the inevitability of all the infections I would suffer if I didn't do as he said.

When there are deep pockets, gaps between the gum and bone (early-mid periodontal disease), bacteria multiply there and typically erode all the healthy tissues, including eventually the bone. I told him I wanted to wait and see and, reluctantly, he did. My dentist recently said my mouth health is amazing, and the gums are in wonderful condition, and it is still a wonder to him considering how little bone there is holding the teeth in. I am happy to share information about the herbs that have been most important to me in reclaiming the health of my mouth. It is an ongoing process of paying attention and caring for it, but infections are now very rare rather than a constant source of pain and depletion of my whole system.

The herbs I love and use the most for maintaining a healthy mouth, and/or to heal infections, strengthen gum tissue, and tighten teeth, are: plantain leaves, witch hazel leaves, twigs, and flowers, yarrow flowers and leaves, echinacea root (and I imagine that flowers and seeds would be helpful too), sage leaves, rosemary leaves, horsetail, oat straw, nettles, pine needles and twigs, roses and rose hips, elder blossoms and berries, and hawthorn flowers and berries. Other herbs I like and use (or have used in the past) are: usnea, burdock, goldenseal, myrrh gum, bloodroot, violet leaves, and white oak bark.

I've also found salt, sesame oil, propolis, and green clay helpful. These can be used in a variety of ways, including, teas, mouth rinses with teas or diluted tinctures, dried and powdered herbs used as tooth powders/pastes, and direct application of softened plants as poultices on swollen tender gums. Herbal teas or diluted tinctures can be put into a water pick to direct the herbs deep under the gum line. If you do this, use the machine on the lowest possible setting, and rinse it out with plain water afterward. When you floss, be thorough but gentle.

There are many other herbs and natural substances that can be used, too, such as baking soda, neem, or cloves, but I am going to write about the ones I know the best, the herbs I've used for myself and clients over the years with great success. Let's delve into situations where these might come in handy, and how best to use them.

Horsetail *(Equisetum arvense).* Horsetail, also called shave grass, is an ancient herb on Planet Earth. Its highly assimilable mineral content is very useful for helping rebuild bone and other connective tissue. Remember that we don't want bones just to be hard, we want them to be strong. Strength requires resilient flexibility to withstand pressure and constant impact. Mere hardness will more likely lead to fractured teeth and bones.

It is best to use only spring-gathered horsetail, since its increasing silica content can be hard on the kidneys as the plant gets older and more brittle. Horsetail is a plant that is best used on and off, rather than as a constant daily source of minerals. Any pain in the kidney area is a signal that too much horsetail is being consumed. Adjust the dosage and frequency of use, and you will be just fine. Horsetail can be a kidney-healing herb, too.

Fresh horsetail can be cooked into soups and then removed, like bay leaves. Fresh horsetail can be steeped in apple cider vinegar for six weeks or more before decanting and adding to food. I don't generally use horsetail as a tincture. I most frequently enjoy it as a simple tea, pouring boiling water over one tablespoon of dried herb and steeping for 15–20 minutes. It mixes beautifully with aromatic (and astringent) rose and elder blossoms for a delicious mouth-healing infusion. When I put horsetail into a long-steeping infusion, I tend to put in a small amount, adding about two tablespoons to one quart of oat straw infusion, for example.

Oat straw *(Avena sativa)*. Oats are well-known for their abundance of highly assimilable minerals that nourish our musculoskeletal system, including our teeth and the bones in our jaw. I steep dried oat straw, including some tops, for about eight hours for a sweet, mellow-tasting brew that is infinitely more satisfying and safer than swallowing a bunch of mineral supplements. This can be used as a daily bone-building tonic, alternating with other mineral-rich infusions of herbs such as nettles (*Urtica* species), red clover *(Trifolium pratense),* red raspberry *(Rubus idaeus),* and alfalfa *(Medicago sativa).* Oat straw can also help with the kind of tension that can lead to temporomandibular joint syndrome (TMJ), which then causes teeth to get ground down. You can add a couple of tablespoons of dried St. John's wort *(Hypericum perforatum)* to increase the muscle-relaxing effects.

Plantain (*Plantago* species). I recommend regular use of plantain leaves to maintain healthy gums. Plantain's nutty, green taste and juicy, chewy texture make it a nice addition to a fresh salad. I also turn to fresh plantain as a first choice for a poultice when infection is threatening or already present. It's a gentle antiseptic, cleaning out infected bacterial pockets, and its astringency helps gums adhere to bone. It is also pain-relieving, always an issue with problems in the highly sensitive area of the mouth.

When a problem is acute and sudden, as opposed to chronic and long-standing, results are often seen very quickly. For example, a woman called me to say her grown son was getting periodontal surgery the following week, and was there anything to be done to help? I told her about my beloved plantain. She went to her tiny Brooklyn backyard and picked a bagful of plantain leaves. He followed her instructions, (that's the really amazing part of the story!)—he chewed up a handful of leaves and packed his mouth with the result, putting it between his cheeks and gums. He did this twice daily, and when he went back for the surgery he was told he didn't need it!

When you don't have access to fresh leaves, you can pour boiled water over dried plantain leaves to soften them. You can also pour boiling water over fresh leaves, but chewing it makes it even more antibacterial (see

Plantain section, page 281). Warning: It may hurt at first to have something touching a seriously infected area. Plantain and most of the other herbs can be combined nicely with internal use of echinacea infusion or tincture (always diluted in tea or water) in the presence of active infection. Echinacea can be used every few hours in 25-drop doses or so, or can be used 3–4 times daily in higher doses of roughly half the person's body weight in drops, or a ½ cup of an 8–12-hour infusion, 4 times daily.

Violet *(Viola odorata).* Sweet blue violet is another poultice I use to soothe inflamed gums. Its salicylic acid content helps it to relive pain and its mucilaginous quality can be a balm for tender mucus membranes/gum tissue. Fresh leaves, softened by chewing, or with boiled water, can be used. It can be drunk as infusion as well.

Witch Hazel *(Hamamelis virginiana).* Witch hazel is a major herbal mouth ally in my repertoire. Rich in tannins, it is highly astringent and anti-inflammatory as well as being a good antibacterial. It's an excellent choice for bleeding gums. The leaves can be used as a healing poultice, as described above. Additionally, witch hazel leaf and/or twig tincture (flowers can be included) has a regular place on my bathroom shelf. I put it onto my wet toothbrush, with or without natural toothpaste, once a day when all is well (and use it more frequently if infection is present) and gently brush along the gum line with it. I often combine it with yarrow tincture for this purpose. Witch hazel can also be massaged into the gums when prepared or purchased as an infused oil.

Yarrow *(Achillea millefolium).* Yarrow is one of my foremost mouth allies. I use the flowers when purchased, or the flowering tops including leaves and stalks when I've harvested them from my garden or from wild meadows. For maintenance, I use diluted yarrow tincture to gently brush and massage the gums as described above, toning and tightening them. Yarrow is a superb anti-infective and anti-inflammatory. Yarrow and witch hazel are two of my favorite wound-healers, and an abscess is like an infected wound in the mouth.

Yarrow is effective both as a tincture and as an infusion (steep for at least an hour). Personally, I prefer the infusion. If there is active infection in the mouth, yarrow will help with both pain and healing. I had

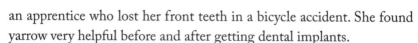

an apprentice who lost her front teeth in a bicycle accident. She found yarrow very helpful before and after getting dental implants.

Yarrow is indirectly useful for building bone. It helps the formation of healthy bone marrow—"yarrow for marrow." Many people with chronic mouth problems suffer from bone loss, and there is a tendency for this to happen to anyone as we age.

· · · · ● · · · ·

The infused oil of St. J's wort can also be massaged into the muscles of the jaw to help relieve jaw tension. If nighttime jaw tension or teeth grinding is a problem for you, you might also try taking St. J's wort tincture (25 drops) with 5–7 drops of skullcap (Scutellaria lateriflora) tincture within thirty minutes of going to bed. It can be a huge help. Chamomile *(Matricaria chamomilla)* works wonders for some people; I find it underrated as an antispasmodic. After a long and arduous dental treatment, it helps relax and relieve a tired, tense jaw that had to be held open for long periods of time. Chamomile is effective used as a poultice around the outside of the jaw, where even steeped tea bags can be helpful, and can also be drunk as a simple tea, brewed for five minutes.

The mouth thrives on good sources of Vitamin C such as hawthorn berries and flowers (*Crataegus* species), pine needles and twigs (*Pinus* species), and roses (*Rosa* species), using both flowers and hips. You could also enjoy elder blossoms and berries *(Sambucus nigra)* for their rich array of bioflavonoids.

I would suggest adding all of these into your diet on a regular basis in the form of long-steeped infusions of dried herbs (except for the pine, which can always be used fresh). Rose hips, hawthorn berries, and elderberries are best when they are steeped, with an airtight cover, for about twelve hours. I steep the flowers for one to two hours, and the pine needles can be steeped for as long as you like. I put one cup of well-cut-up pine needles, and tiny twigs or bark, into a quart jar. It is also a superb antiseptic infusion. The resin of pine can be put right onto an infected area in the mouth for even more antibacterial effect.

I have used both rosemary *(Rosmarinus officinalis)* and sage *(Salvia officinalis)* tinctures in the same way as the witch hazel and yarrow tinctures described above, to brush the gums. However, what I like even more is to dry these herbs and mix them in roughly equal amounts. I sprinkle some of this dried powder onto my toothbrush (with soft, natural bristles), with or without a dab of toothpaste, and brush my teeth with this once or twice every day. This is remarkably effective and nourishing to the gums, as well as being anti-infective and high in antioxidants. Fresh sage leaves rubbed onto teeth help whiten them, and when massaged into the gum lines help gums adhere to the bones and roots of the teeth; in other words, they shrink and close up periodontal pockets.

Old-fashioned warm sea-salt rinses are quite helpful as an antibacterial mouth rinse. I have also had people use powdered green clay as a toothpaste or plaster on the gums. It is powerfully drawing, so make sure it is not too strong for you. If you ever have a sliver of a toothpick or seed stuck in a gum, clay makes an excellent drawing poultice, as does plantain.

Baking soda or peroxide rinses and toothpastes are often problematic for people with sensitive gums. I have seen them cause bleeding. If that happens to you, discontinue them. Goldenseal, myrrh, and bloodroot are commonly used for mouth rinses; I used to use them, but find that generally I don't need such strong plants to achieve optimum mouth health. I like to use plants that are more common and abundant, more gentle and yet still powerful.

When I first investigated herbs for mouth care back in the late 1970s, I was told to massage my gums with sesame oil *(Sesamum indicum)* and drink white oak bark *(Quercus alba)*. Both of those suggestions are valuable. White oak bark tea or tincture helps strengthen the tissue in the mouth. It is rich in tannins and therefore highly astringent, and high in quercetin, similar to the pain-relieving, anti-inflammatory, salicylic acid. At the time I tried to make tea from powdered white oak bark, and found it impossible to drink. Now I use the cut bark as an overnight infusion or the tincture. Sesame oil, naturally antibacterial and anti-inflammatory, is perfect to massage into the gums for maintaining or improving their good health.

As with every other body system, herbs are a piece of the puzzle, not the single magic bullet that takes care of everything. The mouth is one end of your digestive tract, so diet and healthy elimination are also a big part of mouth health. The bio-available nutrients in any edible wild greens and berries will help heal the mouth. Stress, family history, kidney and bone health, general depletion, and environmental factors such as excess radiation all play a part in the health and/or illness of your mouth.

Finally, there are metaphysical or relational factors to consider. The mouth is one of the most obviously interactive openings into the body; it connects our insides with the world around us. Its vitality is connected to our fifth chakra, related to self-expression and speaking one's truth, or perhaps to having been shamed or silenced. So in addition to good oral hygiene, great nourishment, and practicing herbal mouth care, learn to speak your truth, to add your voice and perspective into the mix. Learn to ask for help, to express love freely, to know when to hold silence, and when to shout "no." Learn to let go and howl, or sing, or tone—for healing, and simply to express yourself fully and freely for the sheer joy and delight of it.

8

The Immune-Lymphatic System

Herbs and more for health, acute illnesses and chronic challenges of the immune-lymphatic system; strengthening herbs that tone and nourish you, particularly the body's filter systems, including lymph, liver, kidneys, skin and lungs; anti-microbial herbs to help heal bacterial, fungal, parasitic, and/or viral infections.

Your immune systems are comprised of all parts of the eco-system you know as yourself, and include not only every part of you, from your conscious and subconscious thoughts to your physical body systems, but also how you live and function in relationship with the larger eco-systems that surround you. So perhaps it would be more accurate to talk about your collective of immune systems. We'll focus here, though, on the lymphatic system, the part of the body designed to engage in self-defense and self-protection, as it's the system most clearly connected to what we call "immunity."

The lymphatic system is primarily a fluid system connected to the element Water. It also involves the ground of your being and thus the Earth. It is a remarkably intelligent system that, in addition to its innate abilities, acquires new knowledge through experience. It learns how to identify, tag and neutralize or destroy foreign presences. Your combined internal defenses collectively known as your immune system know how to tell the difference between self and not-self, to know whom and what to eat, engulf, and/or render inert, one way or another.

This system and its health, acute illnesses, and chronic challenges teach you what it is you actually need—emotionally, spiritually, nutritionally, sexually, socially, creatively, etc. in order to feel healthy, vibrantly vital, and alive. And when you're not well, these challenges ask you to find what you need—how much rest and how much activity, for instance, how much giving and how much receiving, and/or what you may need to let go of or embrace in order to heal. And you don't have to do it all at once. Sometimes you just change your attitude, and that helps a difficult situation to shift and change too.

For example, perhaps you have a job you don't like; maybe you're working for a tyrannical boss but because your rent is high and jobs seem scarce, you don't feel it's an option to let go of this job even though it's stressing you out and literally making you sick. You do have options; you can learn and practice ways to help you let go of thinking resentfully about your job and your boss, especially when you're not even there. You can drink supportive, strengthening herbal infusions to help you be present and take care of yourself by nourishing your immune system. This approach will also help you expand your sense of what's possible, so that you can seek and/or magnetize a new and better job for yourself with a boss who respects you.

Knowing your limits, accepting the need for self-care and learning to implement it, and asking others for help, are all vital aspects of healing. Many people feel challenged when it comes to incorporating proper rest, movement, nutrition, and time-out in nature into daily life, but each of these is as vital as herbal medicine. When the immune system gets too depleted, you become unable to continue functioning normally, or in the way that's become "normal" for you.

For example, you may be accustomed to living in a constant "go" mode, and yet end up getting stopped in your tracks because you won't choose to stop yourself and tend to your own need for self-care and fulfillment. Case in point: A dear friend of mine, going into the hospital for exploratory surgery, twisted up her mouth in impatient disbelief, and in all seriousness exclaimed, "I don't have time to get sick. Between the kids and work, I have too much to do!" Happily, she recovered, and has since found that she truly deserves and needs to make time for herself so that she can be well! When she reflected on her situation she realized she no longer found joy or meaning in her job, only security. She went back to school and invested time, energy and hard work to become a science teacher, accepting a substantial drop in her income in exchange for personal satisfaction and a sense of making a difference in the lives of children.

As you go about the busy business of living your life, the immune system can not only become weakened, it can also go awry in the mysterious form of any one of a multitude of autoimmune conditions that challenge people today. Auto-immune conditions such as rheumatoid arthritis, lupus, and multiple sclerosis often offer teachings around investigating and opening to the possibility that you might be working against your core self (often in multiple ways), either through trying to please others or attempting to control impossible situations, whereby you end up hurting yourself. However you are working against yourself, whether by giving yourself away in unfulfilling relationships, or eating food that is really bad for you—or something else entirely—healing often requires shining an illuminating light on yourself and your habits to get to the heart of the matter.

Wherever you enter into the process of healing, whether at the level of spiritual or life insights, nutritional understanding, relationship adjustments, job changes, and/or using herbal medicines to relieve and heal physical symptoms and problems, the healing can and will spread to other areas and continue to strengthen your immune system's healthy responses if you allow it.

Herbalist and educator Paul Bergner once shared an unforgettable story about his grandmother, who had pancreatic cancer. At age eighty-seven, she had lost a third of her body weight, been declared terminal, and given anywhere from weeks to months to live. She had also, it turned out, never fully grieved the death years earlier of someone she loved, and something triggered the realization inside her that she needed to cry. So she cried—for three days. After that, she began to gain weight, and eleven years later died of a stroke at age ninety-eight. Bodies are truly mysterious repositories of all that we are and of the lives we've lived, emotions felt, emotions repressed, and more.

The development of pharmaceutical antibiotics in the mid-twentieth century was a much-heralded breakthrough in terms of creating powerful, potentially life-saving medications for emergency use. However, this is not how antibiotics are used today, even though it is now widely understood that the overuse and inappropriate application of antibiotics for everything from a common (viral) cold to their inclusion as a "preventative-medicine" additive in livestock feed has led to a genuine crisis of antibiotic-resistant pathogens—wreaking havoc on the health of human and animal populations as well as creating chemical residues with long-lasting, destructive impacts on our land and water.

While I would never deny the importance of using antibiotics when they are truly needed, they should not be taken or dispensed nearly as lightly as they are, because they are also dangerous, both in terms of their primary impact, as I'll discuss below, and in terms of the variety of common side effects they engender such as the destruction of healthy gut bacteria, essential for digestive-system health and ultimately for our health in general.

Two-thirds of our lymph is produced in the liver and intestines. Therefore, when the gastrointestinal tract is damaged or impeded and can't function adequately, overall immunity decreases. Of course, you are never really "immune" to anything. It is speculated that everybody's body contains cancer cells and just about everything else that can and does make people sick; but these cells, viruses, etc. pass through you because the body silently takes care of these potential problems every day, filtering them out through the lymphatic and other systems.

A healthy immune system is like healthy soil in a garden. It is the ground of your being, and when well it has the ability to fend off pathogens so that you don't succumb to every virus, bacteria, or pathogenic microbe that passes by or even enters into you. A certain amount of immunity is innate, and then there is the acquired part of immunity that is learned through your lymphatic system's experience with and exposure to various antigens and other immune-challenging triggers, from parasites to fungi to bacteria. It has been argued that an inexperienced immune system sheltered from potential illness triggers is a weak immune system that won't know how to handle a problem when it comes along. Hence, the value of common childhood illnesses like measles (that doctors work to prevent through vaccination) is that they strengthen the immune system and help it learn how to work.

There are also less commonly known, but still too commonly seen, debilitating side effects of antibiotics. Generally, the more vulnerable the individual, such as the elderly and the very young, the more likely that side effects will be harmful and even life-threatening. *Bullous pemphigoid* is one example. These painful blisters can break out anywhere, such as in mucosal linings of the mouth and throat, where they can impede swallowing. This particular side effect ultimately hastened the death of one of my beloveds after she took a single course of antibiotics for pneumonia. The pneumonia cleared up, but her health was never the same, and she lived with many years of painful-to-agonizing outbreaks before she finally made a clear-eyed choice to take her own life—though she loved life as much as anyone I've ever known.

Fortunately, there are marvelous herbal alternatives that can help keep you healthy and allow antibiotics to work for you, if and when you really need them to aggressively stop a debilitating or life-threatening infection. Looking at how herbs help to counter infection and build immunity, as contrasted with how drugs work, can reveal something of the fundamental difference between traditional herbal medicine and modern allopathic medicine.

Essentially, bodies are always oriented toward healing themselves, and herbs work through building up and supporting the naturally protective filtering systems innate in the human design. We'll focus on herbs such as echinacea, burdock, dandelion, yellow dock, poke, and others that generally nourish, support, and/or stimulate the lymph.

Lymph is the clear fluid that contains infection-fighting white blood cells and bathes the tissues of the body. Lymph drains throughout the lymphatic system into the bloodstream, clears up debris and wastes, and targets potential and current threats. The herbs don't take over the job, but they strengthen your lymphatic system so it can do its job better.

Antibiotic drugs work through targeting specific or generalized pathogens, and basically end up (when they are successful) killing the invader, be it bacterial or parasitical—but also severely weakening the host (you). It's as if you say to your immune system, "You are too weak to deal with this anyway, so you're fired. Or, you know what? Why don't you take a vacation while I take these pills or injections; then come back when I'm done and get back to work." But the thing is, the system hasn't been practicing its art, or taking a nice healthful rest—it's simply been undermined, its multidimensional job taken over by a single-dimensional medication.

You have to work diligently and overtime to restore your gut flora after taking antibiotics, and also to send the signal to your immune/lymphatic system that it needs to work on its own again. After using antibiotics there is also a general weakening of your other immune-supportive filters, such as the kidneys and liver, with some antibiotic drugs being much worse in this regard than others.

When herbs are successful in helping you regain your health after becoming depleted of vital energy and therefore more susceptible to repetitive acute illnesses, or after a specific infection (be it viral, bacterial, fungal, or parasitic, since herbs can often be applied more broadly than drugs), you tend to be stronger and healthier than you were before you got sick. With pharmaceutical medication this is rarely if ever the case.

In talking about your "immune" systems, again, we are really talking about the entire body and mind because everything is a relevant part of how you stay healthy or get sick and then recover—or not.

Herbs can be applied like drugs, but that's not how I like to use them, nor how they work best.

It's important to identify which body system or systems are not working optimally, then to feed and strengthen it. Perhaps you keep coming down with lung or bronchial infections and need to strengthen your respiratory system, or perhaps you are susceptible to bladder or even more serious kidney infections, and the urinary system needs tending. If the immune system is working overtime in an autoimmune condition, there are herbs that can help modulate the system rather than attempt to stimulate it when it's already in overdrive.

Another way to perceive the immune system is to think of the lymph working together with the various filter systems of the body, especially the lungs, liver, skin, and kidneys. The other body system that's of primary importance to support immune health, is the nervous system. The state of our "nerves" is deeply interrelated with our immune functioning. (See Nervous System, page 182.)

A healthy immune system begins with mental and emotional wellness, and shows up when someone looks "glowing" or "radiant." This radiance is an energetic aura that is naturally protective. It is created when you are in a state of joy or contentment, for example, or freshly in love, or visiting a favorite beach or forest, or playing with a beloved child or animal.

Next, there is the acid mantle of the skin, the largest organ of the human body, which provides us with external layers of natural defense against bacteria and other potentially harmful pathogens that can enter through the pores. Unfortunately, there is a tendency in modern culture to literally wash away our protective acid mantle with too much soap, which turns the skin alkaline. The worst offender here is antibacterial soap that literally kills the bacteria-fighting layers of our skin! (Please see the chapter on Skin—The Integument System, page 280.)

I prefer to nourish my general immunity with lots of time outdoors, green herbs such as nettles, dandelion, plantain, yellow dock leaves, parsley, kale, broccoli, and more, and a great assortment of wild greens such as lamb's quarters, amaranth, cinquefoil, strawberry leaves, sorrel, oniongrass, and more—as well as with whole foods, good friends, community projects, time to play, meaningful work (even if unpaid), sexual fulfillment, time spent doing absolutely nothing, self-expression, sensual connection, creative outlets, and good quality and quantity of sleep.

Additionally, there are some immune-protective foods I include in my diet on a regular basis such as:

- Berries—support veins and capillaries; immune-building.
- Carrots—liver-nourishing.
- Lemon—cooling, antiseptic.

- Milk thistle seeds—liver-protective, with 2,000 years of recorded use.
- Mushrooms—immune-modulating, anti-tumor.
- Olive oil—an excellent, healthy source of dietary fat.
- Onions and other alliums—immune-supportive.
- Seaweeds—feed all body systems and protect against radiation.
- Sunflower seeds—protective against radiation.
- Wild greens—feed all body systems; high in vitamins, minerals and essential fatty acids.
- Yogurt—for immune and digestive nourishment.

For more dietary suggestions, see My Top Recommended Foods for Vibrant Health, page 426.

. . . . ● . . . . .

Some of my favorite immune-strengthening and anti-infective allies are: echinacea roots, usnea, yarrow flowers and leaves, poke root and berries, plantain leaves, burdock roots, dandelion roots, yellow dock roots, barberry root bark, astragalus roots, nettle leaves and stalks, elder flowers and berries, calendula blossoms, pine needles and twigs, propolis, sage leaves, turmeric root, garlic cloves, basil leaves, thyme, honey, salt, violets, cleavers, nettles, hyssop.

Some immune-strengthening, anti-microbial herbs include:

Astragalus (*Astragalus* species). An immune-modulating member of the pea-family (Leguminaceae) whose root helps rebuild the immune system after depletion; valuable tonic used as tea, in food, and in tinctures. Useful during and after chemotherapy or other harsh treatments to revitalize immunity; moistening, cooling, nourishing.

Barberry *(Berberis vulgaris).* The root bark, leaf, and stem of this non-native invasive shrub is a berberine-rich anti-inflammatory herb, beneficial for digestive system "bugs" and for those who have developed resistance to conventional pharmaceutical antibiotics. It is being used in herbal medicine to help people with tick-borne infections.

Basil. Antiviral, antifungal, antibacterial, and antiparasitic, for the digestive, respiratory, and nervous systems.

Burdock. Provides lymph nourishment; helpful as an antibacterial, antifungal, and antiviral agent; supports kidney and skin health.

Calendula. Vulnerary (wound healing), antiseptic, antibacterial, antifungal, antiviral; valuable for skin, topical and internal use.

Cleavers *(Galium aparine)*. Helpful in a fresh tincture for stimulating lymph; useful for skin and urinary system, including prostate.

Dandelion. Nourishes lymph and liver, strengthens kidneys.

Echinacea. Lymphatic support; supports and nourishes general immune functioning; best combined with herbs specific to the system being helped.

Garlic. Respiratory, digestive, skin, and lymphatic wonder-plant.

Goldenseal. Another berberine-rich anti-inflammatory and anti-infective, this herb is overharvested and endangered in the wild and should only be purchased organically grown.

Hyssop. Antiviral, wound-healing; supports respiratory system; especially helpful for bronchitis.

Lavender. Antiseptic, heals burns (simple or infected).

Lemon balm. Antiviral for herpes, venereal warts, shingles, and colds; calms nervous indigestion.

Oregon Grape *(Mahonia aquifolium)*. Berberine-rich anti-inflammatory; anti-infective.

Plantain. Antibacterial, antiseptic herb for the digestive and lymph systems; supports healthy lungs, kidneys, skin, and veins.

Rosemary. Antifungal, antibacterial, liver-supportive; a cardiovascular, central nervous system/brain tonic.

Sage. Antibacterial, antiseptic, especially for throat and feet.

Salt. Antibacterial; pulls out poisons.

Thyme. Antibacterial for lungs and bronchi; antifungal.

Usnea. Broad-spectrum antibacterial lichen, especially important for respiratory healing from fungal infections.

Yarrow. Antimicrobial, anti-inflammatory, and pain-relieving, especially for the respiratory system, liver, intestines, and skin.

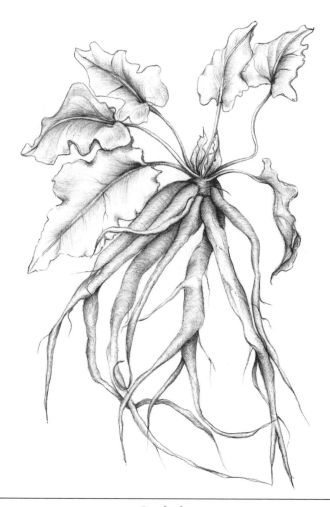

Burdock

Burdock (*Arctium lappa* and other species)

Body: nourishes skin, lymph, liver, kidneys, and gall bladder, and strengthens immunity.

Mind: helps with focused concentration, turns worriers into peaceful warriors.

Heart: helps with centering and grounding.

Soul: connects spirituality with the deep, dark fertility of Earth.

Burdock

I work deeply
To heal your blood within.
I help when cysts and pimples
Erupt on your skin.

Though sometimes I
Can make your skin break out;
I strengthen lymph and kidneys
And give them more clout.

I oil you up
In the healthiest way;
Your joints stay more flexible
And then you can play.

I feed you with
Root nutrients galore.
Cooked with ginger and seaweed
You'll want to eat more!

My roots are sweet,
My leaves are quite bitter.
I'm antibacterial
And I'm no quitter.

Inside thistles,
My seeds are very strong.
I am rich in medicine
And help you live long.

If you feel like
You need a new mentor,

> Trust me and I'll help you to
> Reclaim your center.

Burdock is a biennial member of the large Asteraceae (Compositae) family, originally from Europe but now a widely naturalized weed in the east and central United States. I like to dry burdock roots for infusions and use them fresh as food and for preparing infused vinegars and tinctures.

I was taught to use the late-autumn root as the most potent, medicinal part of burdock. Summer roots can be used successfully, too, but I more often harvest those for food. Herbalist Michael Moore recommended using the spring roots of second-year plants, which makes sense as you are then receiving the gifts of the nutrients that have been stored by the root all winter long. As you can see, there is not just one right way. This got me thinking metaphorically about the potential medicinal benefits of blending autumn-dug and spring-dug roots together.

The autumn burdock root, harvested when the life-energy of the plant is drawing down and sinking into the ground, can reach deep down into the lymph and get into the joints and kidneys, bowels, liver, and gall bladder, and slowly bring sustenance to the life-force and the blood. The spring burdock, harvested when the life-force of the plant is rising up and out of the ground, would stir up that waiting life-force, oil the joints for freer movement, tone the womb, get the blood and lymph freely circulating to move nutrients in and wastes out of the body, and help moisten the mucous membranes of the intestines and strengthen the liver and gall bladder to help slowly and surely regulate elimination through the digestive system.

It's an interesting paradox that a biennial plant like burdock who sends his substantial roots way down into Mother Earth is also a medicine strongly connected with fluidity and the fluid systems of the body, especially the circulatory, urinary and lymphatic systems. But then again, Earth herself is more than three-quarters water, just like bodies, so maybe this is no paradox at all, just another mirror of the cooperation between the elements that make up living beings.

When we look closely into the workings of nature, we can see that cooperation is the strongest life-force there is. We've been taught that tooth-and-claw survival of the fittest and endless competition are the overriding forces at work in nature. But that conveniently divides people and separates us from our greatest power, which is found in community, whether it's a community of cells that join together to create a healthy heart or a community of people who band together to protect a mountain from having its top blown off to provide a questionable notion of profit for a small number of people.

When a woman is growing an embryo into a fetus into a baby in her womb, everything in her body is working cooperatively toward the aim of creating a whole, healthy human being to further the species. Her kidneys will work at 150 percent of normal capacity to filter their blood; calcium will be pulled from her bones if needed to feed the growing embryo; and everything will work to maximum capacity for this creation to occur without harming either the mother or her child. This cooperation is mirrored everywhere we look. A tree struck by lightning falls and becomes food for the ground, a burrowing home for animals, a place for the growth of mushrooms, and a banquet table of insects for birds.

All elements cooperate for the greatest good, so that there is an ultimate orientation toward life renewing itself. This energy is always at work in our bodies, fed and strengthened by herbs such as burdock. It is our natural orientation to heal, to grow, and to thrive. When a wildfire sweeps through Sequoia-tree country, the seeds are given the heat they need to germinate and grow into trees. (Here Fire overtakes Earth, but then Earth is reborn.) When a volcano erupts, lava flows; and when the fire meets the water it creates the newest land on Earth; and that land is fertile and lush, inviting rapid new growth. Soil itself is a living revelation of the cooperation that exists throughout natural systems, constantly adjusting and changing its composition according to the plants that are growing in it, even as the plants are changing their chemical composition to best benefit from the contents of the soil they're growing in. Plants may look passive, but they are not passive at all. Neither are our bodies.

If your lymph nodes get swollen and painful, it doesn't feel good. You feel sick but your body is actively doing its job, confining the metabolic wastes that would overtake your system, holding them in check in your swollen glands while it rallies the forces it needs to heal itself/you. Case in point: In the late 1980s I had a tall, slim beloved who manifested what turned out to be the first full-blown case of tuberculosis recorded in New York City in many years.

I was a fledgling herbalist. After he had spent a year ingesting several potent antibiotics that have become the standard treatment for modern tuberculosis, he was weak and thinner than ever, but declared cured. A month or so later he came to me and showed me a hard lump in his armpit. I discovered that all throughout his lymph system were swollen nodes, with about two dozen hard, various-sized lumps. He went back to the hospital where he had been treated because there was one doctor there whom he respected and trusted. She told him he needed to get a biopsy done right away, as he most likely either had cancer or tuberculosis throughout his lymph. He said, "No, not without talking to my herbalist first."

I was scared, and felt I was in over my head, but I had an instinct that his body was trying to clear itself after all the drugs he had taken, and that his lymph system had gotten overwhelmed. I suggested he take herbs for two weeks and go back for a biopsy if the lumps were still present. He took high doses of burdock root together with echinacea root, because together they are such a great team for catalyzing the lymph system.

LYMPH-LOVERS TINCTURE BLEND

30–60 drops or more of burdock root tincture

30–60 drops or more of echinacea root tincture

These herb tinctures, blended together in hot or cold water, will help the lymph fluid move freely and clear away bumps, lumps and other swellings that indicate wastes and congestion in the system.

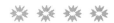

My friend used about 60–80 drops of each herb tincture in water, 4–6 times daily. He began to feel better, and the lumps began to soften and shrink until they were all dissolved. After he went back to the hospital to make sure all was well, he gleefully told me that his doctor said, "Well, either you're a genius or you know a genius!" His doctor was right. The genius he knew was our bountiful burdock (and echinacea)!

Burdock is a powerful protector, and can help transform you from being a worrier into a warrior. It does this by offering such life-enhancing medicine that you become physically stronger and healthier, inspiring you to feel more confident. I've also seen again and again that the more we root and center ourselves in our relationship with Earth, the more we engender a basic feeling of peace and security within—especially crucial in this time of massive personal, social, and environmental changes.

I communicate with burdock as a grandfather plant; when addressed with respect, trust, and gratitude, he will help most deeply. Burdock helps your lymphatic system to be strong and flowing in the presence of all kinds of challenges from teenage acne to lymphoma. Burdock is a fighter, as you can see when you are digging out a root. The roots are canny and, given half a chance, climb under and around giant stones. Perhaps this is the way, symbolically, that burdock approaches swollen lymph nodes and growths—surrounding lumps, swellings, and tumors and then dissolving them over time or slowly but surely pulling them up and out.

Many know burdock (along with red clover and other great lymph-movers) by that quaint, heroic term "blood-cleanser." Blood-cleansers are thought to busily pull out all your impurities and toxins. But your metabolic waste isn't necessarily a toxin, it's simply what your body can't use, and it's meant to be excreted by your filtration systems. The conception of your blood as dirty is not one that feels accurate or self-loving to me. Burdock nourishes and strengthens the challenged filtration system, whether that is the lymph, kidneys, or liver, so that the system itself becomes healthier and can clear away the wastes as it was designed to do. Burdock doesn't take over for your body, as drugs do, which would ultimately weaken it, but supports it in functioning optimally.

Burdock is a great herb for the skin, the largest organ and filtration system in the body. I turn to burdock for many different skin conditions including boils, acne, eczema, and psoriasis. Pimples, rashes, cysts, and boils often will come out through the skin when other filtration systems such as the kidneys, lungs, or intestines are overwhelmed. Burdock is a great helper in all of these conditions, helping both the symptoms and the underlying cause. The problem itself can manifest from something as simple as eating too much sugar and white flour at a holiday party one night or, if those are regular dining choices as in the standard American diet, as a warning sign of deeper problems stirring within the body.

I have seen that sometimes, for some people, burdock makes skin conditions get worse before they get better. When this happens I might switch the person to red clover because it will get the lymph moving and skin-clearing processes going in a gentler way. Or, if the person is willing to handle the discomfort and vanity-challenge of their skin getting worse, it will often be absolutely radiant when they come all the way through the process and out the other side.

I gave a young client at Columbia University burdock root to use for her acne, with instructions to drink 1–2 cups of the infusion daily. The young women in her dorm wanted none of it when she told them about it. Two months later they were begging her to tell them where to buy it when they saw how her skin was clear and glowing.

BURDOCK LOVES SKIN—A SIMPLER'S RECIPE

½ cup dried burdock roots

1 quart water

Put the burdock roots into a one-quart jar. Pour boiling water over them, filling the jar to the top. Wait 8–12 hours and then pour off the liquid, then squeeze out the (now expanded) roots. Drink this hot or cold, sweetened or not, and refrigerate the rest.

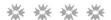

Burdock is an immune tonic that is also safe for autoimmune conditions, since it isn't a stimulant but a complex food-like medicine and a nourishing tonic. I had a situation where I gave a friend burdock root for psoriasis, an autoimmune challenge. When you have psoriasis, your immune system's T cells mistakenly identify your skin cells as "other" and attack them. This attack injures the skin cells, setting off a cascade of responses in your immune system and in your skin, and resulting in skin damage (swelling, reddening, and silvery scaling).

My friend had had patches of psoriasis on her scalp for years. After drinking burdock, it got much worse; it got more intense where she was used to having it, and then began coming out in places she'd never had it before. She was disappointed and angry. My sense when this sort of thing happens is that burdock is reaching deep into the system to help it clear itself. We really want stuff that isn't good for us to be drawn up and out if necessary, rather than to work its way deeper into the body.

I explained this, and tried to shift her herbs for a time to make the process easier on her, but she wasn't open to continuing the herbs. The truth was that she'd never really wanted to use them in the first place. Her boyfriend had convinced her to try herbal medicine because he'd had success with tea and tinctures I'd given him earlier that year. In fact, he was spared an exploratory surgery he'd been told was inevitable—but that's another story.

Within the year, this beautiful young woman was diagnosed with lymphoma. I believe that the burdock was going after the deeper problem when she first took it to help the psoriasis. Eventually, while her doctors were arguing about which chemotherapy she needed for her "incurable" lymphoma, her boyfriend again convinced her to use herbs, and burdock became one of her chief allies for healing herself from this disease. She used conventional medical treatments as well, but her primary herbs before and after chemotherapy were infusions of oat straw *(Avena sativa)* due to a personal connection she had with this plant from her childhood, burdock root *(Arctium lappa),* and red clover blossoms *(Trifolium pratense),* along with tinctures of echinacea root *(Echinacea angustifolia)* and pokeroot *(Phytolacca americana).* She is doing beautifully now, more than fifteen years later.

Poke root is a very intense, stimulating plant medicine for the lymphatic system. It's also traditionally used, especially in the southern United States, for rheumatoid arthritis, another autoimmune condition. Unlike burdock, poke root *cannot* be eaten as a food, although the leaves—properly prepared by cooking and throwing out the cooking water several times—can be eaten when they are very young and green, before any hint of red has appeared in the stalk.

One amazing thing that happened is that this woman knew nothing about identifying herbs, but when I went to her home for a consultation after her lymphoma diagnosis I couldn't help but notice that there was an entire dried poke plant full of purple berries tacked on her wall with push pins, like a poster. She told me that she'd been hiking and felt really drawn to the plant when she saw it. She had not only harvested it but recently worn it to a costume party. I commended her on her intuitive wisdom as I introduced her to the poke plant. Her mouth fell open and her eyes lit up with delighted laughter. That connection helped her to trust plant medicine—and herself—more.

. . . . ⬤ . . . .

Burdock helps your other filtering systems too, especially the urinary and digestive systems. Each of these is biologically brilliant, designed with such absolute perfection that it is evident that we, our cells, and the cavernous black spaces between our cells, are all bits of living consciousness creating and destroying itself all the time. Like skin cells sloughing off by the millions only to be replaced by new cells, we're always dying while we're living. We are fluid energetic matter, though we appear to be individual and contained. No matter. An unintended pun!

The good news is that energy cannot be destroyed—only transmuted and transformed. Science has demonstrated this, but I don't think it has yet come close to describing the marvel of infinite consciousness that we know as the body.

I would consider putting burdock into a recipe when helping someone with almost any kind of cancer. It is an important ally for lessening the side effects of conventional chemotherapeutic treatment. For this purpose, burdock can be used along with seeds from the milk thistle plant *(Silybum marianum)*, also taken as a tincture.

Herbalist Gail Faith Edwards writes that burdock's "profuse mucilage binds with chemicals, heavy metals, and unwanted by-products of metabolic processes, helping them to exit the large intestine quickly." She also tells us that using burdock tincture for two to three weeks after a course of antibiotics will help repopulate our healthy gut flora.

Burdock roots are useful (often combined with dandelion roots) to help regulate blood-sugar levels, whether you are hypo- or hyperglycemic, pre-diabetic, or even diabetic. Burdock and dandelion are rich in inulin (nature's insulin), especially first-year roots dug in the autumn. If you make your own tincture, you will see the inulin in the white, starchy sediment that builds up in the bottom of the jar and is a sign of a good burdock tincture. (Many of my students have forgotten that, and thrown out perfectly good burdock tincture, assuming it had gone "off"—so if you make your own, remember this, and don't do that!)

I've seen regular use of these herbs actually necessitate lowering a person's dosage of insulin. To be crystal-clear, daily use of these herbs when you are taking insulin should be done in conjunction with careful monitoring of blood sugar levels to avoid insulin shock. Your medical practitioners should also be informed and involved in that desired transition to less medication.

Burdock can be beneficial to anyone when used as a delicious food. It is a sweet, mineral-rich root vegetable, like a carrot or parsnip. Fresh young burdock can be eaten raw, slivered into salads—though I personally prefer it cooked into stir-fries, soup, or stew. It is traditionally partnered with ginger, carrots and seaweed, such as hijiki, and it's quite delicious that way. Fresh burdock retains more vitamin C than dried burdock, even when cooked, and it is also rich in essential fatty acids (EFAs).

During burdock's first year, it creates a large rosette of thick green leaves, grey and somewhat fuzzy underneath. During its second and final year, a new rosette appears and then tall, branching flower stalks grow out of its center. Purple thistle-type flowers are followed by the (in)famous burrs that stick to everything, transporting seeds far and wide. I like to harvest and use burdock roots from first-year plants each autumn, after the rosette of leaves has begun to die back. (Note that there will be no flower stalk yet.)

I finely chop the fresh roots and prepare them as medicinal vinegars and tinctures. I also dry the roots for infusions. These roots do not need to be chopped anywhere near as finely as for tincture. You can chop them into two inch pieces, or dry larger pieces of root as you prefer. If the roots are very thick, slice them length-wise down the center to help them dry more easily. You can also buy roots to tincture or dry in a good health-food store that sells fresh, organic produce, or almost any Chinese or Japanese vegetable market where it may be sold as *gobo* or "great *gobo*" in Japanese markets, and *niupang* in Chinese. Dried powdered burdock can also be added to soups or rice, mixed into immune-strengthening honey balls, and/or added to healing salves.

As I've said, burdock works well as a tonic for most of the body's main filter systems—digestion, urinary, lymphatic, and skin. Tonics work like exercise—the more regularly and rhythmically they are used, the better. Just as you'll benefit from exercising once a week every week, more than you will from seven days a week once a year, more benefit is derived from using tonics rhythmically, which can vary from something like one month on and one month off, or one week each month, or for three weeks every spring and fall, to give a few examples. As such, burdock is a great herb for most people at least some of the time, as a vitalizing tonic to achieve and maintain vibrant health and energy. Burdock can safely be used regularly, even daily when called for, for several years, as it works slowly and surely to restore our health and vitality.

The following recipe is an example of bringing together two very different plants and their energies to make a helpful "both/and" remedy.

DEEP-ROOTED EASE BLEND

25–50 drops (1–2 droppers) burdock root tincture

13 drops skullcap leaf and flower tincture

Put the tinctures into tea or water, and drink hot or cold 1–4 times daily.

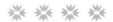

This recipe is a marvelous mixture for combining the deep-rootedness of burdock with the lightening effects of skullcap. Herbalist Kiva Rose's apt nickname for skullcap is "blisswort," and I see it as a plant friend who helps us remember how to center in our natural ease and joy.

I have given this blend to people undergoing challenges, both physical and emotional, for a long time, who are reaching crisis level. I have given it to people who have gone numb, and others who keep breaking into tears and don't know why. I also like this blend when there is a need to deepen someone's trust in being in a body at all. The specific amounts of herbs might be adjusted depending on the person or the situation and the blend will work equally well as an infusion if you prefer.

This recipe will strengthen the kidneys, soothe the nerves, and help relieve various aches and pains. In Traditional Chinese Medicine the kidneys are where our *jing* or essence is stored, and the kidneys are also associated with our fears. I use this blend when there are indications calling for nervous system and digestive system nourishment, as well as for urinary and lymph/immune support. It can be helpful if you overuse your intellect, get stuck in your head, get depressed or self-defeated easily, or find yourself wallowing in self-judgment.

This recipe is useful when you need to cultivate groundedness along with spiritual and/or emotional lightness. It can help you move forward in your life with a sense of calm strength. Skullcap helps you relax and not take everything, including yourself, so seriously; and burdock helps you move more freely from a place of inner stillness.

It may seem paradoxical, yet it is true: When you are stuck in a self-defeating pattern of thought, or something inside you is stuck, as in lymphatic or digestive congestion, you may need a plant like burdock that is deeply rooted and entrenched, planted as solidly in the ground as the mythic sword in the stone. As you take the burdock into yourself and embody it, you slowly and steadily become more solid, centered and grounded, and then everything within you flows more fluidly and freely.

One of the core concepts that attracts me to wise-woman ways of healing is the idea of looking for the "both/and" rather than the "either/or" in our approach to healing. This thinking posits that rather than holding an antagonistic approach to choices, where there is a right and wrong way, everything can be seen as a combination of both. We can use conventional *and* traditional medicine, for example, choosing the most helpful rather than thinking that we *should* do one thing or another.

The following practice is a favorite linguistic self-awareness tool that I suggest you use for taking pressure off. I use it frequently. It is simple and effective, and can help you to slowly yet surely change patterns of habitual self-judgment.

Simple Kindness Practice

Substitute the word "could" whenever you might
otherwise use "should."
For example, when you hear yourself say: "I *should*
(take my herbs),"
Change it to: "I *could* (take my herbs)."

Say both of the sentences out loud, and you will immediately feel the difference. (Really, do it right now!) In the first sentence you are already judging yourself. In the second, you are offering yourself a choice, which is kinder, more truthful, and more empowering. Don't "should" on yourself! (Or anyone else, for that matter.)

Create an intention to compassionately catch yourself saying that you "should" do this or that. Re-state your sentence, aloud, even if it seems inconsequential, such as, "I should do the dishes … call him back now … write that paper.…"

By substituting the word "could" you consciously take back your power, acknowledging that the choice is always yours. The consequences not only reach out far and wide in your life, they also strengthen your immune, nervous, and other body systems.

I invite you to explore the deep sense of peace and groundedness that burdock offers through the simple yet profound ritual of connection that follows. The plant taught it to me when I lived in New York City, and

I've taught it to many others who have also found it helpful. You don't always need to actually *take* the herbs. Sometimes you just need to hang out with them. I've been particularly touched by the positive response of young men to this ritual.

As you proceed, if you feel guided to do it differently, please do—and then I hope you'll share whatever burdock rituals *you* come up with.

My Favorite Burdock Ritual

Find a good-sized first-year burdock plant (though even a tiny one will give you a sense of this). Burdock gets a flower stalk later, in its second year, but the first-year plant will be a rosette of large, green leaves that are grey underneath, have no flower stalk, and grow outward from a common center. Put your index and third fingers of both hands together so that all four fingers meet in the center of the burdock rosette. Close your eyes. Breathe. Take thirty seconds or more.

This ritual is transformative. Burdock knows something worth knowing—how to be still, and know you are. Burdock teaches us to act from a place of peace and inner calm rather than restlessness and impatience.

Here's a story of using burdock root for a sixteen-year-old cat. My apprentice Vivian called me because her beloved cat Honey hadn't been acting like himself. Honey's symptoms were weakness and extreme lethargy. He was also in pain, having trouble urinating, and not eating much. Upon taking him to the vet she learned his kidney enzymes were elevated. Since kidney failure is the leading cause of death in elder cats, this was not good news and, as the vet said, modern medicine has nothing curative to offer in this situation. He wasn't hopeful about Honey's prognosis.

Vivian took him home, and after we spoke she made him an infusion of dried burdock root and corn silk *(Zea mays)*.

KIDNEY-EASE INFUSION

½ cup burdock root

1 cup corn silk

Put the herbs together into a one-quart jar and cover with boiling water. Let them steep, covered, for 8–12 hours. Then strain and refrigerate for use.

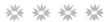

My friend gave the cat the herbs twice a day by filling a dropper with the infusion and squirting it directly into his mouth. I prefer to add the tea on top of (or mixed into) wet food when possible, but she was taking no chances since his appetite was so low and she wanted to make sure the herbs got into him.

I love corn silk for soothing and healing a variety of urinary-tract conditions. It is astringent, antibacterial, and a moistening demulcent. Here we were using the burdock for both its nutritive and immune-enhancing qualities, and to help build and strengthen his kidneys so they would more easily filter his blood and release his urine. The corn silk was in the recipe to help moisten and soothe his urinary tract, relieve his pain and promote healing of the tissue.

Vivian called me about three weeks later to tell me that his kidney enzymes had lowered to normal, and he was doing really well. The vet was surprised when she told him she'd given Honey two herbs to help him heal himself. He even said he was impressed. (But not enough to ask for more information!)

Recently Vivian called me and told me how well they were both doing, and with a smile in her voice added, "We're celebrating Honey's eighteenth birthday today!"

This infusion is a perfectly good remedy for humans, too, to strengthen and soothe the kidneys, bladder and urinary tract, as well as help counter infections. I also use corn silk to help men with prostate challenges such as pain, trouble urinating, and benign enlargement of the gland.

I use the roots of burdock more than other parts, but the leaves, seeds, and peeled flower stalks can also be used for food and medicine.

Burdock leaves are as bitter as the roots are sweet, and provide one of my favorite, effective remedies for a freshly erupted (or about to erupt) itchy poison-ivy rash.

FRESH BURDOCK LEAF POULTICE

Fresh burdock leaves (*Arctium lappa* or other *Arctium* species)
Boiling water

Cook the whole, fresh leaves, after rolling or pounding them a bit, in a shallow pan for 5–10 minutes in just enough water to cover them. Then take the leaves out of the pan, let them cool enough for comfort, and lay them over the itchy area.

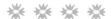

The first time I tried this was for my friend Jackie, who had wiped some summer sweat off her face with her gardening glove, not remembering that she'd been pulling out poison ivy. Ouch! Her face was soon breaking out with a miserable, hot rash, and the burdock was abundant, so I put a large burdock leaf, prepared as described above, onto each cheek as if two loving green hands were holding her face. Her husband laughed at her green cheeks, but she didn't care. She said it was like having her face inside a freezer, which was just the kind of soothing she needed!

I've used this treatment for animals, too. My neighbor's standard poodle Max came in from the woods with a bright pink case of poison ivy that he was scratching and scratching. His human, Jacqui, told me that he would never let me do it, but after one touch of the burdock he stretched out his legs and rolled over, offering me easier access to spread the leaves on his pink belly and flank. My neighbor and I laughed, gratefully!

Burdock leaves can also be gathered fresh to help achy joints. Susun Weed taught me to roll them up and place them in a bottle of vinegar. This works well as a way to store them and keep them ready for use when they are not in season. The leaves can be unrolled and gently heated, or used as is, and placed over an achy hip or other joint for relief. Then, as long as they are not being used over an open wound or infected area, they can be re-rolled and put back in the jar for use again and again, until they are no longer helpful. These leaves, or freshly gathered ones, can also be used as a poultice over an inflamed liver or gall bladder, or for any muscle, ligament, or tendon strain or sprain. I've used fresh burdock leaf, boiled or rubbed briskly between the palms, as a poultice that brings great relief for broken toes. Conventional medicine offers nothing for broken toes, but a burdock poultice reduces the pain and inflammation even as it speeds the healing.

The above poultice you probably don't want to chew up before applying, not only because the burdock leaves are hairy underneath but because they are very bitter to taste. Hold a fresh leaf between your fingers and gently rub the leaf. Then taste your fingers. You will see what I mean, and thereafter you'll be able to correctly identify a burdock plant by taste, as you'll be unlikely to forget it.

You can dry burdock leaves as well, and reconstitute them with boiling water to make a dry-leaf poultice.

DRY BURDOCK LEAF POULTICE OR COMPRESS

Dried burdock leaves (enough to cover the area)

Boiling water

Pour just enough boiling water over the leaves to completely moisten them, and let them sit for about 5 minutes. Lay the softened leaves over the area in need for 20–30 minutes or more (to all day, depending on the situation). For poison ivy, leave the poultice on for as long as it feels soothing. For a broken toe, I might put it on once or twice for 20 minutes during the day, and perhaps sleep with another poultice or compress on it overnight (for other possibilities, see Wound and Bruise Healing, page 471).

You can also make a compress by wrapping the softened leaves in cheesecloth rather than applying the leaves directly to the skin. If you're working with cut-up leaves, this method will make it easier to apply and keep the poultice on.

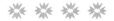

Juliette de Bairacli Levy uses the leaves as a poultice on the skin for burns, and for the fungal infection ringworm. I'm sure the effectiveness of this poultice would be enhanced by also using burdock root internally.

Burdock seeds can be collected from second-year burdock plants after their gorgeous, showy purple flowers have turned into round seed balls that are sharp to touch and contain many seeds. These seeds have a hook-and-loop system that is ingenious for seed dispersal; they attach themselves to anything that passes by, such as hairy dogs or humans wearing clothes, so that they can hitch a ride to a new location. Close examination of such seeds led to the creation of Velcro in the 1940s.

To say it's not easy to harvest burdock seeds is a bit of an understatement. The burrs that contain the seeds have sharp hairs surrounding them, so you don't want to separate them by hand. I put the burrs in a paper bag, roll it closed and whack it repeatedly on the ground to get the seeds out, or use a rolling pin. Fortunately, if you're not up for that bit of fun, they can also be purchased.

Burdock seeds are used for acute relief of chronic skin conditions including eczema, psoriasis, and rosacea. Seeds can be used as tea, tincture, and/or infused oil. To make your own burdock seed tincture:

BURDOCK SEED TINCTURE

Burdock seeds (fresh-gathered or dried)

100-proof vodka

Wide-mouth jar

Fill your jar about 25% full of freshly bruised burdock seeds (or grind them if you prefer) and then cover them with the vodka, filling the jar to the rim. Wait about 6 weeks before decanting the liquid and squeezing out the seeds into it.

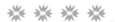

This is a powerful preparation that will strongly encourage the flow of urine. Burdock seed preparations have traditionally been used to both prevent and relieve kidney and bladder stones, sludge or gravel. The root, though, would still be used to help the underlying condition that is causing those symptoms.

You can also make burdock seed tea by steeping a teaspoon of the bruised or ground seeds in a cup of boiled water for 10–30 minutes. Burdock seeds taste a bit tingly on the tongue, like echinacea seeds. Herbalist Jim McDonald says this signifies that the nervous system has been engaged, and will therefore bring a quick response.

It's said that burdock seed preparations, including external use of burdock seed oil, can help hair growth, but I haven't seen that for myself. I have also read that in pregnancy, burdock *seed* preparations are only safe to use in the last trimester.

Here are a few more ways I like to use burdock:

Burdock root vinegar: Apple cider vinegar is a perfect menstruum for extracting the nutrients from burdock's roots and making the mucilage, vitamins, phytosterols and strengthening, cancer-fighting minerals bioavailable. I especially like the vinegar infusions for joint and bone health. It's good to have options, and rotate your culinary/medicinal vinegars as your tastes and needs vary. Add burdock root vinegar to soups, stews, salads, or sautés, or put 1–2 tablespoons in water to drink. You can add honey to taste. Use it in your rotation for at least a year for the best long-term results.

Burdock root/violet leaf/red clover infusion: This trio is important. Each of these herbs is cancer-preventative and can be very helpful for maintaining lymph, breast, and uterine health. Dandelion root could be added, too, or alternated with the burdock root.

One more tip: Burdock is a brown root on the outside, and light-colored on the inside. A lot of people make the mistake of peeling burdock's outer skin—don't! Simply brush off the dirt with a vegetable brush and rinse if necessary. It's perfectly edible.

BURRY BURDOCK RITUAL

Here's a burdock ritual I think is worth sharing because it's so uniquely crazy! I found it in an online article called "Scottish Folk Medicine," and I love that Scottish sense of humor! (By the way, I do *not* recommend you try it.)

> One special ritual with Burdock was traditionally held in the county south of Edinburgh. On the second Friday in August the *Burry Man* paraded around the town of Queensferry and circumnavigated the town boundary dressed in a costume comprising several thousand burrs from Burdock and with flowers at shoulder, hips and knees. He was completely encased in the costume, no provision being made for calls of nature, and was expected to drink plenty of whiskey but to eat nothing while he perambulated from dawn till dusk! It's thought that the intent of the custom was to catch evil sprits in the burrs, the entire costume being burned ceremonially at the end of the day. (Edinburgh Museum Pamphlet #8)

Here we can also see how burdock got the nickname Beggar's Buttons! You could also use the burrs in a magical ritual to symbolically draw something to you—perhaps an opportunity to share your music or art— or to represent something you are looking for such as a new job, home, or opportunity to travel. But I would only do it to draw something I intended to stick with, because with burdock burrs in the mix, like the Velcro they inspired, it will want to stick with and to you!

Dandelion (*Taraxacum officinale* and other species)

Body: supports kidneys, liver, and lymph for skin, digestive, immune, musculoskeletal, and reproductive system health.

Mind: helps with seeing the bright side and having a happier outlook.

Heart: encourages a sunnier disposition, relieves habits of anger.

Soul: deepens awareness of one's interconnection with all life everywhere.

Dandelion

Dandy Lion, so dear to me,
Everywhere for all to see,

Roots and leaves and flowers and seeds
All fulfill our bodies' needs.

There is so very much of you
'Cause we need you, it is true.

You are a doctor with no fees.
Roots for liver; leaves, kidneys.

Flowers ease pain and help lymph flow
And perform a sunny show.

I've heard that seeds are useful, too,
Adding bitters to the brew.

Dandy Lion, so dear to me,
Everywhere for all to see.

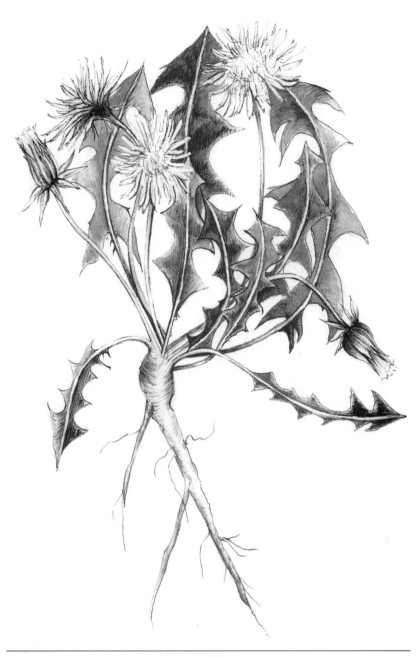

Dandelion

Common dandelions, relentlessly poisoned by homeowners seeking "perfect" lawns, are profoundly healing plants containing vitamins A, C, D, and B complex as well as minerals such as iron, potassium, and zinc. Their leaves have more beta-carotene than carrots, and more calcium and iron than spinach. Dandelions are members of the Asteraceae family, and are often found growing together with burdock in the wild. Rich in antioxidants, carotenes, and phytosterols, dandelion is a nourishing tonic for liver and lymph functioning, acting as a strengthening and restorative ally for the hormonal and reproductive systems.

There is natural latex in dandelion's roots, leaves and flower stalks. This white sap, applied frequently, is an effective topical dissolvent for warts. I had a student who roller-bladed over to Central Park every morning for a couple of months to put some sap on a wart she'd had on her finger for years. She watched as it got smaller and smaller, until it was gone. This is not uncommon; it usually works beautifully. I haven't personally known anyone who is allergic to synthetic latex to also react to natural latex. However, if you do have a latex allergy, start with a small amount and make sure it agrees with you and your skin.

The whole plant has a cooling effect and is bitter and drying. Dandelion roots and leaves stimulate the production of hydrochloric acid in the stomach, necessary for digesting fats and proteins, and helpful for more complete assimilation of minerals such as calcium. It is also a plant rich in inulin (nature's "insulin") which helps to balance blood sugar and promote weight loss when desired.

I use dandelion as a liver tonic, an adjunct to reproductive tonics, and for the lymphatic system. Every part of dandelion is nourishing and medicinal. The roots, especially those dug in the fall, are a time-honored medicine for replenishing and strengthening the liver. Dandelion root can be chopped fresh and cooked into stews or sautés, and eaten in moderation. If too much is eaten, it will act as a laxative.

More typically, the roots are dried for infusions or tinctured in alcohol and used as a healing liver tonic. Even though it may seem counterintuitive to use an alcohol preparation for the liver, the amount of alcohol being consumed in a tincture is quite small. It can be used for a "sluggish" or overworked liver, hepatitis, or cirrhosis. Think of dandelion when someone works with harsh chemicals—a stylist in a hair salon who is regularly exposed to synthetic dyes and nail polishes, a groundskeeper on a golf course who is exposed to pesticides, someone working in a garage or pumping gas regularly who breathes in volatile organic substances, an artist painting with oil paints, or a photographer processing photos with darkroom chemicals. The liver, with hundreds of jobs to do for our bodies on a regular basis, must be aided when it's being overworked. Brilliant as they are, our livers were not designed to assimilate and excrete the volume and variety of harmful substances they are often exposed to, over and over again, throughout our modern lives.

Dandelion root is effective when dried and made into infusions or decoctions. Roasting dandelion roots is fine as a coffee substitute (or drunk in its own right), and is still medicinal, but for more serious conditions I suggest the unroasted root, which retains its full complement of bitter constituents. It is the bitterness that makes it so beneficial to the liver and gall bladder; one of the ways to judge the quality of your roots is by taste. Even here there are alternate opinions; Finnish herbalist and teacher Henriette Kress says that to her, the autumn dandelion roots are sweet!

Dandelion is also a great source of assimilable iron. You can drink dandelion root as a simple, or mix bitter and sweet roots with tart berries, as in this root brew, and many variations are possible. Here's a recipe:

ROOT AND BERRY BREW

    ¾ cup dried burdock root

    ½ cup dried dandelion root

    ¼–½ cup dried elder berries

    ¼ cup dried yellow dock root

    Blackstrap molasses (optional) adds iron and sweetness if you
    are turning the infusion into a decoction

Put the roots and berries into a half-gallon jar. Cover with boiling water. Cap tightly and let sit out on a counter, steeping overnight.

The next day, strain and squeeze out the herbs. This is a very strong (and strong-tasting) medicinal infusion, and I like to drink it as is, but you may want to decoct and sweeten it. If so, put the infusion in a pot on the stove, uncovered, over a very low flame. When the volume of liquid is reduced by half, you have created a decoction that is twice as strong as the original infusion.

This strengthening brew needs to be stored in the refrigerator. 1–2 tablespoons can be taken daily as a preventative tonic. I use 2–3 tablespoons twice a day when there is a low red blood cell count, and anemia and fatigue. It will help digestion, lymph circulation, the skin, and overall energy. It will also help lubricate the joints, and keep the liver and kidneys functioning well. If you find this or any infusion too strong, dilute it with some water and adjust your herb amounts the next time you make it. When you use herbs and wild foods, your tastes will change over time.

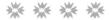

Dandelion leaves are a fabulous food medicine. They are salty, which tells us they are rich in nutrients, and bitter—though not as bitter as the roots—and they are specific for anytime you need to nourish and tone your kidneys. Dandelion leaves are famed for being an effective diuretic that puts potassium back into the body rather than depleting it as pharmaceutical diuretics inevitably do.

I dry dandelion leaves to mix into infusions. I also dry them when they are still on the roots, in spring or fall, to use in infusions. The leaves are a good bitter green, stimulating digestive juices, and can be eaten raw or cooked. I especially like to sauté my dandelion greens with onions and garlic, and season them with a homemade herbal vinegar and olive oil, as in the recipes that follow.

There is a widely believed myth about dandelion greens that I'd like to debunk here—that they are too bitter to eat after flowering in the autumn. Not true! Some of the sweetest, tastiest fresh dandelion greens you can gather are found growing freely in lawns and meadows every autumn. New York City naturalist Steve "Wildman" Brill tells us that dandelion greens are sweetest after there's been a frost. But they're dandelions, so they're still bitter, even when they're sweet!

Here's the dandelion leaf recipe:

BITTER DELIGHT—VARIATION I

1 cup red or yellow onion

2 cups fresh dandelion greens

Olive oil, to taste (use the first cold-pressing of oil, which is expeller-pressed rather than subjected to high heat or chemically extracted; it will be labeled "cold-pressed")

Wheat-free tamari, to taste

Shiitake vinegar, to taste (see recipe below)

Enough water to fill the pot about an inch deep

Dice the onions and sauté them in olive oil until they are translucent and soft. Tear up about 2 cups of dandelion greens and cook them very well (until tender) in about an inch or so of boiling water. Stir them, along with whatever cooking water is left, into the sautéed onions.

Add olive oil and season to taste with liberal splashes of tamari and shiitake vinegar. (See recipe below.) Stir well and serve.

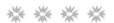

This remedy/dish will stimulate your digestion, make your liver and kidneys hum with health, and nourish your immune system even as it delights your palate. Shiitakes are helpful to the lungs. Like most medicinal mushrooms, they are immuno-modulating, helping to harmonize all the immune functions of the body without chemical stimulation. Onions are rich in health-promoting minerals and vitamins, and are generally one of the most fundamentally basic, immune-nourishing foods available.

Vinegar balances acid-alkaline levels in the blood, which is good for the musculoskeletal system, and as a fermented food is especially healthful for digestion.

The shiitake vinegar works well with the bitter dandelion greens, bringing out and complementing their flavor, and softening it at the same time.

Shiitake vinegar is a delicious medicinal preparation that you can make and take very easily, and a helpful way to make sure you regularly consume these wonderful mushrooms.

SHIITAKE VINEGAR

Fresh shiitake stalks (or whole mushrooms) to fill a jar

Apple cider vinegar

Before or after cooking the mushroom caps for another dish, take the leftover stalks one at a time and, holding each one from the top (where it was connected to the cap) slowly pull the fibers apart by hand, lengthwise, from top to bottom. The fibers separate naturally, like thin threads of string cheese, and it becomes almost a meditation to prepare the vinegar this way. If this doesn't feel to you like the perfect way to prepare them, both physically and energetically, as it does to me, you can simply chop them up with a knife.

Always use a glass jar with a lid made of plastic or cork, as metal will rust. If you must use a metal lid, be sure to line it with a piece of unbleached parchment paper (or use wax paper or plastic wrap) that hangs down just below the bottom of the closed lid.

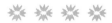

I usually keep two jars of shiitake vinegar within easy reach in the kitchen. One is for current ingestion and enjoyment, and the other is a work-in-progress. For the work-in-progress, I use a wide-mouthed pint glass jar with a plastic lid, and put a temporary masking-tape label on it that might say, for example, "Shiitake mushroom vinegar, started June 4, 2013." I include "working" on the label, too so I can easily tell which jar I am filling.

Each time you cook shitakes, add the stalks to your jar, and keep adding enough vinegar to cover the mushrooms until your jar is full. Then store it in your pantry for a month or two until you're ready to use it. You can make another label now, or when it's ready (or if you're not feeling fancy, just scratch out the word "working"). In our home we always have some jars on the shelf. They've never gone bad. Also note that this preparation doesn't need to be decanted; just use the mushrooms along with the vinegar.

BITTER DELIGHT–VARIATION II
(AKA BITTERSWEET DELIGHT)

Replace the olive oil with coconut oil, and you have a very different-tasting dish. The coconut oil adds its moistening, EFA-rich oils, and its own antiviral, immune-boosting properties to the mix. If you want to add back in a little bitterness, you could use dandelion leaf and/or root vinegar for this variation of the recipe.

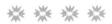

Whichever oil or vinegar you use, it is a tasty, immune-strengthening, and satisfying treat.

For optimum nourishment, use leaves from the wild, including a lawn gone wild, but store-bought or, even better, local farmer-grown dandelion leaves, will be beneficial, too. Be sure that any area you're gathering from hasn't been sprayed with poisonous pesticides. If you have a lawn, let at least some of it go back to a natural, pesticide-free state, and you'll be rewarded with lots of free food and medicine including dandelion blossoms.

DANDELION BLOSSOMS

I once had a dream in which a flowering dandelion said, "I am a light in the darkness." And because dandelion takes to heart her instructions to be available to us, sometimes you'll even see a dandelion flower here or there in the winter. In any season, but certainly most abundantly in the spring, if you are feeling low and need a little yellow ball of sunshine to cheer you up, just look—there she is!

Every year I await the return of these bright yellow disks with great anticipation, and then reward their appearance by promptly popping them right into my mouth and eating them! They are delightful in sandwiches and salads. I pull apart the blossoms and spread the sunny yellow rays throughout the dish I'm putting them into, and they look beautiful in there. If you only want their sweet taste, don't put the bitter green parts of the flower into your meal, just the yellow.

Dandelion blossoms appear to be one flower growing on a single stalk, but look more closely. Each "flower" on that hollow stalk is actually made up of hundreds of individual ray flowers (florets) that will be pollinated by insects (though, if necessary, they can fertilize themselves). These fertilized florets will mature into many seeds within a fluffy white globe. Each seed grows on its own silky "parachute" that will be borne aloft and carried by the wind to spread dandelion goodness far and wide, to the joy of herbalists, children, and wise adults everywhere.

Maria Treben was an Austrian herbalist who passed away in 1991. She shares many inspiring stories of healing in her book, *Health through God's Pharmacy*. She had deep faith in common, local herbs, and used traditional European herbal medicine for everything from paralysis to palsy. She advised people with diabetes to wash the stems, and only then to take off the flower heads and slowly chew and eat five to ten stalks a day, every spring. Dandelions help keep the blood sugar in healthy balance, and she shares that the stalks are especially effective for this in their season. She also says that people who are constantly tired should do this for fourteen days in the spring, and they will be surprised at the good effects. I always suggest eating the stalks and the flowers, unwashed.

If you eat the dandelion stalks, save the flower heads to use in food, tincture, vinegar, and/or infused oil. It is certainly traditional wisdom in many places around the world to gather and eat lots of fresh dandelion leaves and some roots, raw and cooked, for a month or more every spring as a way to enliven the blood, and tone the kidneys, liver, and lymph flow. Dandelions are all about movement flowing freely within the body.

I also make a fresh dandelion flower oil every spring, even though I've had infused dandelion oils last in beautiful condition for five or more years. I love the golden-yellow color of the oil, and it has a magical way of opening up places in the body where emotional tension is stored. It is a favorite ally of many masseuses and masseurs because they don't have to work so hard to help their clients relax. (See page 54 for recipe and special tips on making dandelion-infused massage oil.)

I also tincture dandelion flowers in alcohol, and like to mix that tincture with leaf and root tinctures so I have a medicine made of the whole-plant, bottom-to-top. Sometimes you can harvest the plant and get all the parts at once, which is great, but I like to harvest the roots when they are strongest, early in the spring before the flowers, or later in the autumn.

I also recommend dandelion-flower tincture on its own, as it can be helpful for opening up and releasing bottled emotions, and helps us to look at things with a sunnier perspective. Dandelion flower essence is helpful for that, too.

I've read that dandelion seeds are used in Chinese medicine, but so far I've only admired them. When I'm ready, I'll try them, and that will be a new herbal adventure for me to write about later.

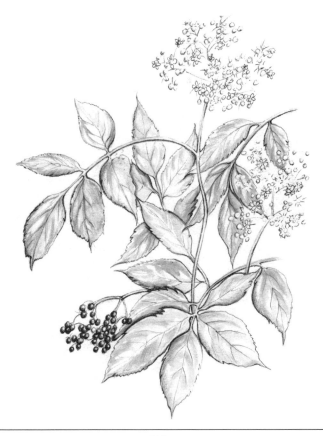

Elder

My Beloved Elder (*Sambucus nigra* and other species)

Body: bioflavonoid-rich, antiviral for colds and flu. Flowers are used
for fevers, ear pain, sinus congestion, wounds, skin, kidney
support, blood and lymph circulation, and berries are rich in iron
and ease chest congestion and coughs.

Mind: increases awareness of the "big picture," enhances knowledge
of interconnection and the unity of all life.

Heart: opens the heart to receive ancestral guidance.

Soul: stimulating, evolutionary plant that offers guidance through
the chaos of transformation.

Elder

What a treasure you are!
Your spirit is strong.
You are Grandma Elder;
You ease so much that is wrong.

You came down from the stars
And up from the Earth,
Mysterious healer
Of inestimable worth.

You have toothed leaves in pairs,
With one on the end.
Your flowers and berries
Make you a great healing friend.

Your creamy-white blossoms
All bob on the breeze
And are brewed and infused
To stop a cough or a sneeze.

When we breathe in the steam
Of fragrant hot tea,
Our sinuses and ears
Won't feel all clogged and stuffy.

Your rich purple berries
Loaded with iron
Help when any new flu
Brings its symptoms so tiring.

Flu, fever, coughs, and colds,
Rough skin and sore eyes,

Gentle guide through chaos—
Grandma Elder, you're so wise!

My first plant ally was the elder tree or, as I like to call her, my beloved elder. It was one month before I formally became an herbal-medicine apprentice, so this was before I knew that a plant ally is a plant or tree that you choose (and are chosen by) for a lifelong relationship. As your relationship with the plant grows and deepens, it becomes a special liaison for your communication with all the other plants, and you can call on it for any type of healing you need for yourself or others.

I was living in New York City, and had a dream that I was being pursued and had gone into hiding. I was getting ready to sleep under a small, wild-looking tree with a rounded crown. I felt safe when I finally got settled underneath it. It was a magical night in spite of the danger, and the tree seemed to have lights sparkling in it. Now I recognize these as the elder's umbels, the creamy-white, nearly flat-topped clusters of flowers that abundantly adorn the tree in June.

When I met my first actual elder tree in October 1985, it was past flowering and fruiting, and was pretty shabby-looking and insect-eaten, yet it unmistakably called to my heart. I felt a clear connection between us, and then recognized it from my dream. Later I learned the legend that if you sleep under the elder tree on Summer Solstice eve, you will see the fairy folks. Did I see them that night in my dream?

Every part of the elder tree is medicinal, but the flowers and berries are the most frequently used and safest parts to use internally. The leaves and bark are purgative, and I don't recommend them for internal use. However, the fresh leaves may be used externally in a simple oil, salve, or liniment for bruises and sprains by steeping the green leaves in olive oil, lard, or rubbing alcohol for six weeks and then decanting them for use. Maud Grieve shares an intriguing compound herbal recipe, stating that the leaves are:

> ... very cooling and softening, and excellent for all kinds of tumors, swellings and wounds: Take the Elder leaves ½ lb., Plantain leaves ¼ lb.,

Ground Ivy ⅛ lb., Wormwood ¼ lb. (all green); cut them small, and boil in 4 lb. of lard, in the oven, or over a slow fire; stir them continually until the leaves become crisp, then strain, and press out the ointment for use.

Elder leaves are also famous as a natural insecticide, made by infusing the dried or fresh leaves in boiling water and then applying the tea to the body and/or clothes when it has cooled. It's said that strewing the leaves also deters mice and moles. I'm looking forward to trying this in our gardens this summer, as our cat isn't able to keep up with all the creatures who come by for free samples!

I've used mainly the blossoms and berries, and can speak more about their medicine from my own experience.

ELDER BLOSSOMS

Elder blossoms are antiviral and can be used for head colds, for problems with skin, ears, eyes, or upper-respiratory tract, and as an anti-infective generally for any of those systems. I also like elder blossoms for healing the tummy if there is queasiness or nausea from post-nasal drip.

Elder blossom (infusion or tincture) is the first herb I reach for when there is fever. Remember that fever is not an illness but a healing response to an illness. If the fever is necessary for healing, elder won't bring it down, but it will regulate the fever mechanism, bringing it down when the time is right. It's one of my favorite plant medicines for upper-respiratory congestion, as it's so helpful in opening clogged sinuses. (Upper respiratory refers to the nose, sinuses, and throat. Lower respiratory refers to the bronchia and lungs.)

EASY ELDER FLOWER INFUSION

1 cup dried elder flowers

½ gallon water

Pour boiling water over the dried elder blossoms in a half-gallon glass jar. Cap it tightly and let it sit out for about 2 hours. Strain out the herbs and squeeze them to get every drop of goodness.

This infusion can be refrigerated and gently reheated on a stovetop. I often pour it into a stainless-steel thermos to drink throughout the day. You could also put it in a pitcher with ice if it is a hot summer day. This infusion is safe for anyone from infants to elders, and you don't have to be sick to enjoy it.

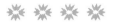

Elder flowers are important for conditions such as sinusitis and common allergy symptoms. I think of drinking elder infusion when I want mucus to flow more freely out of the sinuses, releasing acute congestion of stuffy nose, red, watery eyes, and painful ears. Elder flowers ease sinus headaches, and generally help the body to release fluids and cool down.

Elder is expansive, moving things out from the center. When you look at the tree, you can see that the flower and berry umbels expand outward too. Even elder's branches are arching and reaching out from her center. Elder is classified as an astringent and is somewhat drying, but I find her flowers subtly moistening to skin and internal mucus membranes. One of the most effective ways to use elder flowers is as a slightly astringent yet moistening steam for sinusitis and common allergy symptoms.

ELDER FLOWER STEAM

½ cup dried elder flowers

1½ quart or more water

Put elder flowers into a 3–4-quart soup pot. Add 1½ quarts or more of cold water. Cover and bring to a boil. As soon as it boils, turn it off and let it steep, covered, for about 10 minutes.

Set up a place where you can sit comfortably at a table with the steaming pot of elder on a heat-protective mat in front of you. Put a large towel over your shoulders so that you can pull it closed tightly underneath your chin. Pull the rest of it up over your head (tie your hair back first if needed) and put your face over the steaming pot. Please be careful, as the steam can burn you if you come too close to it or if you let your nose touch the hot water. Put the towel down around the outside of the pot and then circle your arms over the towel, holding them closely around the pot while the towel acts as a "potholder" to protect your arms. If it's still too hot, you can lift up your head and/or the towel. You want to be able to relax over the pot and breathe deeply to open your sinuses and relieve chest congestion.

There are additional benefits to an elder steam. The first is that it will make your skin glow radiantly. The second is that if you have ear pain, stuffiness, or infection, the elder steam works wonders. When you are under your towel, tilt your head from side to side, "breathing in" slowly and deeply through each ear as if you had a nostril there, and imagine the steam flowing through your sinuses from one ear all the way through your head to the other. Even if only one ear hurts, or especially if there is an infection in one ear, always treat both ears; otherwise the condition is likely to migrate back and forth from one ear to the other.

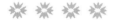

If you look at labels in a health food store, you'll notice that a lot of beauty products, especially for skin, are made with elder blossoms. Elder nourishes the capillaries, increases circulation, and oxygenates the body including the skin. It's known to reduce or prevent wrinkles. Elder blossoms are also used as a wash to soothe stressful skin conditions like burns, cuts, wounds, and ulcers. It can be used for sunburn, too. I've used it successfully, both as an infusion to drink and in full-body baths, for eruptive skin conditions that are infectious—specifically for measles and chicken pox, where its antiviral, immune-enhancing properties coupled with its skin-clearing effects have proven invaluable time and again. I like to mix it with nettles for this use.

In much of Scandinavia, birthplace of the legend of Elda Mor, the healing woman who lives in the elder tree, the flowers are used far more frequently than the berries, often even exclusively.

ELDERBERRIES

Contemporary studies have focused substantially on the antiviral and immune-strengthening properties of elderberries. Original research in the 1980s from Hadassah hospital in Jerusalem was the first to show that elderberries are more effective against flu than any known flu medication. I use the berries as an iron and vitamin-C tonic, and for colds, flu, and lower-respiratory viral infections. I turn to elderberries for coughs and chest congestion, especially the kind that starts out as a head cold and then moves down into the chest. Elderberries can also be used to improve the flavor of less tasty infusions.

EASY ELDERBERRY INFUSION

1 cup dried elderberries

½ gallon water

Pour boiling water over the elderberries in a half-gallon jar. Cap it tightly and let it sit for a minimum of 8 hours. (I prefer a longer steeping time, about 12 hours.) Pour off the liquid, squeezing out the berries as much as you can between your hands, or wringing them out in a piece of cheese-cloth. Refrigerate and/or reheat the infusion as described in the Easy Elder Flower Infusion recipe. Compost the berries.

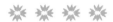

I also like to powder dried elderberries in an electric seed grinder (you can use a mortar and pestle if you prefer) and then store the powder in a glass jar to be used in or on food for the extra iron and immune nourishment elderberry provides. It also tastes good in sauces. You can make a honey spread with this, too.

POWDERED ELDERBERRY HONEY SPREAD

1 cup elderberry powder

2 cups honey

Grind dried elderberries to make the powder. Put them in a jar and pour the honey over them. Stir until the powder is saturated with the honey. This is ready to be used right away, and provides a powerful remedy for cold and flu that can be taken alone, spread on toast, added to tea, or whatever your imagination comes up with.

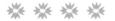

I was inspired to try herbs as powders by English herbalist Anne McIntyre, and to use the herbs in honey by medical herbalist Paul Bergner. I prefer not to cook this honey spread so that it doesn't lose any potency.

You do not need to refrigerate honey preparations or tinctures. You can buy elderflower or elderberry tincture, or make your own.

EASY ELDERBERRY TINCTURE

Fresh elderberries—enough to fill a jar

100-proof vodka or brandy

Wide-mouth glass jar of any size

Fill the jar with the elderberries so that it is full but not jammed tight. For example, a pint of tincture would take about 1–1½ cups of berries. (You may use elder *flowers* for this tincture, but you'll need about 2 cups of fresh flowers for a pint jar, as they are much lighter and less dense than the berries. The other amounts and guidelines remain the same.) Pour vodka— from glass bottles only, please—over the berries. Fill the jar to the top, and then cap it.

Wait at least 6 weeks and then pour off the liquid, squeezing out the berries as thoroughly as possible, one handful at a time with or without cheesecloth; or use a small herb press designed for home use. (See Resources, page 514.)

Before I continue, Elder would like to speak for herself:

I like to have my feet wet. That tells you something about me right there, and I'll get to that in a minute. Do you notice how my bark is so many different textures and colors? It's always changing. See how it's covered with nipples, like a generous mother? I can easily sacrifice my branches and my limbs, which get brittle in the winter and can snap off in high winds. Most of the year I'm moist, juicy and flexible, so I do grow new limbs back readily enough. All the elements are inside me, the same as they are inside of you. I need earth, water, sunlight, and air, just like you.

Remember how I said I like to have my feet wet? I especially like wet places, and I can help you with cold and dampness too. If you get wet and cold and develop symptoms of the common cold in your head or in your chest, use my flowers for your head, and my berries to help your bronchia and lungs. My flowers love to soothe and ease open your sinuses so you can breathe in and out deeply again. That's one way to open yourself, to shift your consciousness, to awaken to a larger perspective. And that's my deeper purpose.

You know it's the time of your Earth's evolution when women need to lead the way to a transformed world culture—not without men, of course not, but guiding them as mothers, sisters, daughters, loving partners and leaders. We elders are here to help in this time of vast transformation. Remember that we are your natural guides through chaos. It all seems terribly urgent from your perspective, with your illusory sense of time. And it's true that every choice you make matters. We also want you to get together and laugh about things, to gather and sing and celebrate each other's lives. This will help you own your power and effect change, more than you know.

I am here to hold and mirror the energy of sacred space. Respect everything in the material world, for the divine is contained in every aspect and facet of existence. Self-respect is one of my primary teachings.

I've lived on Earth for a long time, but I don't come from here. I come from the stars above and the stars below, within the Earth. Wherever the dimensional bridges are, there I am. You intuitively planted me in the in-between place, didn't you? Between the forest and the field. I am your guide through chaos. I am maiden, mother and crone, both elder and younger. I cover and hold the magical, multidimensional passageways to other places, star places, and places deep under the ground. In our groves we join together to create a container for the chaos that transformation requires you to travel through. We offer you our guidance to help you journey. Come sit here with us or, even better, underneath us.

We elders are guardians between this world and other worlds, and we help you to connect with your ancestors.

We also remind you that wherever you go, there's nowhere to get to but *here*.

Humans often say, *"I'm getting there,"* as in, "please be patient with me," but since what you really need is to be fully present wherever you are, try saying, *"I'm getting **here**,"* aloud, and feel the difference!

Remember, your path is always under your feet.

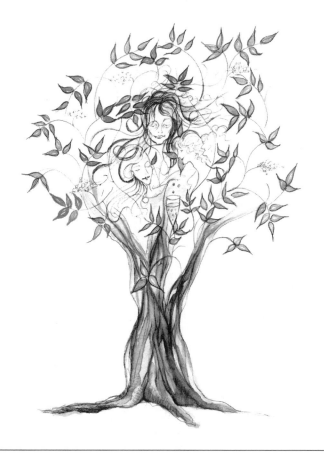

Elder Tree

Here are some additional recipes featuring elder blossoms and elderberries:

TOTAL ELDER INFUSION EXPERIENCE

1 part dried elder blossoms

2 parts dried elderberries

There are three ways I make this infusion because sometimes one way feels easier to me and sometimes another. They all work well.

Method 1:

Pour boiling water over ½ cup of flowers in a quart glass jar. Cover. Steep for 1–2 hours.

Pour boiling water over ½ cup of berries in another quart jar. Cover. Steep for 8–16 hours.

Decant the two infusions. Before decanting, you can put the elderflower infusion in the refrigerator when it is cool enough, then wait until the berries are ready and decant them both at the same time if you prefer. Mix the infusions together and you have a delicious, bioflavonoid-rich healing blend that brings together the medicinal and nourishing qualities of both flowers and berries.

Method 2:

Put 2 cups of elder berries in a half-gallon jar.

Put ½ cup of elder blossoms into an unbleached coffee filter. Staple it closed (my silly joke is to always use organic staples!), and add this to the jar. Cover with boiling water.

You will need to fish the filter out of the jar after about 2 hours, and squeeze it into the infusion when it's cooled down enough to handle. Both of these methods can be applied to any infusion recipes where the herbs being blended require different lengths of time to steep to their perfection.

Method 3 (Lazy Herbalist Method):

Ignore the proper steeping times above, and put your ½ cup of flowers and cup of berries into a half-gallon jar, then steep overnight. My father taught me this method because he found the other ways too much trouble. To my surprise and in spite of how I was taught elsewhere, it works really well for elder and some other flowers such as linden and hawthorn! I'm not trying to confuse you, dear reader; I'm simply wanting to show you the variety of things that happen in real people's kitchens when they get their herbs home. There are a lot of "right" ways to make your herbal medicine! You can experiment and find out what you prefer, or follow what I present. Either way, the healing powers of the herbs will help and delight you!

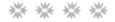

SOS (STRENGTHEN OUR SINUSES) ALLERGY RELIEF POWDER

1 part dried elderberries

1 part dried goldenrod leaves, stalks and flowers (any *Solidago* species)

1 part dried nettles leaves and stalks

Grind the herbs finely in a seed/coffee grinder that's reserved for your herbs. Combine them in a jar for ease of use. Take from 1 teaspoon–1 tablespoon daily in hot or cold water, yogurt, or honey. Or sprinkle atop oatmeal, applesauce, or other food. Using local raw honey will add to its effectiveness. A second daily dose, or even a third, can be added if needed.

For a small animal such as a cat I suggest giving ⅛–¼ teaspoon daily. When I grind up the freshly dried herbs, I put them together into an 8- or 16-ounce glass jar for daily convenience. You could make this blend as an infusion, but it may work best as a powder because you're consuming the whole plant.

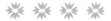

This powdered herbal blend is a tasty blessing during airborne (pollen-induced) allergy seasons. It strengthens and nourishes the immune system, and acts as a natural antihistamine. Regular use, especially before the season in which your allergies act up, will decrease your need for allergy medication. Coupled with other healthy practices, this blend is so strengthening it can altogether eliminate your need for pharmaceutical allergy relief.

I've also used it to great effect with animals (mixed into wet food) and people of all ages. Any cat or dog I've given this blend to has liked it. The first cat I gave it to had been sneezing excessively for years. After 1–2 months of use, her sneezing stopped and has never resumed!

ELDER BLOSSOM DELIGHT—VARIATION I

1 tablespoon dried elder blossoms

1 tablespoon dried nettle leaves and stalks

½ teaspoon dried hibiscus flowers (Malva species)

Put the herbs in a saucepan and pour 2 cups of water over the herbs. Bring to a gentle boil, turn down flame, and simmer for 10 minutes or so.

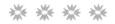

This delicious recipe has a touch of tartness from the vitamin C-rich hibiscus. The hibiscus also brings a bit of moistening balance to the astringency of nettles and elder. If you like, you can steep this brew longer, up to 2 hours. Bioflavonoid-rich elder, vein- and artery-strengthening and elasticizing nettles, and all three herbs rich in iron make this a healthful, delicious brew that is good at any time of day. At night it will soothe you; yet if you drink it in the day it will help provide good, focused energy. When you taste it, you probably won't need any other reason to drink it!

ELDER BLOSSOM DELIGHT—VARIATION II

½ cup dried elder blossoms

1½ tablespoons dried hibiscus flowers

¾–1 cup dried alfalfa leaves and flowers

You can cook these as in Variation I, or put the herbs into a half-gallon jar and just steep for 2 hours (up to overnight).

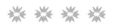

This bioflavonoid- and carotene-rich tea blend is nourishing and tonifying to numerous systems in the body including the kidneys, nervous system, and musculoskeletal system. The alfalfa is a good source of protein (as is generally true of any legume), and adds a rich storehouse of vitamins such as vitamin A, vitamin B1, vitamin B6, vitamin C, vitamin E, and vitamin K, along with fortifying minerals such as calcium, potassium, iron, and zinc. This will aid the immune system in helping you through a cold.

ELDER BLOSSOM DELIGHT—VARIATION III

Add ¼ cup dried (or ½ cup fresh) sassafras leaves

Add golden (dried) or green (fresh) spirit-lifting sassafras leaves to Variation II to make the infusion even more beneficial for clearing lymph, skin, and lungs.

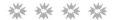

Adding sassafras will increase the cooling, soothing moistness of the remedy, which is beneficial if there is hot, dry congested mucus in the chest. The sassafras leaves also yummify (yes, I made that word up) this recipe, and almost any remedy, adding to the "delight" of Elder Blossom Delight. Steep this blend overnight before decanting it.

ELDERBERRY ELIXIRS

Elderberry elixirs were widely popularized in recent years by the wonderful herbalist and prolific writer Kiva Rose Hardin. Elixirs are a marvelous way to get the maximum benefits of elderberries and enjoy a taste treat, too. An elixir recipe, much like the cordial recipes shared by the late Adele Dawson, beloved author of *Herbs: Partners in Life*, is made by mixing honey (or another sweetener) and alcohol (often brandy) with the fresh or dried herb, and waiting for alchemy to take place. (See recipes below.)

I've been inspired by Adele and Kiva to make many varieties of cordials and elixirs, but a simple elderberry elixir remains a perennial favorite in our house (and anywhere else I take it)!

FRESH ELDERBERRY ELIXIR

Fresh elderberries

100-proof vodka or brandy

Buckwheat honey

Fill your jar completely with fresh elderberries—whole, mashed, or cut-up. Pour vodka or brandy over about ¾ of the berries, and finish filling the jar with buckwheat honey. Gently stir it all in together until all the berries are covered and steeping in the mixture. Let your brew sit infusing for at least 6 weeks, and alchemy will happen.

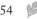

Decant it by pouring off the liquid and thoroughly squeezing out the berries. Use by the tablespoon for a cold or flu, to increase your circulation, or for general antiviral immune-system strengthening.

Additional options to add (per pint, approximately): 1 vanilla bean or 1 tablespoon vanilla extract, 1 bruised cinnamon stick, fresh ginger, five-spice powder, grated cacao bean, etc. These optional ingredients can also be added to the following recipe.

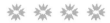

DRIED ELDERBERRY ELIXIR

Dried elderberries

100-proof vodka or brandy

Buckwheat honey

Fill any size wide-mouthed jar ½-full with dried elderberries. Cover them with brandy from ½–¾ full, and fill the rest of the jar with the rich, dark honey. Once again, let your brew sit infusing for at least 6 weeks—or as long as you can stand to wait! Alchemy will happen.

This recipe is almost as good as using fresh berries. Adele Dawson used to say of her cordials, "Test your character by waiting three weeks." My favorite additional ingredient in my elderberry elixirs is a vanilla bean. (See directions for working with vanilla beans on page 465.)

There will be more on all of the above, including elderberry syrup, in the section on the respiratory system. (See page 239.)

HERBAL RESPONSES TO A FEW MORE IMMUNE-SYSTEM CHALLENGES

Here are a few remedies and recipes that have proven effective for helping the body stave off illness from bacterial, viral, fungal, or parasitic infections.

There are numerous kinds of Staphylococcus bacteria, all commonly known as staph. Infections, especially of the skin, are most commonly caused by a strain known as *Staphylococcus aureus*. It's said that 25–30%

of healthy adults have some staph bacteria on the skin or in the nose that don't cause any harm. However, if the normal defenses of the body, beginning with the acid mantle of the skin, are depleted, then the staph bacteria can lead to infection. A staph infection can be mild, moderate, severe, or life-threatening, depending on the condition of the person who has the infection.

Staph, a Gram-positive bacterium, can get inside the body and cause sepsis, and symptoms such as fever, chills, and low blood pressure. It often infects surgical wounds, among other potential problems. The most common symptoms, though, include boils and other red, pus-filled wounds and lesions on the skin.

Additionally, we now have what are commonly called "superbugs" that are resistant to various antibiotics such as MRSA (methicillin-resistant *Staphylococcus aureus*). At first, these were only contracted in hospitals, but the Center for Disease Control reports that about 12% are now contracted elsewhere and known as community-associated MRSA, or CA-MRSA. This variety of staph is more threatening, and only 1% of the population carries it on their skin without illness developing. Younger people are most vulnerable to these community-borne infections right now, with the average age of exposure and infection being twenty-three.

To avoid staph infection, first tend to the foundation of your health with real, whole food, regular movement, time outdoors, and good hygiene (especially washing hands, but not with antibacterial soap), and cover any open wounds. Then, thankfully, our herbs can be of great benefit in these situations.

Here are the recipes I created for my dad when he had a hospital-introduced MRSA infection. In this case it resulted in a boil on the buttocks that was so painful the man couldn't sit or lie down without pain. This was still true after two different rounds of antibiotics. The first recipe below is for internal use, and the second is for external use as a wash or, in his case, in a sitz bath.

There are many herbs that can be effective in helping us heal from serious infection caused by our vulnerability to infectious microbes, including parasites, fungi, and viruses. And in the case of Staph bacteria, this is very good news because the antibiotics used against MRSA are not always successful now. These new strains are called VRSA (vancomycin-resistant *Staphylococcus aureus)*. Each of these acronyms refers to the bacteria by the pharmaceutical medicine that doesn't work against it, and over time, unfortunately, I imagine more of these acronyms arising.

Our herbs are timeless and time-tested, and we will always need them. They need for us to be in good relationship with the land we live on. This is vital. It is yet one more reason to care for and about the health of our land and water. We need to preserve our most precious assets and resources, and fully understand that these aren't the things that cost us the most money, such as our cars, houses, and electronic gadgets, but rather the fundamental elements that support life on Earth and surround us with such natural beauty.

MRSA TINCTURE BLEND
(for internal use)

Indigo root tincture

Propolis tincture

Echinacea root tincture

Plantain leaf tincture

Usnea lichen tincture

Combine equal parts of these tinctures made by a reliable herbalist or herb company (or you). Take at least 2–3 droppers, or 50–90 drops, three times daily (depending on the person and the severity of the infection) until all symptoms are completely gone.

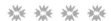

It is likely that even two or three of these herbs will be enough, and that other anti-microbial herbs could be substituted depending on what is available and known by you—or, better yet, harvested by you. Other herbs that come to mind are roses, rosemary, basil, and pokeroot. The above recipe is simply one sample formula that proved entirely effective, and is made mostly of plants that I know and have some relationship with.

MRSA INFECTION SOAK RECIPE
(for external wash)

2 tablespoons white oak bark or leaves

1½ tablespoons dried calendula blossoms

1½ tablespoons dried rose buds or blossoms

1½ tablespoons lavender flowers

1 tablespoon plantain leaves

1 tablespoon elder blossoms

1½ teaspoons rosemary leaves

Mix the herbs together well each time you make an infusion to bathe a wound, boil, etc. Pour one quart of boiled water over the dried herbs in a quart jar; cap it and let it sit steeping for one to two hours. For larger amounts, simply increase the parts proportionally. This recipe is for one quart of infusion to add into a sitz bath. Double the amount of each herb in this recipe to make a ½-gallon infusion for a full bath.

If the infection is everywhere on the skin, and/or systemic, use a ½ gallon of infusion in a cool or tepid bath. Sit or lie in it for at least 20 minutes. Adding seaweed could be quite remarkable for both soothing and immune-boosting effects, though I haven't tried that yet. I might add a cup of kelp to the recipe next time.

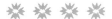

Common fungal infections include ringworm, athlete's foot, jock itch, and yeast overgrowths such as candida and thrush. As with any infection, you are more susceptible to fungal infections when your immunity is low, whether from illness, stress, overwork, poor diet, lack of sleep or support, etc. They are also a common side effect of antibiotics.

Fungal infections have a tendency to lodge in the skin or respiratory system. They thrive in warm, moist conditions. Because of this I prefer powders and washes over oils for external treatment of fungal challenges, because oils hold in moisture. Internally, a combination of infusions and tinctures can be taken, depending on what's going on, and with whom. Harsher fungal infections lodged in the lungs may require more intensive herbal treatments.

FUNGAL INFECTION POWDER

1 part rosemary leaf, dried and powdered

1 part calendula blossoms, dried and powdered

¼ part green clay powder

Combine equal amounts of powdered rosemary and calendula, and add a bit of green clay to the blend. Dust the infected area with this powder frequently.

FUNGAL INFECTION FOMENTATION AND INFUSION

1 part rosemary leaves

1 part calendula blossoms

External washes, called fomentations, are also beneficial. Make these without the clay, and use whole herbs rather than powders, steeping them in boiled water for about a half-hour. Separate into two containers, one for drinking and one for washing. These can be refrigerated, too, for ongoing use.

For the fomentation, dip a clean washcloth or piece of flannel or muslin in the preparation, and wash the infected area well. Let it dry naturally. Apply the powder afterward. Wash the cloth fully with soap and water and dry it before using again or, better yet, use a new cloth or clean rag.

The infusion can be drunk hot or cold and, depending on the severity of the fungal infection, can be drunk two to four times daily. It can be used on its own or with additional herbs or tinctures added, as discussed below.

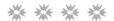

Rosemary and calendula both have considerable antifungal gifts, and are the first herbs I turn to. Other herbs that are effective in antifungal powder blends are: neem leaves, lavender flowers, yarrow flowers, garden sage leaves and flowers, and red clover blossoms, among others.

White clay can be used instead of green clay, though green clay is more medicinal while white clay is more commonly used in non-medicinal dusting and cosmetic powders. If you like, cornstarch can be mixed equally with either clay to give any powder (medicinal or not) a smoother, silkier texture.

What to take internally may depend on where the fungal infection is lodged. For respiratory fungal infections, I almost always use the lichen usnea as a tincture. This lichen is a symbiotic life form, a combination of algae and fungi, and is often found hanging from trees near the ocean. It is also good for healing in the presence of all Gram-positive and -negative bacteria, including strep and staph. Red clover infusions are helpful for fungal skin infections, as well as lung infections. Garlic is useful for digestive infections. Black walnut hulls are famous in the herbal world for taking care of toenail fungus, though I'd suggest using it as a fomentation rather than the frequently used oil. (By the way, infusing black walnut hulls in olive oil does make a nice citrusy-smelling, hair-darkening hair oil.)

Here's a recipe that worked quickly to help heal a mom who had thrush on her nipples, and her baby who had thrush in his mouth.

ANTI-THRUSH REMEDY FOR MOM AND BABY

> 1 tablespoon dried basil leaves
>
> 1 tablespoon dried calendula blossoms
>
> 25 drops (1 dropper) usnea tincture
>
> 1 teaspoon yogurt (optional)

For the baby: Pour boiling water over the dried herbs in a cup and steep for up to 30 minutes. Mom should drink it 20 minutes or so before nursing. In between nursings, a spoonful of the tea can be mixed into a bit of yogurt and swabbed inside the baby's mouth.

For the mom: Bathe the nipples in the tea, and let them dry naturally. Drink 3 cups of the tea daily with a dropper of usnea tincture in it.

Other options instead of usnea tincture could be bee balm (*Monarda* species) or yellow dock root (*Rumex crispus*).

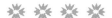

This young mother had come to see me, at her wit's end, after different rounds of various antifungal medications had failed to work. She and her son had been seriously uncomfortable for months. Not only that, but antifungal drugs tend to be especially harsh on the body. I talked with her, educating her about the simple herbs that could be her allies, and she used the washes (fomentations) and teas along with the usnea tincture.

In about a week they were smiling, free of thrush.

There is much more that can be written about strengthening the immune system with herbs such as plantain, garlic, calendula, milk thistle, yarrow, elderberry, red clover, garlic, and lemon balm, but there is more about these and additional herbs in other sections in *The Gift of Healing Herbs,* on skin, respiratory, digestive, and kitchen medicine.

For now, please remember, in addition to external factors: Illness is nourished by fear, isolation, and self-judgment, while love, community, and joyful self-acceptance nourish healing. Which do you choose to feed, and which do you choose not to feed? The choice, as always, is yours. And though it's personal, it has an impact in the world as well.

This is something I often have to remind myself when I fret about being "unproductive" for taking time to take care of myself, especially if I'm doing that as preventative medicine and not in response to pain or fatigue. (I still tend to get to it only when there's an obvious need—but, hey, I'm growing, too!) It's worth reminding yourself that every helpful thing you do for yourself helps everyone, because self-care is one of the most productive things you can do with your time. It's not only kind and loving—it's smart, and gives you a solid foundation from which to help others.

The Musculoskeletal System

Herbs and more for health, acute illnesses, and chronic challenges of the musculoskeletal system; how to nourish, tone, and strengthen the muscles, bones, joints, cartilage, tendons, ligaments, connective tissue, and spine.

The musculoskeletal system is comprised of smooth and striped muscle tissue, ligaments, cartilage, tendons, joints, and bones. This system makes up our basic physical structure and our ability to move within it, and is thus aligned with the Earth element. The musculoskeletal system provides a sense of stability as well as freedom of movement, or our perceived lack of freedom to go, do, or be according to our heart's desire. Our hearts are muscular, too, made of unique tissue that combines smooth and striped muscle tissue. Regular, rhythmic physical movement is one of the keys to the health of this system.

The health of our musculoskeletal structure is directly impacted by our diet—not only the nourishment we take into ourselves, but how well nutrients are assimilated and wastes are eliminated. This connects this system to the element Fire, having to do with digesting and assimilating life with passion and joy.

This system is also dependent on the electrical impulses of the nervous system for messages that are sent via neurotransmitters to direct much of its workings, including the rhythmic beating of our hearts. And like the nervous system, this system needs a complex array of minerals including calcium, magnesium, silica, and others. Minerals are strong, solid substances that work together synergistically to nourish and grow the bones that, along with our joints and their supportive ligaments, tendons, and cartilage, form our skeleton.

The skeleton is a perfect mirror of component parts all working together, like the minerals that help form it. An adequate supply of the roughly twenty essential amino acids that are converted into the diverse and complex structures we call protein is another key to the health of this system and, in fact, of every cell in the body. Protein makes up about fifty percent of the weight of every cell.

The health of our bones is interdependent with the health of our kidneys, also connecting this system with the element Water, related to flowing nourishment and releasing wastes freely. The kidneys not only filter the blood, they also process the minerals, helping them become suitable for our optimum use. One of the jobs of the kidneys is to balance calcium and phosphorus levels in the blood so that calcium isn't pulled out of our bones to supply a lack elsewhere.

The voluntary skeletal muscles that stabilize our joints are directly dependent on our breath, more so than our smooth muscles. This links this system with the element Air, which helps to circulate movement. So we see that our musculoskeletal system, most obviously linked to Earth because it links *us* to Earth, is truly an amalgam of all the elements.

It is not uncommon to see people with musculoskeletal challenges, such as so-called "bad" backs (though bodies never react well to being labeled "bad") struggling with a need to control things or people, feeling insecure in their physical situation, oppressed and entrapped by obligations, responsibilities and duties, and/or feeling that they don't have any way to get the help they need. As with other body systems, these patterns are often set at a young age and may still be acted out in the body long after their relevance is gone. Even if the onset of a particular stress to this system is from a recent accident, you can still discern a pattern when you turn a helpful eye and an open heart toward such a discovery.

This system's health, acute illnesses, and chronic challenges often offer teachings around flexibility and fluidity, being open to change, and being receptive to receiving help from others. Learning how to ask for help from people and the universe, and being willing to humbly accept your vulnerability, is often a teaching here, too. Valuing mind over body can come into play here. When you are generally "in your head" you don't pay as much attention to your body, and can injure and stress yourself from either overuse (pushing too hard and not respecting your body's limits and need for rest, sleep, good food, etc.) or underuse (being too sedentary in a way that has currently become the norm for many people, and yet is unnatural and unprecedented in human evolution).

Releasing undue burdens, taking on too much and then needing to get stuff "off your back," or taking on too much responsibility and feeling the weight of the world "on your shoulders," are commonly connected with pain in those areas.

It can't be stressed too much that these are generalities, and not true for all of the people all of the time. Also, within these broad categories, there is room for the enormous range of unique expression that human beings are capable of.

In this chapter we'll explore some of the most nourishing herbs for building bone, strengthening muscle and improving joint and spinal flexibility; but first, let's look at how herbal medicine can help with healing common injuries of the musculoskeletal system. I've been able to help a fair number of people avoid surgery that they were told was their only option. The way I look at it, even if they hadn't been able to avoid the surgery, the herbs would still have helped them achieve as full a healing as possible, thus improving their final outcome.

One example is a torn meniscus in the knee. This is a common injury that can be brought about in any number of ways, usually when the knee is twisted with full weight on it, or when gradual degeneration of this cartilaginous tissue has made it more vulnerable. Meniscus tears can be mild to severe, and while mild tears are often treated with ice, medication, and time to heal, the moderate or severe ones are generally considered to require surgery. That isn't always the case, though. The body is always oriented to heal itself, and given the right support it can and will often do just that.

Some of my favorite musculoskeletal system allies are: red clover blossoms, comfrey leaf, lobelia, horsetail, poke berries, goldenrod, motherwort, St. John's/Joan's wort, oat straw, mullein leaf, stalk and root, arnica flowers, yarrow, black birch bark, and ginger.

Avoiding or Aiding Surgery with Herbs

RECIPES TO HEAL A TORN MENISCUS
Infusion for internal use:

1 cup dried comfrey leaf (see note below)

1 cup dried mullein leaf

½ cup dried horsetail (above-ground parts)

Mix the herbs together in a half-gallon jar and fill jar with boiling water. Steep overnight. You may wish to sweeten this with honey.

Drink about 2 cups daily until you're completely healed. If you're under a doctor's care, confirm this by x-ray. Additionally, be assiduous about applying herbs topically, too. See below.

❋ ❋ ❋ ❋

Note: You might choose not to use comfrey internally. Though it has a venerable history as a nourishing, healing herb throughout the world, it has been recognized in recent laboratory studies that comfrey contains "potentially liver-toxic pyrrolizidine alkaloids (PAs)." It cannot be sold for internal use, and the FDA recommends not drinking it at all. There is much scientific and herbal debate about this, so if you plan to drink comfrey tea or infusion, do your own research, look at all sides of the story, and ultimately make your own informed decision.

Comfrey is rich in mucilage and has a special gooey, glue-like component called allantoin that makes it extremely healing to tissue. It has also long been my favorite herb, used both internally and externally, for sore, inflamed, and/or injured knees. I find it to be remarkably effective for healing cartilage, making it a natural for the knees.

Larger leaves and comfrey stalks are more medicinal than younger leaves, and generally the mature plants contain less PAs. Some say certain species of comfrey are safe while others are harmful.

You can prepare this recipe without the comfrey, or you might add a half-cup of dried Solomon's seal root, though it works differently and I have limited personal experience regarding its use. I've recently planted it in my garden, and I see it in the woods now and then, but am only beginning to get to know it. Many herbalists including Matt Wood and Jim McDonald write glowingly about this herb's abilities to heal tendons and ligaments.[1] Whatever you choose to do, make sure to include comfrey *externally* for healing a torn meniscus, as in the recipe that follows shortly. There is no debate about the safety of comfrey when used externally.

I use fresh comfrey leaves for poultices, and dry the leaves for poultices, compresses and infusions. I prepare infused oil from the fresh leaves and roots. I also eat the lovely, bell-shaped purple or pink flowers, as they are very sweet.

I was taught to use comfrey leaf as an everyday nourishing infusion, but I listen to my mom who always said, "When in doubt, don't." So I still use it, but not as abundantly as I once did, focusing on it now more for specific healing uses and repairs than for daily nourishment. In a case like this, you might choose to use only it until you are healed.

I read a message of caution in those fiberglassy hairs that cover the leaves and stalks. My personal understanding is that the harmful chemicals make up a tiny percentage of a mature comfrey plant, buffered by its other constituents. These constituents include not only the previously mentioned allantoin but a great array of minerals and protein that are vital to the musculoskeletal system and so much more.

On a personal note, when I was ill with some serious liver challenges I felt drawn to drink comfrey leaf infusions, so I did. I grow comfrey in my gardens; it benefits the soil and the bees, and provides a healing presence. I find comfrey strengthening and use it sparingly but without hesitation for musculoskeletal and sometimes digestive healing. Meanwhile, all agree that comfrey is one of the foremost tissue-healing botanicals on Earth, benefiting skin, muscle, nerves, bone, joints, cartilage, and tendons.

Mullein is included in this recipe because its leaves, roots, and flowers support healthy joints, helping to nourish and re-enliven the synovial fluid. Mullein leaf is also rich in the essential nutrient magnesium. If magnesium is deficient, the body will rob calcium from the bones to feed the blood. Without enough magnesium, bones become brittle and joints less flexible.

Mullein leaves are velvety, earning them the name "velvet dock," and yet they're a little scratchy, too. They're spongy, perhaps like the protective, spongy cartilage found in our synovial joints (joints such as knees and elbows, where there is movement between two bones). Sometimes I include mullein's leaf stalk too. Its tall presence growing straight up from the center of rosette of leaves makes me think of the spine running up the center of our backs.

Mullein leaf, flower, and root are valuable not only for doing "repair work" but for nourishing and strengthening numerous aspects of the musculoskeletal system. Mullein can be a fine infusion to include as part of a regularly rotation of nourishing infusions that you drink for healthy vitality and sparkling vibrancy.

Horsetail (*Equisetum* spp.) is a great healer of connective tissue. It is one of the richest sources of bio-available silica. Silica forms the matrix for many of your body's tissues, including bones, cartilage, tendons, ligaments, and blood vessels. Horsetail, like comfrey, will rebuild the structure of the body and aid in the assimilation of the vital mineral nutrients mentioned earlier. It also helps by providing boron and potassium, and nourishing and tonifying the kidneys.

Horsetail is an ancient plant. It predates the flowering plants, and reproduces by spores, like ferns. Thank goodness it's still here, as it's one of our great connective-tissue healers, improving strength and flexibility in joints and in the spine.

POULTICES AND/OR OILS FOR EXTERNAL USE

Fresh or dried yarrow flowers and leaves (and/or infused oil—see page 54)

Fresh or dried comfrey leaf (and/or infused oil—see page 54)

There are no safety concerns with external use of comfrey. Apply comfrey as a poultice for optimum results. If using a fresh leaf, pound it and then cover it with enough boiled water to soften it. Let it steep for ten minutes. First put a generous amount of comfrey and/or yarrow oil all over the knee and general area. Next, wrap the leaf or leaves around the knee and cover with a good-sized piece of flannel, held together with a safety pin or two. Or just sit with your feet up, with a soft cloth wrapped around the poultice, for 20 minutes or more and let the poultice do its magic.

If you're using dried leaves, follow the same process except that you won't need to pound the leaves. If they're cut up into pieces, put them into a piece of cheesecloth or a muslin bag and pour boiling water over them, enough to completely cover them. Let them steep for about ten minutes. Squeeze the excess moisture out of the leaf bundle, wrap that around the knee, and secure it with safety pins. Leave it on for at least 20 minutes. Repeat as frequently as possible each day, using a fresh poultice each time, for a minimum of 2 times daily.

Whenever you are not using a poultice or compress, apply the oils every time you think of it, all around the entire knee area, and add St. J's wort oil, too if you need additional pain relief.

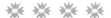

I know a lovely young man who was a doorman at the building where I met with my New York City apprentices for seven years. We used to exchange friendly greetings when I arrived, and often talked again after the class before I headed home—not about herbs, just books, baseball, city living, or whatever came up.

One day I came in and he wasn't his normal cheery self. He was obviously in pain, and I saw that he was limping. A pair of crutches was leaning against the wall. I asked him what happened, and he told me he'd fractured a bone in the bottom of his foot and there was nothing medical doctors could do to help him. I'm not sure if it was one of the metatarsals or the calcaneus bone, but it hurt a lot. He was told to ice it, stay off it as much as possible (unwelcome advice for a New York City doorman), endure the pain, take pain medication as needed—and that time would heal it eventually, as much as it could.

I told him I could offer him a better plan if he was open to it, and he was genuinely interested. So during the class that night, we put together a few herbs and tinctures for him, some to use internally and others to make into an infusion for soaking his foot. Our hostess Diana generously added two quart jars to make the infusions in, so he'd be able to start without delay. She knew that one of the keys to good healing, with the least amount of repercussions later, is immediacy of treatment. I gave him the tinctures, dried herbs, and jars on my way out, along with specific instructions to follow for the best results.

Diana, a former apprentice and incredibly dear woman, who doesn't "work" as an herbalist per se but shares her herbal knowledge and wisdom freely to help everyone she knows, had sent her then nineteen-year-old daughter to me for a consultation years earlier. Heather was scheduled for "necessary" foot surgery after an injury. After we spoke, she decided to use herbs for two months, and then see whether she'd made progress or surgery was still needed. She was glad to put it off—and who wouldn't be when the doctors had said that even after the surgery she would probably never be able to run, ski, or play tennis again! But the surgery never had to happen; her foot healed completely. She and her mother were overjoyed.

Given her age and housing situation, I had her simply add St. John's wort, comfrey, and yarrow tinctures into a bucket of warm water to soak her foot in, and also drink "tincture tea" instead of brewing any infusions.

Here is the recipe that my apprentices and I put together for the doorman.

FOOT SOAK FOR A FRACTURED BONE

1 cup or more comfrey leaves

100–120 drops (about 4–5 droppers) St. John's wort flower tincture

100–120 drops (about 4–5 droppers) yarrow flower and leaf tincture

(Variation: You may substitute an infusion made with ½ cup each of dried yarrow and St. J's to a quart of water for the tinctures. This will be a very strong infusion, stronger than you would make it for drinking.)

Make a strong comfrey leaf infusion, leaving it to steep overnight. Then strain and squeeze out the herbs, and gently warm the infusion for the foot soak, though it will be equally effective at room temperature if you prefer. When it's ready, stir in the tinctures. Soak one or both feet in the mixture for about 20 minutes, 2–3 times daily.

I know, only one foot has the broken bone, but the other foot often compensates, so it's nice to treat it well too—and besides, it feels good. However, soaking the foot with the broken bone is all that is required. This soak recipe could be used for any bone break or bone bruise that you can reach by soaking.

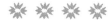

I told the young man about the warnings regarding internal use of comfrey, and that he could drink it or not as he felt comfortable. He drank about 2 cups of the mixture daily, using 2 droppers (about 50–60 drops) of each tincture per mug of comfrey infusion.

When I came back one week later, the doorman met me with a big smile. He'd done everything suggested, and was extremely pleased with how much better he felt. So was I! He said he was barely feeling any pain. He assured me he would continue to practice his self-care.

As his healing progressed to completion over the next month, he told me that his doctor said he'd never seen anything like the speed with which he'd healed. Less than two months later, there was no sign of inflammation, he had no pain, and an x-ray showed the break was perfectly healed. Bravo! I give him a lot of credit for following through on his herbal care. And thanks to that, he could stand a full workday without pain!

By the way, we didn't give him tinctures rather than dried herbs for infusions because we thought they were better—nor are infusions necessarily better than tinctures. Either option, or a combination, will work equally well both internally and externally. It depends on the herb, the person, and the situation. In this instance, we used what Diana had in abundance to share.

One of the basic tenets of healing in the wise-woman tradition is to make use of what you have available. If you can only get one or two out of three herbs called for in a recipe, just start with what you have. And I suggest using the best-quality herbs you can gather or afford. Additionally, learn to grow and harvest them, and wildcraft your own herbs. Yarrow and St. J's are wildflowers that grow freely as weeds. I also plant and grow them in my gardens, along with comfrey.

Comfrey's ability to heal tissue (including broken bones) has earned it the nickname "knitbone." Yarrow and St. J's wort are two of the very best herbs for relieving pain and inflammation. They will be discussed again in the section on Wound and Bruise Healing (page 471). Each of these herbs is anti-inflammatory and pain relieving, and the St. J's has a special affinity for reducing inflammation of the nerves. It also helps nerve repair when they have been damaged, whether from impact or illness.

Please realize that when a pharmaceutical painkiller relieves your pain, it's simply masking it. The danger of this is that you are tempted to do everything as if you are not in the midst of a healing process, which can increase the severity of the injury and make it worse. When an herb like yarrow or comfrey reduces the pain, it happens at a natural pace because the injury itself is actually healing. These herbs reduce pain through healing, not masking. There *are* herbs that can mask pain, and that can be a blessing (see Indian pipe, for example, page 214), but it's wise to use them carefully and to remain mindful of what's really going on in your body.

I created the following recipe to help my illustrator Karen Flood's sweet nine-year-old Labrador retriever Willow, who loved to romp and play but had become severely debilitated by Lyme disease. I adapted it from a blend that helped me get my full movement back after my own various tick-borne infections left me with a lot of stiffness, pain, and fatigue. Just like me, even after her full courses of antibiotic treatments, Willow didn't get her health back. Willow's main symptoms were arthritic inflammation and pain and, because of that, lethargy and decreased movement.

ANTI-INFLAMMATORY
HONEY BALLS OR PASTE
(for tick-borne infections resulting in arthritic symptoms)

3 tablespoons turmeric powder

3 tablespoons hawthorn berry powder

3 tablespoons ginger powder

1 tablespoon honeysuckle powder

1 tablespoon slippery elm powder

Additional slippery elm powder for final rolling of the balls,
and for coating your palm while making them

Mix all the dried powders very well, smoothing out any lumps or clumps. If you are powdering any of the herbs yourself, make sure they are finely ground. Slowly add honey to the powders, working it all in together very well, to get a paste-like consistency.

Take a teaspoon or so of the mixture at a time and form it into small balls about the size of a cherry.

Once they're formed, roll the balls in the additional slippery elm powder.

Here's an alternate method that works really well for turning the paste into honey balls, which I learned from my student Mavis from Ghana: Coat your palm with the slippery elm powder, then take the paste into that palm, and making a loose fist, shake your hand exactly as if you were about to roll dice. It's fun, and they come out rather beautifully!

Sometimes I like to make the paste into a larger ball, from lemon- to baseball-sized, keep it in a tin or glass jar, and then simply pull off between ½–1 teaspoon or more as needed twice daily. For a small animal I'd use about ⅛-¼ teaspoon twice daily.

Use the honey of your choice. As always, local, raw honey is preferred. This paste doesn't need to be refrigerated. The honey balls can be dried in a low oven, but I've never felt the need. If they are a bit too soft, add more powder and rework them, or drying can help.

These balls keep very well in a tin or jar. I wrap them in unbleached parchment paper inside the tin or jar. They travel well, too.

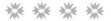

Karen reported that after one or two anti-inflammatory honey balls, Willow literally began to jump up and dance for the next ones. Karen said that soon she began to run around; she happily told me, "She's playing like a puppy!" Not only did this mixture help Willow, but I've since then used it to help other four-leggeds affected by Lyme disease to reduce pain and regain their health and energy.

In addition to being anti-inflammatory, the mixture is liver-supportive, antibacterial, and pain-relieving through the combined benefits of ginger, turmeric, and honeysuckle, and circulatory- and digestive-enhancing and soothing by combining those three with the hawthorn berry and slippery elm bark. The honey brings its antibacterial goodness to the medicine balls, and honeysuckle in particular has a way of getting into our deepest nooks and crannies, where the spirochete bacteria like to hang out and do their ongoing damage if left to their own devices. Honeysuckle helps the lymph cells find the spirochetes, and overwhelms them with its sweet and powerful antibacterial gifts. Many years ago I meditated with this plant and she told me, "I'm so sweet I get in everywhere I want to go!" So true—and a darn good thing, too. The medicine seems to work in our bodies the way the vines grow on the earth, reaching into crevices and other hidden places.

I've now started using various versions of this paste for humans, other than just myself, and it's been helping us, too! One of my current clients who is using honey balls makes them with coconut oil rather than honey as he has a bad reaction to any sweetener at this point. I'm very excited to be sharing this recipe when so many people in my area of the world and elsewhere are debilitated by tick-borne illnesses and the arthritic symptoms that follow the infection.

Because of the prevalence of ticks here where I live (in the north-eastern United States), and my love of gardening and walking out in the woods, I've had quite a lot of personal experience with them, and have been infected several times. I've also helped clients, friends, and students who've been infected. I feel that antibiotics alone are definitely not enough. Herbs alone are enough for some people if they are very diligent with them over a long period of time, and have a strong enough constitution, and were basically healthy before the infection. The most prudent course of action if an infected tick has bitten you is to take both antibiotics and herbs.

All of the herbs in this paste, especially the honeysuckle and turmeric, as well as the weeds, Japanese knotweed and Teasel, are primary herbs for healing from tick-borne infections. I think it is wisest to work with a practitioner to custom-tailor a recipe that matches you and your symptoms. To say the least, it is not something to take on lightly because the repercussions of potential symptoms can be profoundly debilitating.

If you choose to take antibiotics, focus keenly on maintaining healthy bacteria in your gut, and restoring your gut flora with fermented foods such as yogurt, kefir, miso, sauerkraut, and pickles for as long as it takes to restore it fully, and then continue them less intensively. It can take people a long time—longer than you might think—to fully recover their gut flora as discussed in the chapter on the digestive system.

Nourishing the Musculoskeletal System

Nourishing the musculoskeletal system is as important as nourishing any other. The best way to do this is with food, herbs, and exercise, although some supplements may be necessary, depending on the person, the history, etc. Mineral-rich infusions are vital for nourishing ongoing musculoskeletal health. The following are some I particularly favor.

Red clover infusion is a great source of bio-available minerals that support excellent musculoskeletal health. Nettles are rich in iron and calcium, and also feed the kidneys. Oat straw's array of vitamins and minerals builds bones and increases flexibility in the joints, as well as relieving pain. I mentioned mullein for magnesium and much more. Alfalfa and red raspberry are both great sources of calcium. Horsetail heals connective tissue and tones the kidneys. *Artemisia vulgaris* is rich in minerals that nourish the nervous system, and also the joints and connective tissue. You can drink these infusions individually, as simples, rotating them. You can play with different combinations of two or three herbs together.

Use herbs that you like—that way you'll remember to drink them. Also, please feel free to experiment. Sometimes an infusion that you don't like when it's hot may be perfectly palatable to you cold, or vice-versa.

JOINT AND BONE BLEND INFUSION RECIPE

¾ cup dried oat straw (stalks and usually some seeds)

¼–½ cup dried horsetail

¾ cup dried red clover blossoms

Put the herbs together in a half-gallon jar. Add boiling water to the top, and cover tightly. Steep overnight. Decant the infusion and squeeze out the herbs. Refrigerate to store. Heat and/or sweeten with honey if desired.

Drink the infusion freely, 1–4 cups daily. Rotate your herbs, using simples and different combinations as desired or needed.

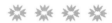

Another vital source of nourishment for the musculoskeletal system comes in the form of mineral-rich herbal vinegars, including plain apple cider vinegar. These are enormously helpful for providing nourishing bioavailable minerals. Pick mineral-rich herbs to infuse in good-quality apple cider vinegar, and then use these freely in your food, or by the tablespoon in water if you prefer that.

Vinegars that I love and use regularly include infused artemisia vinegar, lemon balm, white pine or red spruce needle, nettle, dandelion leaf and root, burdock root, concord grape, grape leaf, lady's thumb (*Polygonacea* species), violet leaf, and more.

Recently I had a client drink two tablespoons of artemisia vinegar daily in water, and the back pain that she had woken up with every day for years simply disappeared. Recipes and suggestions for various herbal-infused vinegars are found elsewhere throughout *The Gift of Healing Herbs*.

Eating wild greens provides an abundance of vitamins and minerals for muscles and bones. All wild greens are good sources of calcium, and many offer abundant essential fatty acids (EFAs), so helpful for our joints. Purslane *(Portulaca oleracea)* and evening primrose (*Oenothera biennis* and other species) are particularly high in EFAs.

Learn one wild plant at a time, and incorporate it into your meals. Learn unusual uses for familiar garden plants. For example, I go into the garden for our salads and cooking greens, gathering wild strawberry leaves, cinquefoil leaves, dandelions, evening primrose leaves, artemisia leaves, chives, garlic mustard, violet leaves, various wild mustards, and more. The only one of those I actually planted is the chives; the rest are provided by nature.

Vitamin D3 is not only essential for proper immune functioning, it is also essential for our bodies to be able to assimilate calcium. It is hard to get enough vitamin D from sunlight alone, and impossible if you constantly use a sunblock. Oily fish such as sardines and mackerels are good additional sources of vitamin D, and a good-quality liquid supplement is a reasonable option to consider.

Also, please remember to make use of the simple arthritis remedy made with apple cider vinegar and honey (see page 420).

Herbal oils can also be helpful for pain relief and inflammation. I love infused rosemary and ginger oils, combined or used separately. They both stimulate warmth and increase circulation. Ginger is particularly helpful for relieving inflammation.

Sometimes a person's condition is hot and inflamed—joints look red, and they need a cooling herb more than a hot one. In those situations I often turn to black birch oil. It soothes and cools down inflammation, but still ultimately brings back circulation to the area. I also use wintergreen *(Gaultheria procumbens)* liniment by infusing fresh wintergreen leaves in rubbing alcohol or apple cider vinegar. Wintergreen is a classic cooling herb that's used more externally than internally, often for inflammation in the joints. Its leathery leaves suggest to me that this isn't an herb to take internally on a regular basis, but it is fine for periodic or occasional use. I use infused pine needle oil, too. I find it somewhat neutral, a little cooling, and toning to the blood vessels and capillaries, helping the blood circulate more freely and bringing oxygen to smooth-muscle tissue.

The following is an herbal-oil recipe originally created to help my mom when she was in a lot of pain. She had lung cancer that had metastasized to the bones. The recipe has since helped many people, myself included, with varying degrees of nerve and muscular pain from injury, post-surgery, or just from overdoing it at yoga, gardening, or at the gym or from too many hours spent sitting still at a desk or in a car, plane, or other mode of transport.

ROBIN ROSE'S EASE OIL
(for external use only)

1 cup fresh coltsfoot leaves *(Tussilago farfara)*

1 cup fresh comfrey leaves and stalks

1 cup fresh lobelia leaves, stalks, flowers and seedpods

1 cup fresh St. John/Joan's wort leaves stalks, flowers and buds

1 cup fresh yarrow leaves, stalks and flowers

½ gallon olive oil

My favorite way to make Ease Oil is to gently cook this herbal blend in a half-gallon of cold-pressed olive oil for about 3 days, and then pour it into jars. Leave it to sit with the herbs infusing in it for several months.

I use roughly equal parts of the herbs, depending on what's available, and I prefer to use them fresh when possible, though well-dried herbs are an acceptable option. The directions for cooking this oil are the same as those given for A–Z Oil (see page 367), which can also be helpful as a warming stimulant. When you're ready, squeeze out the herbs and be sure to remove any water from the bottom of your jars that may have accumulated after they sit for 24 hours or so.

Store the oil in a cool, dry place. Pour off into smaller bottles or jars for easier usage. Gently shake the usage bottle before applying the oil. Use it liberally, and as frequently as possible for maximum healing.

You've got options for making this oil, too: You can buy or make infused oils of each of these herbs, then combine them together. You can make it with a combination of dried herbs, fresh herbs and/or infused oils. You can even make it in a crockpot if you like, on the lowest possible setting, making sure it doesn't bubble and boil.

I originally learned from the writings of herbalist Maria Treban that coltsfoot, better known as a cough medicine, is also a specific for bruising. I've confirmed that by using it for myself and other people in poultices and oils, which is why I now I include it in Ease Oil.

The comfrey leaves and stalks are tissue-regenerative for skin, bones, tendons, ligaments, and cartilage, and both the comfrey and coltsfoot give Ease Oil an added dimension as a bruise-healing oil. The lobelia is a profound anti-spasmodic and sedative, quieting cramps and providing relief from painful spasms. St. J's is one of the best all-around anti-inflammatory, pain-relieving nerve medicines, and it will help regenerate damaged nerves. Finally, yarrow is one of my favorite herbs for its anti-inflammatory, pain-relieving properties. It is perfect for bruises.

Ease Oil can be used topically as long as there is not a deep wound, in which case it's better to use other forms of herbal medicine besides oils.

Ease Oil is already quite potent, and anyone I've ever made it for has asked for refills; it can also be enhanced by adding tincture of St. J's and/or lobelia after it's finished, but only in the smaller usage bottles, so that the oil won't spoil. Add approximately ½ teaspoon of tincture to each ounce of Ease Oil. It doesn't necessarily need to be made stronger by adding tinctures, but it is an option.

You can also personalize it by adding a tincture to fit the need it is addressing, or just to experiment and learn. For example, herbalist Bonnie Rogers, one of my former apprentices, added arnica tincture to Ease Oil to help her husband after a motorcycle accident, and it was very effective in relieving his pain and bruising and speeding his healing.

Post-Surgical Healing

I'm going to conclude this section on the musculoskeletal system with one of my favorite healing stories. In 1995 I moved out of Manhattan to a small mountaintop cabin about an hour upstate. I became fast friends with Zack, a sweet black Labrador retriever who lived next door with my landlords.

I liked walking in the deep woods, and Zack wanted to accompany me everywhere I went. The problem was, he had been hit by a car nearly a year before I moved in, and put back together with quite an array of steel pins, rods, and wires. The first recommendation had been to put him to sleep, but his people cried mightily and said absolutely not, so the veterinary surgeon worked his magic.

Now, Zack's spirits were as good as ever, and he did the best he could, but he would get tired and I imagine he was always in pain. He'd still go on walks with them and with me, using his tail for balance the entire time he walked. He would twirl it 360 degrees, around and around, like a non-stop propeller. He only had the use of three legs. One of his front legs was permanently held up in the air at shoulder height because of the steel rods implanted in his shoulder.

I asked his humans if I could try to help him with herbs, admitting that I'd never worked with any situation like this before, and they enthusiastically accepted. So I began to make him tea and herbal compresses, and to my surprise, he would not only come running when I called him, he would lap up the tea and lie down quietly for the herbal compresses. I was amazed, and I learned a lot from Zack. I only used three herbs, both internally and externally, first in combination, and then switched to using them one at a time.

POST-SURGICAL MUSCULOSKELETAL HEALING INFUSION

½ cup comfrey leaf

½ cup red clover blossoms

½ cup oat straw herb

Let the herbs steep in boiled water from several hours to overnight in a quart jar, and then decant them by pouring off the liquid and squeezing out the leaves. For Zack I put some of the tea out in a bowl at room temperature. You, however, can take this infusion as usual, by the cup, after straining it and squeezing out the leaves. Store the rest in a refrigerator.

※ ※ ※ ※

Zack lapped this tea up over the course of an afternoon. I repeated this most days that I was there, maybe three or four days a week, and most of those days he would drink it. Occasionally, he wouldn't, so I'd feed the plants with it.

MUSCULOSKELETAL COMPRESS
(for external use)

⅓ cup comfrey leaf (mullein leaf is another good option)

⅓ cup red clover blossoms

⅓ cup oat straw herb

Pour boiling water over the herbs, and bring it back to a boil. Turn down the flame and simmer, covered, on a very low flame. After a few minutes, turn it off and let it infuse for at least 15 minutes before use.

Retrieve the herbs with a slotted spoon or sieve, and press them out while draining so they won't be dripping. Wrap the herbs in cheesecloth or another thin, porous cloth to make a compress.

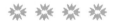

I did this, and pressed the compress gently to Zack's shoulder and underneath and around it, for as long as he would let me, sometimes as long as 10–15 minutes, twice daily, when I was around and had the time. As long as my hand stayed on top of the compress, he was pretty content. I also applied a fomentation, washing the leg and the whole area with a soft cloth dipped into the infusion.

If you're working with a cat, you're lucky if he or she will give you two minutes! However, when they are sick or injured, even cats can be surprisingly responsive to herb compresses.

Now and then Zack would back away from the compress when it was offered, and instead of trying to force it on him, I watched and learned. He helped me learn more viscerally that animals, like children, have instinctual body wisdom that we adult humans would do well to learn. Instead of repeating a treatment on "automatic pilot," there are times when it's healthier to take breaks. I did some research and learned that comfrey can sometimes be too cooling when used repeatedly, so I took it out of the mix and once again he stretched out languidly to receive his compress, now made from oats and red clover. Today I might add mullein to this mix, and/or soak a whole mullein leaf in the tea and apply it that way, as a poultice. (See Mullein Mélange, page 486.)

If you listen to your body and your intuition, they'll guide you well. There are countless ways to develop listening skills. Some helpful and classic practices include: dancing and drumming, sitting and walking meditations, *t'ai chi* or *chi kung,* painting or journal writing. It's important to find what works for you, and even the time of day or night that works best for you. Whatever you choose, the commonality is that they all offer an opportunity for quieting the mind, and slowing down enough to be present and able to listen for inner guidance—and guidance from the plants themselves.

Animals and small children don't need practices. They simply trust themselves. I began to put out Zack's herbal infusions as simples, so he could choose only the ones that were best for him in that moment. This approach generally works really well with animals.

One day, after about four months, my landlords, Zack, and I were all taking a walk together. I noticed and pointed out that though his tail was still moving continuously, it was sweeping from side to side to side, like non-stop windshield wipers, only moving 180 degrees instead of 360. I somehow knew this was a sign he was healing, as if he only needed half the help now.

Sure enough, little by little during the next weeks, I saw that every day his right front paw was coming closer and closer to the ground. Finally one day it touched earth. I was overjoyed. Another day he put weight on it, tentatively. Then he walked on it, seeming quite pleased with life. His tail was wagging like a normal tail on a happy dog. All his humans were thrilled.

About one week later, his paw was back up in the air, around his shoulder. My landlords were upset, and accused me of harming their dog—how quickly we forget! I urged them to take him back to the vet and see what was going on.

At the vet's office, x-rays revealed that some of Zack's bones had knit back together so beautifully and completely that they'd pushed the steel rods out! The ends of the rods were poking against his skin, causing him pain. The vet made very small incisions, and pulled out every rod he could reach. He couldn't remove them all, as some were so deeply interior it wasn't practical, and it was complex, with wires wrapped here, there, and everywhere. However, Zack walked on four legs after that for the rest of his life, and I believe that the herbs helped reduce some of his inevitable scar tissue too.

Next, a beloved student, now a doctor and herbalist in San Francisco, used the same protocol with the same results. She had had similar repair work done on her knees during several surgeries in previous years, resulting in extensive scar tissue and stiffness on a daily basis. After using the herbs, she was able to get several of her largest pins removed, and though she still had some scar tissue and the arthritic stiffness that comes with that, she gained more comfort and mobility in her knees than she'd had in a long time. She even went back to enjoying yoga and dancing.

We tend to think, because it's what we've been taught, that many injuries to the musculoskeletal system are irreversible, and that once the damage has been done, that's the end of the story. But the story actually does goes on, and many injuries thought to be permanent are not. Everything is free to change. And although we can't re-grow limbs, herbs can often help us regain strength, mobility, and flexibility if we allow our thinking to be flexible enough to embrace that possibility.

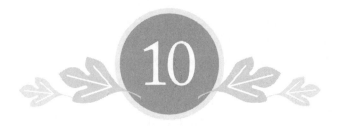

The Nervous System

Herbs and more for health, acute illnesses, and chronic challenges of the nervous system; building strength, soothing stress, lifting spirits, and relieving pain to bring heart, mind, body, and soul into a state of more peace, equanimity, and equilibrium.

The combined central and peripheral nervous system consists of a complex network of nerve cells and fibers that coordinate the relationships among all body systems. Its healthy functioning plays a pivotal role in our overall mental and physical health.

Every part of the body contains nerves except for cartilage and the nails on our fingers and toes. Each nerve cell, called a neuron, has multiple branching dendrites extending from its body, collecting impressions and information, and a single axon that transmits messages to the dendrites of other neurons across a space called a synapse. Consider this fun fact: The longest axon in the body runs all the way from your big toe to your brain to deliver information for you!

We are all sensory beings, abuzz with impulses, feelings, and sense impressions. Humans are sensual, naturally inclined toward taking pleasure and delight in our senses. Unfortunately, the teaching that this is somehow immoral and that we can't trust our senses has been heavily promoted over centuries, and successfully implanted into individuals and entire cultures. It has led to lots of struggle with what is natural, rather than the sheer delight in living that is our birthright.

As you heal yourself with natural medicine in the form of food and herbs, an additional gift is that the plants begin to reawaken your senses, and with that your trust in your own perceptions grows. It is both empowering and liberating to trust your own senses. (No doubt that's why it has been so frowned-upon.)

This interior Internet, governed by the brain and spinal cord, operates 24/7 and guides how you relate and respond to messages from within and outside yourself. Electrical impulses travel from cell to cell, conducted through the fatty myelin sheath that coats every axon. These electrical impulses stimulate neurotransmitters—chemicals that help complete the connections between nerve cells across synaptic junctions. The nerve cells interact with immune, digestive and endocrine cells. Endocrine glands secrete hormones (such as adrenaline and cortisol when you feel excited and/or threatened) in response to the lightning-fast messages being delivered all over the body by the nervous system.

Just as you have a conscious and subconscious mind, you have a voluntary and involuntary nervous system. The involuntary (or autonomic) nervous system controls functions that, unless you are taught through meditation and other practices to affect them, are generally outside your conscious control—functions like heartbeat, respiration, dilation of pupils, and the release of digestive and other hormones from the glands.

The autonomic nervous system is divided into the sympathetic and parasympathetic nervous systems. The sympathetic is the part that reacts to stress, while the parasympathetic part of the system is the more peaceful responder, and works when you are at rest and relaxed.

These days, your sympathetic nervous system works overtime as stressors rarely let up, either actually or in the imagination. You worry about paying bills, sickness, and environmental pollution. You get steamed up over a traffic jam that's making you late, or corruption in a local bureaucracy; or you read the paper and feel fearful about the state of the world in general. Stress hormones are aroused—but no release follows. Stress responses are supposed to move in cycles that rise and fall. They are designed to be protective, not dominant.

Stress hormones divert energy from the viscera of the body to the periphery so that, when you need it for survival, vital energy moves away from digestion and internal healing to the arms and legs to help you fight or run from a real threat, such as an assailant or a wildfire, or perhaps to lift an impossibly heavy object off of someone you love. Thought processes in the new frontal cortex are sacrificed in lieu of activating the oldest part of the brain that stimulates survival mechanisms and reactions. When a woman lifts a tree or a car off her child, as has happened, or runs into a burning building to rescue her aged grandmother, she isn't thinking logically about whether or not she can do that; she just does it.

As you can see, this system is brilliant, and it's designed to help you adapt to present needs and circumstances in an instant. But it has not adapted to the kind of ever-present stress you live with today. This is why it is so important to nourish, calm and strengthen the nervous system, both for personal well-being and because this helps you find the intelligence and power to respond creatively and collectively to the real threats facing all of us.

When you join with others in community and become actively engaged in finding and implementing creative solutions to the challenges of our time, it begins to satisfy the sympathetic nervous system that you are not in immediate danger. Joining with others in common cause strengthens and supports you and can be fun, too. Seeking creative, intelligent responses to the threat rather than reacting in primal fight or flight mode lets your nervous system go off high alert. Your immune and digestive systems can return to their normal work. This, in turn, allows you to think and function more clearly, to connect with others more openly, and makes more vital life-energy available to help you find viable solutions.

As mentioned in the section on the digestive system, the intestine has its own (enteric) nerve network. So the advice to never discuss politics or religion over dinner makes sense! The parasympathetic nervous system controls digestion, but if the sympathetic nervous system is aroused, the parasympathetic shuts down, diverting energy in an attempt to prioritize your survival even in situations where your survival isn't actually at stake. It is both a psychological and physiological connection. If you feel anxious and/or argue while you're eating, your stomach and other muscles will tighten up and you won't be able to digest your food easily. At the same time, if you have gas pain and indigestion, it's going to cloud your thinking and influence your emotional mood for the worse.

Unfortunately, this describes many Western people's regular state of being. People in our modern culture complain that it's not possible to keep up with their own schedules and are often looking to catch up, whether on sleep, downtime, paperwork, time with friends and family, or whatever it is they really want to do or feel they have to do. It's common to hear people bemoan the fact that they feel as if they are always running and not necessarily getting anywhere, and many of us regularly eat "on the run." A family sitting down to a meal together without watching television has become a rare phenomenon.

The constant stream of information coming at us from the media, cell phones, and the Internet is part of the challenge. Staying perpetually plugged in to virtual reality and cyberspace keeps you from being fully present to where you are and whom you're with and, as importantly, to who you are in relation to the real world of nature—the cycles of night and day, the seasons, the waxing and waning of the moon, the birds and animals, the insects, and what's going on and growing in your own backyard. These relationships are vital for the health of your nervous system.

It can be healing to lie down in a hammock, look up at the trees, and remember that it is enough just to be. Rest is a necessary part of healing this system—a very necessary part.

Simple Mantra for Relaxing the Nervous System

It is enough just to be.
It is enough just to be.
It is enough just to be.

This is one of my favorite mantras to recite when my mind is working on overdrive. Say it aloud at least three times, as above, while taking slow deep breaths. Experience the wisdom of it. Feel yourself releasing tension out of your mind and body. Don't worry—you won't stop doing what you need to do. You'll simply do it from a more relaxed state of being. Remember, you are a human being first, not a human doing!

The health, acute illnesses and chronic challenges of the nervous system often offer us teachings around flexibility and adaptability, around where and when to hold firm and when to go with the flow. Another teaching of this system revolves around how to be present with what is—the actual state of having your mind and body in the same place at the same time (one of my own ongoing challenges).

Simple Mantra to Become Fully Present

Mind and body in the same place at the same time.
Mind and body in the same place at the same time.
Mind and body in the same place at the same time.

This mantra is not only calming and strengthening to the nervous system, it is one of the great teachings that nervous-system challenges offer us—true embodiment, true presence.

. . . .

Feeling tense, nervous, anxious, and overwhelmed, with or without a specific cause, are classic symptoms of a depleted or overtaxed nervous system. Exhaustion is another symptom, as is chronic muscle pain.

Herbal medicine can help with all of the above, but herbs alone aren't enough. Learning to quiet the mind and rest in the spaciousness of the present moment is vitally important. Connection with the Earth is essential. Presence, calmness, responsiveness and resiliency are the attributes of a healthy nervous system.

The nervous system is connected to the elements of Air and Fire. The neurons crackle with electricity, firing their messages through the Air/ spaciousness of the synaptic junctions, connecting one neuron to the next and the next. (Air embodies inter-being.) These messages provoke movements, feelings and responses to sensations that are all part of Fire/

assimilating and digesting life with passion and joy. Part of it is also learning to release the thoughts, people and situations that provoke feelings of weakness and depletion, anxiety and worry, and rob you of your sense of fun (Fire includes eliminating whatever doesn't nourish), leading to exhaustion.

You can build the strength and health of your nervous system with the help of whole foods, especially fruits and vegetables that are rich in B and other vitamins, and a full array of minerals and chlorophyll, and with herbal nervines, tonics, adaptogens and nourishing infusions. Whole foods and appropriate herbal medicines help you respond to persistent stress with more aplomb. Not coincidentally, many nervous-system herbs help the immune, endocrine and digestive systems, too.

Like any other electronic network, this electrical system needs some Earth to ground it. That's where minerals come in. The rock-like substances of the Earth, such as those found in graceful, flowing oat straw and dancing, fluidic seaweeds, help form and feed this system. And if you can get some of those minerals from grounding root medicines like burdock and dandelion, so much the better.

The nervous system depends upon and thrives on minerals. Calcium makes up about fifty percent of its requirements, and the other fifty percent is made up of many different minerals, such as potassium, magnesium, phosphorus, iodine, copper, silica, boron, and more, all bound together in nature's harmonious ratios that match our cellular receptors perfectly. It is impossible to feed the nervous system with supplements or pharmaceuticals as well as with herbs and foods. Our cells simply don't recognize supplements the same way they recognize food. I'm not saying there isn't a time and place for supplementation, just that it is not optimal.

The nervous system responds well to self-care in all forms, including getting enough sleep, herbs, food, meditation, yoga, dancing, singing, spending time in nature, working at something you care passionately about, putting time aside just for you—time to play, and time and space to enjoy the simple pleasures of good relationships. It also responds positively to receiving nurturance, and especially to feeling cared about by others, even by just one other being.

I use all forms of medicine for this system, from helpful affirmations and meditations to physical and energetic exercises, to nervine tinctures such as motherwort or skullcap, adaptogenic infusions such as holy basil, tonic syrups made from herbs like violet and dandelion, and smoke recipes that combine herbs such as lavender, damiana, and artemisia. I favor infusions of herbs such as oats, roses, linden, and lavender that can be taken internally and also used as footbaths and full-body baths for nourishing and soothing the nervous system and easing emotional pain.

I use stronger sedating herbs when there is a specific need for them, usually in response to extreme pain. I almost never use very stimulating herbs as an answer to exhaustion, preferring to build the system more slowly and safely with infusions and mineral-rich vinegars of herbs such as nettles, dandelion, and violet. For pain relief from acute or chronic pain, I use herbs that are pain-relieving, anti-inflammatory, anti-spasmodic, and nerve healing, such as yarrow, oats, and St. J's wort. Lobelia, an anti-spasmodic, nervous system sedative, can also be very helpful, internally and externally. (Please note there are cautions about internal use of lobelia—see Respiratory System section, page 239.)

There is a wonderful maxim: "Don't believe everything you think." This is funny and also wise. The nervous system is profoundly influenced by what we believe, consciously and unconsciously. This is true of all our systems, but I think it's easiest to see in this one. If I hear strange sounds and believe an intruder has entered my home, my heartbeat will quicken, my muscles will tense up, and adrenaline will start pumping. If I soon hear a familiar "meow" and now believe my cat has come in through his own door and knocked something over, my involuntary fight-or-flight response will dissipate.

Many people, familiar with the relatively new science of genetics, believe that their genes reveal and determine their fate; but this is an incomplete understanding of the complexity of who and what we are. Genetics reveals the patterns of the past as well as potentials of the future, but genes are malleable and continue to evolve just as everything else does. They evolve in relationship to what we believe as much as in relation to what we eat, how we move or don't move, how we relate to ourselves and others, and so much more. This was once only the province of spirituality (or, if you prefer, quackery) but now it is being seen and studied scientifically. There is a science even newer than genetics, aptly called epigenetics ("beyond genetics").

Epigenetics shows us, in ways that match the most startling revelations of particle physics, that energy never dies and that we actually create our bodies and our health, moment to moment, according to what we believe. (See the Resources section for more information.) This is how the placebo effect works, and it's what makes "nocebos" so powerful. Nocebos happen when you are told nothing can help you. You believe it, and that negatively impacts your physiology, making you sicker. People with nervous-system challenges are likely to be diagnosed and treated accordingly, whether with herbs or pharmaceuticals.

Once you believe your diagnosis, you can get stuck in it. I asked a client what could happen if she stopped believing that she had obsessive-compulsive disorder. She couldn't even imagine it. A few years later, she has healed tremendously with the help of real food, herbs, and lots of support, and is currently living a healthier, happier life without the label, without the drugs, with new friends and a significantly restored relationship with nature.

. . . . . ● . . . .

Some of my favorite herbal allies for the nervous system are: motherwort, skullcap, St. J's wort, lavender, mullein flowers, cherry blossoms, California poppy, flowers of linden, rose, mimosa, and chamomile, peach (all parts), violet leaves and flowers, wintergreen, black birch, yarrow, lobelia, hawthorn blossoms and berries, sassafras leaves and roots, nettles, borage, alfalfa, and oat straw.

Oats *(Avena sativa)*

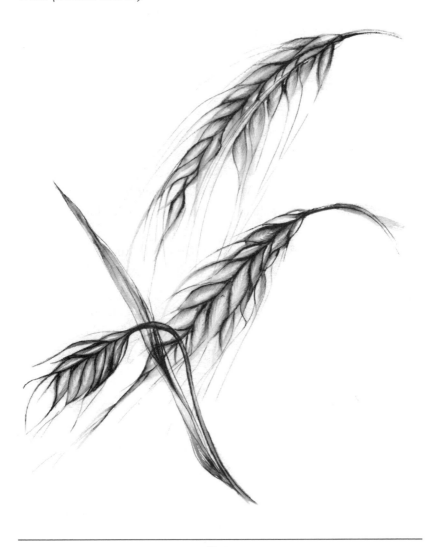

Oats

Oat Grass Moving Meditation

Read this through a few times; then close your eyes and do
the ritual without worrying about the words, or have someone
read it aloud to you. Or record it in your own voice: Speak
slowly and leave time to respond. Enjoy a soothing cup
of oat straw tea to complete your simple ritual.

This ritual is best done outdoors, barefoot. It can be shared with
children, with friends, or be done on your own. If you can't be
outside, stand barefoot on your rug or floor. If music is helpful
to you, put some on. Close your eyes and settle into the present.
Relax. Now, imagine you are out in a meadow.

You are a tall stalk of grass, oat grass, and a soft gentle breeze is
blowing. Feel how your body naturally wants to sway in the breeze,
and let your flowing breath become the breezes you sway to.

Feeling downward, feel shallow roots grow down where your
feet once were. Feel them reaching, grasping the Earth, holding
tightly to the soil, feeding and being fed by it.

Your grass roots are *strong*.

These roots in Earth create a living anchor to support your
fluidity, your flowing dances above the ground.

You are tall oat grass, top-heavy with milky seed, swaying and
dancing with gentle winds or even gale-force winds.

Feel yourself dancing with the winds of change as beautiful,
fluidic oat grass, with your roots anchored in the Earth,
holding you from underneath.

When you're ready, imagine the air getting calmer, growing still,
inviting your oat grass-stalk body to come to center, to stillness.

Draw your roots back up into you. Your anchored roots become
free feet again as you regain your human shape, feeling more fluid
and connected than before, with the blessing of *Avena sativa,* oats.

I mostly use oats as an indispensable infusion. This is a superb, nourishing herb for your nervous, glandular and digestive systems, and also for skin. The green oat stalk, including its few leaves and the grain as well, is harvested and sold as oat straw or oat grass.

Oat tops, which are the unripe seeds in their milky stage, are also harvested and sold separately. The tops are considered to be more specifically anti-depressant. I use them in tincture form for acute situations, as in the first example below.

Oat straw has more Vitamins A and C and is lower in calories than the tops on their own. Some herbalists consider the tops the *crème de la crème* of the plant, but I generally prefer the whole plant. I find infusions of straw and tops more deeply strengthening to the nervous system than the tincture, more calming and uplifting in the long run.

Here, though, is an example of using oat tincture in a different way. The following recipe includes oat tops. It was created for more extreme situations, and has proven to be very effective. I call it:

SUPER-SOOTHER OAT TINCTURE BLEND

> 1 part fresh motherwort tincture (leaf, stalk, and flower)
>
> 1 part fresh California poppy tincture (leaf, stalk, and flower)
>
> 1 part fresh oat tops tincture
>
> 1 part fresh skullcap tincture (leaf, stalk, and flower)

Combine the four tinctures together in equal proportions.

Add 25–75 drops into water or infusion, as needed. This is a recipe to use for a finite period of time, not for years on end.

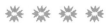

These tinctures are all made with aboveground parts of the plants. Reflecting on this symbolically, I found myself thinking that perhaps they not only soothe us but help us to rise above the ground when we feel we are sinking under it, as if we were dying.

I have used this blend in a variety of situations. It was first created to help a friend who found herself the primary caretaker for her much-beloved husband, first through an illness as it progressed, and then through his slow and only partial recuperation from surgery. She found that this blend helped her handle what life had thrown to them with more patience, even calm and grace—not easy for a fiery Aries woman!

Later, she told me this medicine "saved" her when she had the flu. It was the only thing she could (or wanted to) consume and keep down. I was surprised to hear about this use for the blend, but I took note!

Perhaps most exciting, I used this blend to help a wonderful man who'd become a drug addict to get his life back. Pete generously invited me to share his story.

After ending a five or six-year addiction to OxyContin, which he had been crushing and snorting, he had been on another drug called Subutex for eighteen months, this time by prescription. By the time I came onto the scene, he was preparing to go off the Subutex and had been reducing his dosage slowly and significantly, but already felt like hell and wasn't sure what his chances of success were. Everyone he knew who'd tried to come off it had failed. The withdrawal symptoms from Subutex are extremely difficult.

Pete wrote:

The drug that I initially was addicted to for five or six years is called OxyContin, a synthetic-opiate pain-reliever. Oxycodone is its active ingredient. Before that, I was dabbling with Percocet for a bunch of years, which is oxycodone with acetaminophen (the active ingredient in Tylenol), which has a lower dosage of oxycodone

Once I decided to get off of those drugs, I was prescribed Suboxone (often called Subox or Subs). Actually, I was prescribed Subutex, which is the same drug without an inhibitor. That meant that if I wanted to party I could, without getting sick. I made sure to get that one … typical drug-addict behavior. But as luck would have it, I stayed true and didn't party.

I was on the Subutex for about eighteen months. It worked well in getting me over the psychological addiction of crushing pills and snorting them, since it was taken sublingually. However, it too is an opiate. In trying to get off of it, I realized how strong an opiate it is. I started with three milligrams per day, and eventually got down to one a day. However, in my research, I found that one milligram of Suboxone or Subutex is equivalent to twenty milligrams of oxycodone! So when I stopped it was cold turkey from months of taking one milligram of Subutex, or twenty of oxycodone. Not easy.

The herbs that I received from you did certainly help a lot, particularly the drops. I used them during the day and to help me sleep. The teas were great, as they were quite soothing. Their psychological effects cannot be overlooked, as there was a sense of calm after taking them, knowing that, in time this would be over. And, as it happened, it worked. I am now fine … at least no longer addicted to oxycodone, and sleeping just fine, and functioning just fine. The overall effects of having taken those drugs for so long has certainly left its mark, but with time I believe that too can be reversed.

The drops he mentions were Super-Soother blend. He used the larger dose at night when he was having a terrible time sleeping, and it finally helped him. The teas I brought him were oat straw and chamomile. These gentle plants are potent relievers of pain. Antispasmodic and calming, they also helped his sleep.

I give him all the credit in the world for his own recovery, as he was ready and willing to get off the drugs he was hooked on. However, he truly had grave doubts about his prospects, because he had no model of success for this, only of failure. The reassurance that the herbs would help him over the hump made a huge psychological difference, and the herbs obviously made a physical difference as well. For a while Pete tried to interest the friends he used to party with to see me and use herbs to help themselves, but no one followed through. We're all free to choose.

When my friend and former neighbor hit his lowest point, he had lost his music and his business. Later his house was foreclosed on. He'd moved away, and when I was writing this section of the book I hadn't seen him for over a year. Suddenly, out of the blue, I ran into him. In answer to my questions, he smiled hugely and told me about some big changes he was making in his living situation. He affirmed that he was drug-free and is now sharing his music with the world from a healthier place within himself. I couldn't be happier for him. We parted with a hug.

BASIC OAT STRAW INFUSION

Put 2 or more cups of dried oats into a half-gallon of water. Boil gently for about five minutes, then pour everything into a half-gallon jar, cap tightly, and let sit out overnight on your counter.

In the morning, squeeze out the herbs into your infusion, getting every last drop out of them that you can. Then compost the spent plant material that has given its all into your infusion.

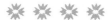

You may notice that oat straw is included in many of my herbal infusions, especially those suggested for daily sustenance. I believe that unless you suffer from celiac disease and can't digest any gluten at all, this is an amazingly healthful herb. It is a regenerative endocrine system tonic. Almost everyone I've seen, even those like myself who are gluten-intolerant (but not allergic), have a fine response to oat straw infusion.

I recommend boiling oat straw to get the most out of it. Therefore, when oats are in any mixed blend, boil the oats along with the water that you're going to pour over the other herbs in the jar for overnight steeping, as described in the infusion recipe above.

Oats are rich in B vitamins and minerals such as calcium and magnesium that soothe and strengthen the nervous system. I consider oats to be adaptogenic. Oats are one of the plant medicines that will alter how you respond to stress in the short and long term. They soothe immediately, but also build resources for the long term. Oats help to improve synaptic functioning and communication between the nerve cells, so they are indicated anytime there is damage to the nerves or a slowdown of the system, as in accidents and degenerative nerve diseases like multiple sclerosis.

Improving the functioning of your nervous system and the health of your glandular system also improves your sexual responsiveness. Oats increase your awareness of sensation and sensitivity to pleasure, and the deep nourishment they provide gives you the stamina and strength you need to enjoy the sexual experiences that drinking regular oat straw infusions will encourage you to desire.

Oats are also an excellent food medicine for the skeleton, building healthy bones and joints through highly assimilable minerals and proteins. Oats bring flexibility as well as density—something we need for long-term bone health that bone-density tests not only can't show but can actually be misleading about: A healthy bone has resiliency, but a dense bone may or may not be resilient.

Oats are anti-spasmodic and can help with pain, especially pain that comes from tension or overuse of muscles, tendons, and ligaments such as from gardening all day or doing yoga or any exercise without warming up first.

I call the following blend my:

PERSONAL SUSTAINABILITY INFUSION

¾ cup dried red clover blossoms

¾ cup dried nettle leaves and stalks

½ cup dried oatstraw

Boil the oats in a half-gallon of water. Put the dried herbs into a half-gallon jar and pour the boiled oats and water over them, filling the jar to the rim. Cap tightly. Steep the brew overnight. In the morning, or after 8 hours or so, decant the infusion by pouring off the liquid through a strainer or cheesecloth and squeezing out the herbs before composting them.

Store this tea in the refrigerator, as it is high in protein and will spoil rapidly if not refrigerated.

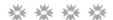

This is one of the most frequently drunk infusions in my home, and one I often recommend to friends and clients. I usually take one bag with the three herbs pre-blended in it to make infusions when traveling. It is a safe, nourishing tonic and replaces the need to take expensive, hard-to-digest vitamin and mineral supplements.

This three-herb blend tastes delicious and goes down easily hot or cold. It offers optimum nourishment for a healthy and strong immune system, builds blood and bones, and increases the suppleness of veins and arteries—all while soothing and strengthening the nerves and muscles, improving the digestive and sexual-reproductive systems, relieving muscle and joint pain, and healing skin rashes.

This is an all-purpose excellence blend, with so many gifts that I'm going to simply summarize them—nettles for strength and stamina, red clover for calm clarity, and oats for sexy suppleness.

Speaking of recipes, oats are delicious and healing on their own but also provide a nice neutral-to-sweet base that mixes well with other herbs. Here are a few more ways I love to enjoy my oat straw:

Oat straw/alfalfa—nourishing and strengthening to the nervous and immune systems; rich in minerals and vitamins.

Oat straw/rose—soothing, calming, heart-opening, and skin-healing.

Oat straw/linden—calming, anti-spasmodic, pain relieving, and moistening.

Oat straw/lemon balm—uplifting; soothes digestive distress.

Oat straw/lemon verbena—calming, delicious; delightful nervine.

Oat straw/lavender—gentle, soothing; brings sweetness and stability. The last five of the six blends above can be used to prepare a lovely herbal bath. I do, however, have great respect for the healing power of a hot oat straw bath all on its own. It soothes and smoothes skin while it relieves joint and muscle pain and melts away mental and emotional stress and tension. Add a half-gallon of oat straw infusion to your full bathtub, and soak for at least twenty minutes to enjoy the full benefits.

St. J's Wort (*Hypericum perforatum* and other species)

One of my favorite nervines is St. J's wort. I turn to this bushy, yellow-and-red flowering herb for loosening up muscular tension in the neck and shoulders, and for soothing and repairing nerves, more than for its most celebrated contemporary use as an herb for mild to moderate depression, though it's definitely helpful for that, too. St. J's invites you to join her on the sunny side of the street, psychologically speaking, and to join her physically in the sunny meadows where she likes to grow. Speaking of sunshine, St. J's is considered a specific for Seasonal Affective Disorder, or SAD, when depression (or simply a case of the blues) is directly correlated to a lack of adequate sunlight. (Check your vitamin D levels too.)

I suggest starting with about fifteen drops of tincture in a cup of warm water or tea made with any nervine you like. You might add it into skullcap tea if you are ready to go to sleep, into chamomile tea if you are having belly cramps, or into linden blossom infusion to help with sadness and grief, and to help you relax and get ready for a good night's sleep.

You can also use St. J's flowers as a tea or infusion, though the lovely blossoms turn a bit bitter as they steep. When I add them into infusions, I use them sparingly.

I consider this weed (wildflower, if you prefer) an invaluable asset for the nervous system. It is one of the herbs I take care to always keep in my green treasure chest of herbal medicines. I keep dried St. J's flowers on hand for infusions and soaks, as well as plenty of the rich, red tincture and infused oil that I make from flowering tops of the fresh plants. If I haven't made enough to last me until next year's harvest, then I buy some from another herbalist or herb company that I trust. I also take a bottle of tincture and another of infused oil with me when I travel, to help with aches and pains from sitting too long in a car or plane, or hiking all day, or dancing all night.

St. J's is a restorative tonic for the nervous system. This means that the longer you use it the less regularly you will need it. It strengthens and calms the nerves. Studies have shown it to be at least as effective as chemical anti-depressants, without the side effects and without inducing dependency. In fact, it's also helpful when releasing chemical or other addictions, as it helps the liver to excrete drugs. (To the liver, all pharmaceuticals are basically processed as poisons.) Because of the way that St. J's helps the liver to detoxify the body, it is best to take it several hours before or after other pharmaceuticals in general, and not at all when it is contraindicated, as for a selective serotonin re-uptake inhibitor (SSRI) like Paxil or Celexa. Herbalist Gail Faith Edwards suggests using skullcap 4–6 times a day for weaning yourself from those drugs before starting St. J's.

The dosage depends on the sensitivity of the person, and may vary if St. J's is being blended with other herbs in a recipe rather than being taken as a simple. As a simple, I usually suggest about 25–30 drops of the tincture in water or tea, 2–3 times daily.

I find St. J's especially useful when tension, including tension of mental/emotional origin, is manifesting physically, such as in tight shoulders, shoulders up around the ears, or a perpetually stiff neck. Sometimes I like to alternate it or mix it with motherwort tincture (15–30 drops per cup) when there is a strong emotional component behind the tension.

St. J's helps repair nerve damage that has resulted from accidents, illness, injury, or surgery. Here is a recipe that I used for someone who had serious nerve damage after an auto accident. The exact combination of herbs can vary depending on the needs of the person.

NERVE REPAIR RECIPE

½ cup dried oat straw

½ cup dried yarrow flowers (stalks and leaves can be included)

½ cup dried nettles (stalks and leaves)

½ cup dried St. J's leaves, stalks, and flowers

¼ cup dried sage leaves (flowers can be included)

Put the oats and cold water in a pot and bring them to a boil for a few minutes. Pour the boiling water and oats over the rest of the herbs in a half-gallon jar. Steep them overnight or for about 8 hours. Strain out the plant material and drink 2–4 cups most days, until the blend is no longer needed.

My friend had such severe nerve damage after her car accident that one day she was in her kitchen and didn't realize she was burning her fingers on a hot electric stove until she smelled burning flesh. She hadn't felt a thing. When she told me this story, I asked her if she was willing to let me try to help her with herbs. She didn't really think it would help, but she felt she had nothing to lose and did it anyway. She found that she liked the infusion, so she kept drinking it for quite a few months. She got a substantial amount of sensation back even though she'd been told that would be impossible. She also found that other areas that had been in constant pain were much less so. She had suffered from daily headaches since the accident and these too were greatly reduced in frequency, duration, and intensity. As I've said before, side effects from herbal medicine tend toward the positive!

For nerve repair in feet, I would also suggest taking baths or foot baths in this blend. Even once a week would help hasten and deepen the healing. Additionally, massage St. J's wort oil (as she did) into the affected areas as frequently as possible. No matter where the nerve injury is manifesting, have someone massage St. J's oil into your spine at least once a day (or do it yourself as best you can if that's truly your only option). This herb, as you can see, is truly a blessing.

St. J's is also a great anti-inflammatory for the nerves (and adjacent muscle tissue). The longest and largest single nerve in the body is the sciatic nerve that runs from the base of the spine, down the leg, to the foot. Sciatic pain, called sciatica, can be quite intense, impacting both muscles and nerves along the spine, lower back, and legs. St. J's is specific for this condition and here you would use it internally, as tea or tincture, and externally, as infused oil, as frequently as you can. Sciatica can also present as numbness or tingling sensations and St. J's will help in those instances, too.

St. J's is reliable for viral conditions such as herpes (see Skin section, page 300). If it is taken and applied right at the tingly beginning of an outbreak, it will sometimes keep the sores from manifesting. When there are outbreaks, it relieves pain and helps to prevent scarring even as it increases the speed of healing. St. J's is specific for healing all manifestations of the herpes virus, including the painful nerve condition known as shingles. I often combine it together with the lovely lemon balm *(Melissa officinalis)*.

Lavender (*Lavandula angustifolia* and other species)

There are many species of lavender, and any aromatic species can be used. I grow *Lavandula angustifolia* in my garden for harvesting, and usually grow a few different varieties to experiment with. Lavender is not an herb that grows wild in the northeastern United States.

Lovely lavender calms the nervous system, heals burns on the skin, and disinfects harmful bacteria in the digestive tract. You can drink the tea, wash burns with it, cook with it, and even put it in your bucket to wash your floors and walls. This will not only act as a disinfectant, it will smell lovely and bring a peaceful vibration into your home.

Lavender is a physical ally in so many ways. Scientific research has shown that it contains a class of molecules called monoterpenes. One of these is perillyl alcohol, which has been shown to help stop cancer cells from dividing. Lavender is also a spiritual ally, helping bring ease and sweetness into our lives.

Use dried lavender flowers and leaves for teas, infusions, baths, oils, sprays, honey balls, or as part of a smoke blend. You can make a soothing lavender bath by adding a half-gallon of lavender tea into your bath water, or grinding dry leaves and flowers and mixing them with sea or Epsom salts. Add one tablespoon or more of this mixture to a bath. Do what's pleasing to your senses in terms of how strong or mild a lavender aroma you like.

If you are adding essential oil of lavender to a bath, make sure to add it (5–10 drops) after the bath is filled so that it doesn't dissipate and waste the oil. You can also make your own fresh lavender flower and leaf infused oil. If you use that in your bath, add about a tablespoon when the bath is about half full, and swirl it around to blend it in. It creates a fragrant, beautiful blend and helps in situations on the whole continuum from simple calming to post-traumatic stress healing.

Lavender tea is pain-relieving, muscle-relaxing, anti-depressant, and helps to soothe an aching or breaking heart. For any of these last purposes, it can be used alone or combine it with oat straw.

LAVENDER/OAT STRAW SERENE-A-TEA

1 cup dried oat straw or tops

⅛ cup dried lavender flowers

2 quart jars

Boil the cup of oat straw (or tops) in one quart of water for about 5 minutes, and then put the oat straw and boiled water into a quart jar. Top up with more boiling water if necessary to fill it to the top. Cap jar and let it sit overnight.

    Put the dried lavender into the other quart jar. Fill the jar with boiling water. Cap and let sit for 20 minutes. Decant it, squeeze out the herbs, and refrigerate the lavender infusion until the oats are ready.

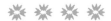

Because these two herbs require such different lengths of time for steeping, it's easier to make them separately than to combine them. It also allows you to boil the oats, which brings out more of their flavor and nutrients. Please don't over-steep lavender. I consider 3–5 minutes of steeping to yield a nice beverage, and precisely 20 minutes to yield a medicinal-strength infusion.

After you've decanted the infusions, combine them for a sweet, soothing blend to deeply nourish your whole being. Drink this when you feel worn down emotionally, when your digestion is upset because you feel frazzled, or simply because you'll enjoy it.

It's good iced, too.

Lavender helps with tension headaches and anxiety. Herbalist Kiva Rose shares this observation and advice: "Lavender is appropriate as a nervine when a person is anxious, confused, and has a wrinkled forehead that can't relax. The forehead will give it away every time."

Another lovely way to use your lavender is as an infused honey (see page 388). This helps with agitation, the blues, and bitter grief.

Lavender tea helps ease insomnia. It is a relaxing, restful sleep herb. It's theorized that chemicals in lavender interact with the reticular activating system (RAS) in the brain that controls the wake-sleep cycle to induce restful sleep. That may be—or it may be the lavender-hued woman who rises up out of the plant to stroke your hair like a loving mother (probably right over the area of your reticular activating system) who soothes you to sleep. Or perhaps it's both, and they are different expressions of the same effect!

You can put a small bag of dried lavender under a pillow, and spray lavender water onto pillows and other bedding for restful sleep and especially to relieve nightmares. I've had very good results using lavender for children and adults with nightmares.

Here are two easy spray recipes:

LAVENDER SPRAY—VARIATION I

Lavender essential oil (French lavender or whatever species you prefer).

Spray bottle

Water (use bottled water only if truly necessary)

Fill a 2-ounce spray bottle (preferably glass) almost full with fresh water. Add up to 10 drops of essential oil. Shake gently.

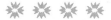

This potion doesn't need refrigeration, and will keep for a long time. When it gets low, you can simply add more water and then lavender oil, as needed.

There are many grades of essential oil available for purchase (see Resources, page 514). You can't make essential oils at home without special equipment. I use these highly concentrated oils sparingly, and for external purposes only. Make sure you use genuine essential oil as opposed to fragrance oil. It is more expensive, and more effective. Essential oils are extracted from different parts of plants by a variety of methods, whereas fragrance oils are manufactured for scent and are often synthetic.

LAVENDER SPRAY—VARIATION II

Dried lavender flowers

Quart jar

Spray bottle

Water

Put ⅛ cup of good-quality dried lavender flowers into a quart jar. Cover with boiled water. Cap and steep for 20 minutes. Decant promptly, squeezing the flowers to retrieve the last of their oils.

Fill your spray bottle with the lavender infusion. Keep refrigerated when not in use to prolong the shelf life of this preparation. You can also add one drop or more of the essential oil to help preserve it.

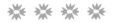

Whichever version you prefer, these sprays are indispensable aids when traveling, whether by plane, bus, train, or in your own car. I carry a bottle with me almost everywhere. (On a plane you can currently carry up to a three-ounce bottle in your ziplock bag of liquids.)

In any public place, your lavender spray will calm and refresh you, and lift your spirits. Its antiseptic oils will also help to disinfect germs. You can spray it on your hands and face. It's very lovely, and people almost never object to it. In fact, more often than not, they ask for some too. I'm sure you'll find other creative applications.

The following stories illustrate some of these creative applications:

I had a student who was working as a bartender. She had been doing that for a long time, and though the money was good she was totally fed up with some of the behavior she had to deal with at the bar. She created her own lavender spray, and when necessary she would lean over the bar and spray it into the face of an overly inebriated, amorous male customer. To her surprise, the first time she did this, not only did it work to stop the man in his tracks without offending him but the guy liked it so much that he started asking her questions about herbs! (She went on to create a successful herbal-product line.)

I once offered my lavender spray bottle to a surly store clerk who, in answer to my questions, told me she had a terrible headache. I had her spray it on her face and neck, and massage some into her temples. By the time I left the store fifteen minutes later, she was smiling. She told me she was astonished to find that her headache was gone. Hooray for lavender!

If you find yourself in a traffic jam and are getting upset (which has never yet been shown to make traffic move any faster), try a little lavender spray to help you calm down and relax. Remember, being present with what is rather than mentally struggling against it not only strengthens and heals the nervous system, it helps clear your thinking so that you might come up with an alternative route, or decide to listen to a tape or CD in the car that you've been meaning to get to. Or perhaps imagine that you are in the car with a dear friend, and this is the only time you are going to have together for the next few years. Feel how content you would be with that traffic jam.

Sometimes, as in that last active imagination exercise, you have to start by tricking yourself into accepting what is by adding an imaginary dimension that makes it an appealing scenario. It's all the same to your nervous system. Remember that bodies are innocent and believe everything you tell them. If you think, "This is terrible!" the nervous system reacts accordingly. If you think, "What a gift!" the nervous system responds with delight.

I tried this once in a completely frustrating, unexpected, middle-of-the-night traffic jam on the Throgs Neck Bridge in New York City. My friend and I sprayed lavender and decided to breathe into the moment exactly as it was, and see what might happen if we chose to trust it.

Neither of us has ever forgotten what happened next. We looked around us, as if with new eyes, and to our delight we realized we were able to count seven bridges including the one we were on. It was very beautiful. As we began to truly revel in the experience we wouldn't have had if we weren't stopped dead in traffic, the cars in front of us magically began to move, and the traffic jam was soon over!

Dried lavender flowers are great to use in sleep pillows and dream pillows. Any herbs used for a pillow must be thoroughly dried to prevent mold. As I mentioned earlier, children with nightmares will benefit from lavender. A pillow can be crafted as a creative, empowering, self-healing project with your children. If they are too young to sew, they can still hand you threads and lavender flowers, and help you make the pillows. They can choose colors or the fabric they love best, and it can be a round, square, or whatever-you-like shaped pillow. I remember crafting my very first dream pillow. It was shaped like the crescent moon, and was white on the waxing side and black on the waning side, with tiny pearl beads and silver stars sewn onto it.

SIMPLE SLEEP PILLOW

Felt, cotton, rayon, flannel, hemp, or silk fabric

Lavender flowers

Stuffing (see suggestions below)

Needle, thread, scissors

Use any (preferably natural) fabric for your pillow. Cut two pieces of material into the size and shape you want, and then put them inside-out and back-to-back. Sew them together, leaving one seam open. Turn the pillow fabric right-side-out now. Mix the lavender flowers into the stuffing material, and fill your pillow to the desired fullness. Then sew up the final seam. Decorate if you wish, and—*voilà!*—you've made your own herbal sleep pillow.

It can be put underneath, alongside, or inside the pillowcase of your sleeping pillow, where the weight of your head will release the fragrance. You can also bring out the lavender fragrance by squeezing your pillow and, optionally, adding a few drops of lavender essential oil to the outside of it when it needs refreshing.

You can use standard polyfill stuffing from craft stores. I've used that for years, and it works well, especially for getting the herbs blended into the fibers; but it is a synthetic petroleum product, so if you like you could use something more natural. If you are not up to gathering and drying your own plant silk (from milkweed pods, for example) you can use tiny pieces of cotton or wool fabric scraps, or cut-up pieces of old socks or T-shirts. You can also purchase kapok silk. I've seen it sold by the pound online. It is like down, but comes from the seeds of the sacred ceiba tree and makes a lovely, silky stuffing. (See Resources, page 515.)

Here are some variations for this pillow:

If you want more than one herb in your pillow, other herbs that encourage calm, restful sleeping are catnip or marjoram leaves, and chamomile or rose blossoms.

I put hops flowers *(Humulus lupulus)* into pillows for people who have a lot of trouble falling and/or staying asleep. Female hops flowers are cone-shaped, sticky, and contain a fragrant yellow resin called lupulin. These flowers, called strobiles, are the part of the vine used in herbal medicine and in brewing beer.

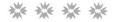

Occasionally taking 15 drops of hops tincture or a cup of the bitter tea before bed can help, too. Some herbal practitioners have cautioned against internal use of hops when struggling with depression. I haven't seen that, but in any event, there is no problem associated with having the flowers in a pillow.

SLEEP PILLOW TO WARD OFF NIGHTMARES

Make the pillow in the same way as described above, but blend the lavender with more protective herbs such as agrimony leaves, roses, rosemary leaves and flowers, and/or grandmother cedar leaves *(Thuja species)*. Other possibilities include angelica leaves and/or seeds, calendula blossoms, and thyme leaves. You could even sew in a protective hawthorn thorn embedded deep in the center of the stuffing, but make absolutely sure it can't come loose and poke through the pillow.

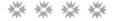

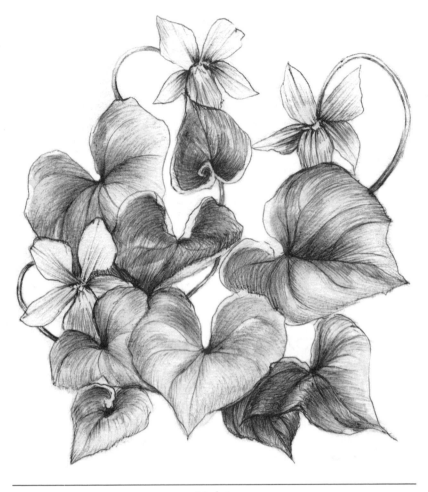

Violet

Violet (*Viola odorata* and other species)

Body: pain relief, lymph support; anti-inflammatory rich in salicylic acid; nourishes nerves, dissolves lumps, reduces edema, relieves dry coughs, helps with digestive and reproductive system cancers.

Mind: serenity; helps one see the sweetness in others.

Heart: heals grief and anger.

Soul: invokes your natural essence of joy.

Violet

My leaves are green,
My petals bright
In colors ranging
From yellow to white.
Most famous, though,
Are my purple flowers,
And though I am small
I have great healing powers.

I'm not bragging;
That's not my way,
So though I am shy
Please hear what I say.
I have gifts, yes!
I'm abundantly blessed,
And for pain relief
My lovely leaves are the best.

You can dine on
My heart-shaped leaves.
They cool you softly
Like a summer breeze.
Or chew them up
And lay them on a cyst
Every single day,
And it will not long persist.

I specialize
In moistening.
I soothe and I smooth

Your lymph, breasts, and skin.
I heal with love,
As all the green plants do
Remember that *I*
Am another part of *you.*

Sweet blue violet is the plant so in love with life that she flowers twice—
once just for fun, and once to set seeds!

The "false" flowers are the ones most people are familiar with. They
are the lovely purple (or lavender, white, or yellow), irregular, five-petal
flowers that first appear in the springtime. They are delightful to see; their
beauty is set against an abundance of shiny green leaves that uncurl from
the center to slowly but surely reveal their valentine heart-shape. Often,
a little bit of curl remains at the very outer edges of the heart.

If ever there was a plant that speaks to its connection to your heart,
it is sweet blue violet. Not only does violet help your body dissolve cysts,
lumps, and bumps, this plant's soothing nature can help you dissolve the
red-hot burn of anger, cool the draining white heat of frustration and
resentment, and relieve the simmering roil of feeling stuck in separation
when ruled by your judgmental mind.

Violet leaf infusion or tincture is the remedy to use if your head is
aching in response to over-thinking, or to feeling angry and frustrated
with someone. Violet leaf nourishes the nervous system and provides pain
relief due to its salicylic acid, the anti-inflammatory chemical related to
aspirin. Violet is one of the sweetest-spirited plants I know. I harvest a
lot of this prolific weed, as it's difficult to buy really good-quality violet
leaves. To make the infusion, cover about two cups of dried violet leaves
with boiled water and steep them in a half-gallon jar overnight.

Once in Central Park, my weed-walk group and I were squatting to
look at low-growing violets when a man mentioned that he had an ache
up and down the back of his neck and the bottom of his skull that had
been plaguing him for months. I had him chew up a few violet leaves. He
liked the taste so he swallowed them, then chewed up more for a poultice!
(That never happens with a band-aid, now, does it?) His girlfriend helped

him to spread the poultice over the back of his neck and up to where the top of his spine met the base of his skull. We stood around while I told the group some plant stories, and then asked him how he was doing. He was truly amazed at the degree of pain relief he had gotten in less than ten minutes, and the people on the walk with him witnessed how powerful these wild little plants underfoot can be.

Violets are also delicious to eat. My former apprentice Eileen, who was the first person to introduce herbal medicine into a contemporary medical clinic in New York City, told me this adorable story. Her little nephew was caught by his mother eating the violets in their backyard. His mother was frightened by this, and told him to stop. Eileen told me that he stood up straight, put his hands on his hips and with great dignity (as only a five-year-old can muster) he said, "Mommy, Auntie Eileen showed me these, and told me how to make sure they were violets. I can show *you*. I'm being very careful."

And then, all adult logic aside, he shouted with great enthusiasm, "Besides, Mommy, they are DELICIOUS!" Case closed.

I find violet leaf tincture, tea and oil very helpful for many kinds of grief, especially hot grief in response to loss. I also eat the cooling, shade-loving leaves in salads all summer. Violet doesn't flat-line your emotions the way pharmaceuticals often do—in fact, quite the opposite. Violet brings a gentle touch to grief so that it can be felt, cried through, accepted, and healed. Herbalist Kate Temple-West uses violet "for grief that masquerades as anger."

Since sweet, cool-you-off, moist, juicy violets help you see the sweetness in others, they are invaluable in difficult relationships where diplomacy is called for. But because violets truly help you see the person's sweetness under whatever gruff exterior they present, you won't necessarily feel as if you are trying to be diplomatic; instead, violet simply helps you to express your sincere, honest feelings.

Here's a beautiful violet story that a wise-woman herbalist shared with me back when she was my apprentice:

"I felt as though I was facing an impossible catch-22. I would do nearly anything for my husband, including help care for his difficult, hypercritical, thorny mother, but the question was how to do this in the face of our very challenged and strained relationship. She was the only person in my life from whom I had consistently received negativity, laced with an overriding sense that I could never please her. But I was the only person that she wanted in the ICU upon exiting surgery for the removal of a cancerous lung. What did she want from me? I wasn't sure, but imagined it had something to do with my comfort in navigating the medical bureaucracies, my energy-healing skills and, most of all, I believe she wanted to feel my compassion and love.

"Desperate for guidance on herbs that might reconcile my wish to show true kindness as well as protect myself and preserve my integrity in this situation, I called Robin for help. Violet was Robin's immediate suggestion, and I set off to the park in search of a fresh patch. When I found it, I sat down beside the plant and shared my challenge. It didn't occur to me till weeks later that this was the first time that I was as consumed in conversation with a plant as I would be with a friend—but I was fully aware that violet was there speaking with me, gently offering her wisdom, her care, and her protection of my heart (as a human friend would do).

"This ultimately allowed me to find a way to offer kindness and compassion to my mother-in-law while preserving my sense of safety and my boundaries in this situation. I asked violet's permission to take her with me, and I placed some of her oil over my heart as I boarded the plane, drank some tincture as I headed to the hospital, and kept her within reach throughout my stay. To my surprise, truth to tell, I was at peace during this entire care-giving mission, and felt stronger as a result of it.

"After returning to NY, I visited violet (which is now part of my weekly routine) and thanked her for her teachings and protection. As I sat with her in meditation, she told me that the gentleness of heart that I showed to my mother-in-law was a practice I should be applying toward myself in daily life. This is a new way for me to be, and a lesson that violet continues to share."

Tennessee Williams wrote, "The violets in the mountains have broken the rocks." Indeed, sweet blue violets will slowly, gently, and most assuredly break through the stony encasements you carefully construct around your heart. My perception is that she doesn't exactly break the rocks so much as melt them with kindliness, soft strength, and friendliness, until the boundaries have melted away and your heart is free. Violet helps set your heart free to do what it is designed for—to love freely and fully yourself and all those you regard as "others" but who, when seen through the eyes of the heart, are found to be another part of you.

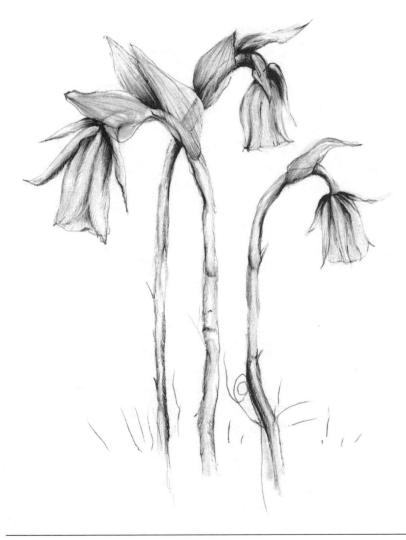

Indian Pipe

Indian Pipe *(Monotropa uniflora)*

I admire and deeply respect this unusual plant, devoid of chlorophyll, that is known as Indian pipe. To quote herbalist Dr. Ryan Drum, "it is an epi-parasite, a plant that parasitizes parasitic tree fungi."

Indian pipe is completely white and blackens easily when bruised. It often has a pink tint, and more rarely grows to be deep red. The stem and single flower are waxy and resemble a spine with a nodding, relaxed head. The first time I saw it, and many times thereafter, I had the intuitive impression that wherever this plant was growing in abundance Native American people had gathered together to meet in councils. Interestingly, in an article by Dr. Drum, he says that the coastal Salish people associate it with places that wolves have marked as their territory.

Indian pipe is a powerful sedative nervine. According to Dr. Drum, it has been used to stop seizures and convulsions, and to help those with mental disorders and chronic muscle spasms. Herbalist David Winston recommends this herb to help "reduce the perception of pain," and he makes an excellent tincture that I've used when needed (see Resources, page 510).

Personally, I observed this plant with awe in the northeast woods for over twenty years before I actually harvested any, even though I had apprentices who harvested this plant under my watch because they felt drawn to do so. I wasn't ready.

When Indian pipe called me, though, the call was powerful and unmistakable. I was walking alone in the woods in Massachusetts and heard/felt/sensed a presence that said, almost as if with words,

"Sister, you've visited me for so long. Come, please, harvest me for medicine—it's time you got to know me more intimately. I help those in extreme pain, and you never know when you will encounter those who need my gift."

I sat quietly with the plant, and continued to listen.

"I am half in this world and half in the other world—the underworld, the overworld, and between the worlds. See how I'm pale, devoid of color? Like human skin when you die, when the blood stops flowing and the heart stops beating, the color of blood flows out of the body, no matter what color your skin had been before, it pales. I will show you how to harvest me. Do it today if you can. Wander to different patches of me and gather me. You will see how I turn purple, the color of spirit. I am spirit medicine, ghost pipe, corpse plant. I am good to know."

Later that year, I needed the tincture for a friend undergoing a slow recovery from a terribly painful back surgery. Over time his surgeon and doctor said they had never seen anyone healing as well from this kind of surgery. The herbs he was using were helping him, including Indian pipe. As long as there is rain, Indian pipe is plentiful in the woods where I live, the more rain, the more Monotropa. Indian pipe should not be harvested in a region where it's rare.

I continued to explore Indian pipe over the next few years, smelling it, meditating with it, and experimenting with different tinctures, sometimes from the whole plant and other times from the cut-up plant, sometimes including the below-ground parts, and other times not. Indian pipe always brought me in touch with another dimension though I stayed completely cognizant of my physical body and surroundings. Once, when I tasted the plant without really being completely present (my mind had wandered briefly), I felt nauseated. When I was fully present, that never happened. It's not a plant I would ever eat for food, nor am I suggesting you try it. I was tasting tiny amounts in order to learn more about it.

I take the tincture in water by itself or mixed with other herbal tinctures such as anti-inflammatory St. J's *(Hypericum),* anti-spasmodic Lobelia, or a mineral-rich, strengthening nervine such as skullcap. The dosage needs to be adjusted to the person and the situation. A few drops might be enough or someone could use up to 25–50 drops in water.

I generally use Indian pipe for physical-plane pain, but it can also help when you need to place a foot onto the other side briefly, into another dimension.

I used this plant to help my beloved cat Pandora when she got very ill, and eventually to help her pass over. I made a bath for her with ten drops of tincture in warm water, dipped a cloth in it, and bathed her fur with the mixture while I cried. It clearly soothed her and relieved her pain.

The night she died I also took some, as I was guided to do, to be able to journey part of the way with her.

According to David Winston, Indian pipe acts much like an opiate drug in that it helps separate you from the sensation or awareness of pain. That can be a true gift.

This mysterious ghost plant tells the truth; it is a good ally to get to know, both in living and in dying.

Healing Herbs for Heartache, Heartbreak, Grief, and Shock

Hearts get broken. They always have, and they always will. The only heart that can't be broken is the heart that is already completely open.

We are often told we have to "just let it go," whatever "it" is. While you can let experiences settle to the back of your mind and heart instead of the forefront, what has happened has happened. What you've seen, you've seen. To where can you let it go? These painful events are part of you, part of what makes you who you are. Experiences that hurt so badly when you're going through them ultimately awaken your compassion and foster the deepest healing and reconnection.

You can consciously partner with an herb using a specific intent to reconnect to and open your heart, to remember how to put love first. I counsel people who have been trying to let go and yet feel totally stuck, that the task is not to let go but to allow their own heart to expand in order to hold the pain and not be engulfed by it—to metaphorically grow the heart so that the pain can be there, held in their love, which is so much greater than they can imagine.

I realize this is not easy. It requires courage, clear intention, and support. It asks for your willingness to release attachment to your story, to your interpretation of events. Along with this flexibility of mind, it requires clear seeing, which is to simply see what is without blame.

. . . .

Some of my favorite herbal allies for heartbreak and heartache, shock, and grief are: lavender, rose, hawthorn, motherwort, linden, and violet.

Other supportive herbal allies are sassafras, burdock, nettles, and holy basil. I also like chamomile, mimosa, and cherry blossoms. Soothing nervines that are helpful to get to know are California poppy, skullcap, orange blossoms, and oat straw. Flower essences play a part here, too, as do herbs that match a specific individual in a specific situation. Always use the best herb available rather than none at all when there is an immediate need. Very often even one herb is enough to be comforting, grounding, and/or uplifting. You could go to your kitchen cupboard and make a cup of thyme or basil tea, and benefit immediately and tangibly from the physical, mental, and emotional tension-relieving qualities of these plants.

MAGICAL GIFTS OF SOME NERVOUS SYSTEM-HEALING HERBS

Borage—gladdens the heart and mind; courage.

Burdock—deep-rootedness, grounding, centering in self/body/Earth; trust when one has lost one's mooring; works well with dandelion.

California poppy—helps sleep, soothes pain, relaxes physical tension.

Dandelion—helps release anger, dispel fear of darkness, brings light.

Hawthorn berries, flowers, leaves and thorns—heals the heart on every level; lifts spirits; helps claim body as sacred space.

Holy basil—clears vision, helps you adapt to change.

Indian pipe—for physical pain; death medicine to help someone accept crossing over; in life, opens you to dance across the dimensional divide.

Lavender—eases heartbreak; adds sweetness, reassurance.

Linden—grief-relief after death or divorce; expands perception of multidimensional magic.

Motherwort—comforting, calming, strengthening; brings courage; works well with skullcap for shock.

Nettle—strength; healthy, respectful boundaries; helps express anger; electrical reconnection, rewiring personal power grid.

Oat straw—grace and flexibility; soothes heart tension that's been taken in physically.

Oat tops—eases depression and withdrawal symptoms.

Orange blossoms—sensual soother; re-awakens sexuality and desire; warms up a cool libido in both women and men.

Rose—healing after betrayal or death of beloved; helps you to see and respect others' perspectives.

Sassafras—spirit-lifting, joy-inducing; brings lightness and laughter.

Skullcap—profoundly soothing, nourishing, restorative, and sedating.

Violet—helps you see the sweetness in another; eases grief, releases anger.

. . . .

In addition to the possibility of large-scale shock and grief in a communal calamity such as an earthquake, volcano, or flood, or a senseless murder or terrorist strike, there is the more everyday nature of heartache and heartbreak.

In our personal lives, our hearts get broken again and again. Parents or children disappoint us. Husbands, wives, girlfriends, and boyfriends leave us. Lovers we trusted cheat on us. People get sick. People die—even children. We lose our homes, our animal companions, and as we age and grow we lose not only our youth but also many of our most prized illusions. We realize that not only will we die, but everyone we know and love will die, too.

Because this isn't healthily woven into the fabric of our culture, we don't know how to handle that knowledge. To one degree or another, we inevitably begin putting psychic armor around our hearts in response to life's large and small disappointments, and begin closing ourselves off to the goodness, power, and naturalness of our loving.

But people don't all react to heartbreak the same way. One person might not even know her heart is aching because she keeps so busy working or fighting for a cause in order not to feel anything. Another person might sleep all day and night, while for another not being able to sleep could be his worst symptom. One person is spitting mad, and another just wants to die.

These different responses can help determine which herbs might be best for a specific person and situation. When your heart is aching, it can feel like a heavy stone (linden), completely numb (hawthorn), or as if it's burning and shooting laser beams of anger out at an injustice, another person, or your own self (violet). Or you can simply feel so tender and raw that you feel you must hide your heart and loving nature away for safekeeping (lavender, motherwort, skullcap, rose).

In their own way all of these reactions, even planting yourself in front of a television set for hours on end, are ultimately expressions of self-love, of trying to protect and care for yourself the best way you know how. But these and other methods are inadequate for the long run because they function more like temporary escape valves. When you don't face the pain within that's calling for your attention and often for the release of healing tears, none of your strategies will work for long. Whether you are drowning yourself in alcohol or repeatedly bicycling a hundred miles a day so as not to feel your painful feelings, the heart will still have its way with you—and the way of the heart is to open, accept and love.

You are designed to open to your loving nature. This is part of your personal and social evolution, and right now is the pivotal moment. You are being called to move from being led by the small, excluding mind to being led by the spacious mind and the inclusive heart. Common to all people is the fact that, where there is pain and grief, heartache and heartbreak, the heart is being invited to open.

More than once, I've heard a person who has recently lost a beloved one "confess" with shame and confusion that they felt more open than they had ever felt in their lives. When a beloved dies, or you are left by a lover you thought would never leave you, it can touch you so deeply that it tears right through all your normal defenses and pulls your heart wide open. The invitation (and it's not such an easy one to accept) is to keep the heart open after the shock wears off, and to remember and reaffirm that life itself is still good.

Author Alice Walker said, "My heart feels like an open suitcase. It has been broken so many times it feels like it has just sort of dropped open."

I have cultivated this metaphor as a guidepost for my own growth. I imagine walking through an airport or bus terminal carrying my heavy suitcase full of aches and betrayals, grievances, fears, and disappointments. When my heart is broken yet again, my suitcase gets so overstuffed that it simply falls open, and my resentments, bitterness, and despair come tumbling out all over the floor. It looks like a mess, and feels awful. But is it?

Breathe. Feel. Drink rose tea. Feel again. Take a lavender bath. Sit quietly. Everything has changed.

Alice Walker continues, "Instead of that feeling of having a thorn through your heart, you have a sense of openness, as if the wind could blow through it."

Now empty, the heart is wide open. It becomes totally available to shine out love and joy to friends, strangers, even supposed enemies, because all are seen as part of you, and part of your oneness with all that is. You can fight it, but ultimately you can't help it. It's how we're designed to evolve. The spiritual heart refills and empties, again and again, just as the physical heart's chambers refill and empty as it beats and the blood circulates through your body.

It seems amazing that plants can help us with any of this, much less all of this, yet they can, and do, every day. I will share several stories to illustrate. But first, consider:

The herbal allies are not only helpful but will also become ever more necessary for individuals and masses of people in situation after situation for the foreseeable future. They are a much healthier alternative to anti-anxiety and anti-depressant pharmaceutical drugs—or I should say that the new and barely understood pharmaceuticals are a more dangerous option than time-tested and reliable herbs. Change is upon us now, and as we labor to raise the consciousness of our Earth family and birth our new way of being in this world, there will be much dying-off of the old. There will be much destruction, and seeming madness. We will need our herbal nervous-system strengtheners and tonics even more than we already do. Fortunately, they are here!

In times like these, which plants will help you find your lightness of heart and your spaciousness of mind? Which will help you open to the beauty that is within and all around you, and to the joy and loving-kindness that is your true nature? Let's begin with lavender.

Beautiful purple-hued lavender is a healer of heartbreak; it is one of her specialties. I have had women and men drink simple lavender tea after terribly painful divorces to regain their equilibrium. Sweet, gentle lavender with her powerful healing scent is up to the job. When someone's treatment of you has led you to become confused and anxious about your own self-worth as a human being, lavender tea offers a profound easing of that anxiety. My sense is that she opens the crown chakra to help you connect with Spirit, and engages your child-self's delight by smelling so sweet.

There is great complexity in this seemingly sweet, innocent plant. I remember one time when I suggested daily lavender tea to a powerful woman to help her cope with the aftermath of a nasty marriage and divorce. She looked at me as if wondering whether I was a fraud or merely incompetent. "You don't understand," she said, "how ugly we're talking. You don't understand at all." I assured her that though that might be true, I nonetheless strongly felt that lavender was the right plant to help her begin to heal. She decided begrudgingly to try it.

Now, twenty years later, she has become an herbalist and is married to her soul mate, and told me that not only had it been the perfect plant ally for her then, it is still the plant that she reaches out to for comfort when her heart is aching and she is struggling with low self-esteem. It has become her cherished friend.

I think lavender also likes to be called upon to help when you need to regain confidence and the feeling of being attractive. If you are grieving the loss of your youth, as Western culture teaches you to do, drinking lavender tea or taking an oat/lavender bath can help you realize that your beauty is simply different now. If you are a woman, your attractiveness may shine more from your calm sparkle and easy laughter than from your perky breasts; and if you're a man, your magnetism may spring more from your easy-going ways and calm self-confidence than from your rock-hard abs. Lavender is so reassuring that she helps you replace anxiety with true self-knowing and assurance, which is always attractive.

Speaking of attractive, we have the famed and exquisite rose. Thorny, prickly rose—especially wild rose—opens the heart to love like no other plant I know.

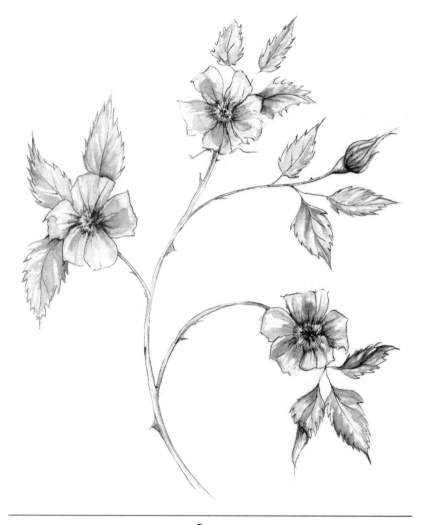

Rose

Rose (*Rosa* species)

Body: hormone balancer; cools liver fire, helps digestion, aids circulation; skin soother, kidney and heart tonic.

Mind: opens and soothes, helps you to respect other perspectives.

Heart: inspires self-love, deepens your relationships with others.

Soul: sweetens the soul, increases love of life, heals ancient wounds.

My Dearest Rosa

Wild blossoms of pink and white,
And fragrance that brings delight,
Sweetening the day and night.

Open petals, scratchy thorns—
If animal you were born,
You'd have soft fur and sharp horns.

Cooling the liver of fire,
Relieving the mind of ire,
Spirit soars ever higher.

Waking libido and love,
Trust in Below and Above
Brings more peace than any dove.

Soothing skin and heart as well,
Making heaven out of hell,
Ringing like the clearest bell.

It's almost as if rose is saying, "Look at these prickly, protective thorns, at your service. Go ahead and love. Open your heart. It'll be safe. I'm here."

For sheer heart-healing delight. I highly recommend glycerites (and infused honeys) of both roses and rose hips.

Try it and see. Make your own or buy some from a rose-intoxicated, earth-loving herbalist. (See: Resources pages 509–510.)

ROSE BLOSSOM GLYCERITES

Gather roses in their season. (Where I live, I gather rose flowers in June.) Fresh flowers can be gently pulled apart and then fill a glass jar of any size with them. Pour vegetable glycerin (see: Resources, pages 509–510) slowly over the herbs, poking them with a chopstick to insure that all the petals get fully saturated. Fill to the top and cap and label your jar. Wait at least six weeks before decanting. Pour the viscous fluid through a cheese-cloth strainer atop a sieve and then squeeze out the herbs in the cheesecloth as completely as possible, manually or with an herb press. (See: Resources, page 514).

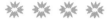

ROSE HIP GLYCERITES

Gather frost-ripened rose hips in their season. Where I live, I gather rose hips after both light and hard frosts in October and November. They get sweeter the longer you wait. Gather them, carefully—those thorns are no joke! I use scissors for these and snip them off multiflora bushes mostly (and trim the remarkably prolific bushes at the same time with a pair of heavier clippers). Cut and/or mash up the berries and fill your jar with them. Follow the chopstick-poking, capping, labeling, and decanting directions above.

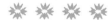

These preparations don't need to be refrigerated. They can be stirred into water or tea. Drink quickly though, because they fall to the bottom of your cup. They can be added to vodka tinctures to sweeten them, add about 25% to your vodka tincture of roses. They can be put over yogurt or oatmeal or onto anything on which you might use honey. Enjoy this sweet, heart-healing medicine, at its sweetest! And if you prefer, or additionally, you can follow these same recipes and make rose blossom and hip infused honeys, too.

Turn to rose tea if your heart is aching from fighting with a beloved—your husband or wife, child, parent, or best friend—and no one will back down. Think of rose when you are aching with frustration from feeling unseen, unheard, or misunderstood. Rose will help you and the other person open to each other's point of view. How does rose do it? How does she help you *want* to respect the other person's perspective, to put love and kindness first? I have no idea, but she does! I've seen it again and again, even if one of the people has no interest in doing that, and no confidence in herbal medicine!

I was once having a disagreement with a student who had made a commitment and then broken it. She expected me to accept her decision with no consequences to her, and I expected her to accept consequences and understand my point of view. We were both trying to convince each other that we were the one being reasonable and clearly correct, and the other wasn't.

I finally took a deep breath and expressed that we weren't getting anywhere, so why not take a break, drink some rose tea to soothe our hearts, and perhaps open ourselves to the other's point of view? We could make another appointment to address our seemingly irresolvable dilemma. She agreed to this plan.

When we spoke again, nothing had changed but our attitudes. It didn't seem that there was any way to settle the situation without someone walking away unhappy and feeling like they got the short end of the stick. But a third alternative arose that had simply never occurred to me before, and when I proposed it and she accepted, we both felt good about it! We were both so relieved to have found a way forward, and are still in touch to this day with deep regard and affection for one another.

Rose is magical. Unlike lavender with its soft touch, rose isn't so easy to handle. Her prickly nature is part of her medicine, and it increases as she ages. She gets more powerful and thorny with time, and yet her blossoms stay just as intoxicating and delicious, her hips just as sustaining and fortifying.

Perhaps this too is a mirror for us on a multitude of levels. Good relations necessitate caring about one another, but they don't necessitate being so nicey-nice that people walk all over you. Rose requests that you value yourself, and helps you to keep your self-respect in all your relationships, particularly the intimate ones. When necessary, you can show your thorns. After all, your body is sacred space, and if you don't act that way, no one else will either.

If a relationship has ended, especially through betrayal, and if your heart feels damaged, any use of rose will slowly but surely help your heart to heal, and your self-love to rebirth itself. Take a rose bath, drink rose tea, or use rose honey or rose glycerin. And speaking of thorns, no heartbreak-healing plant is more audaciously thorny than hawthorn.

Hawthorn (*Crataegus* species)

This is one of my favorite healing trees of all; she is a wise old elder. Hawthorn presents a complex, even contradictory picture. She is skinny and gnarly, twisted, and usually though not always a fairly small tree. Yet however you use hawthorn you'll find that she brings big power, magic, and medicine with her. I think of her as rose's sexy grandma, and she is grandmother to all who call on her.

In the spring, her blossoms burst open—white with touches of red and pink, and a smell that some describe as reminiscent of decay and some describe as divine, musky, and sensual. (I vote for divine, musky, and sensual!)

In all seasons, hawthorns of every species—and there are hundreds—are covered with thorns, less along the trunks and more along the branches. The longest hawthorn thorn recorded was four and half inches long. After flowering, the haws (berries) slowly but surely turn from green to red, coming to their full ripeness after a hard frost. So with her sexy flowers, nourishing berries and long thorns, hawthorn's message seems to be mixed: "Come hither! Go away! Come hither! Go away!" But I think her true message is more like:

> Come hither with love and respect in your heart
> And I will share with you forevermore!
> Come hither with lust and greed for my gifts
> And I'll pierce you right through to the core!

Hawthorn has a magic I've seen time and again, where her largest thorns can be completely invisible—until they are not, because you have been painfully pierced! This is a tree rife with metaphorical meaning and medicine. Hawthorn's thorns are a reminder to be awake and attentive, to hold your healthy boundaries and sacred space while keeping your heart open. Hawthorn exemplifies a wise saying I often quote from spiritual teacher Stephen Levine: "You can throw someone out of your house without throwing him out of your heart."

Hawthorn's medicine helps when you are having trouble letting go of someone who is clearly not good for you, or when you "hate" someone you used to love, poisoning yourself more than it hurts him or her. Hawthorn's potent, thorny medicine helps you say "No" to someone else and "Yes" to yourself, without shutting down your heart.

I include hawthorn berries in almost any heartbreak recipe I put together. Hawthorn strengthens the heart, and helps it drop barricades as it opens wider. Hawthorn lifts the spirits, especially when used regularly. It's as if hawthorn helps you see through the eyes of the heart where, as the Sufi saying goes, "all masks fall away."

I often include hawthorn's flowers as well as her berries— flowers for feminine softness, sensuality and multidimensional magic, and berries for being "of stout heart," improving circulation and stamina. Flowers also help when someone needs to reclaim the sovereignty of their own sexuality.

In terms of lingering or ongoing depression, I've noticed that for some people it's the flowers and for others the berries that help them shift from down-heartedness to a more steady equilibrium and cheerfulness.

Mimosa *(Albizia julibrissin)*

Mimosa is a common "weed tree" in the *Leguminosae (Fabaceae)* or pea family. Like all common names, 'mimosa' can be used to refer to different plants and trees in different regions, but this species is the only one I am writing about as it's the only one I have personal experience using.

Herbalist David Winston (see Resources, page 510) makes a lovely tincture called Grief Relief™ that contains mimosa bark along with hawthorn and rose.

I prefer to use mimosa's flowers. The following recipe is one that I love to make and to take.

I make each fresh flower tincture separately, and then blend them together.

TRIPLE-BLOSSOM TINCTURE BLEND

1 part rose flower tincture

1 part hawthorn blossom tincture

1 part mimosa blossom tincture

Add 25–30 drops or more as needed to a cup of hot water for a healing tea. It is soothing, comforting and uplifting to the emotional heart, and awakens the spiritual heart. I give it to people who've been shafted, to those whose spirits run low without warning, as well as to those who've suffered one loss after another. It not only helps bring you back to life, it invites you to enjoy a more expansive version than the one you'd been living.

Mimosa blossoms are among the most beautiful flowers on Earth. Gazing at them softly can be healing to an aching heart. When I lived on busy, treeless West 14th Street in New York City, I used to walk four blocks south and half a block east toward Fifth Avenue, and then simply stand still under a beautiful little mimosa tree growing out of the sidewalk on the small, charming, west village street. One of mimosa's nicknames is "silk tree" because she is so silky-smooth and soothing.

Whenever I felt an aching longing for nature or for like-minded companions, the mimosa's flowers—soft, feathery, gossamer balls made of silky strands of pink magenta and glimmering gold—would almost always bring me back to delight. I had no idea that I could make tea or other medicine from them. Here's a simple and delicious recipe:

MIMOSA FLOWER WATER

Gather three to four cups of fresh mimosa flowers from the tree and place them in a half gallon glass bottle or pitcher of fresh water. Wait 2–3 hours. Serve as is or on the rocks, and drink to your heart's content.

This drink is delectable, with a subtle aftertaste that is worth tuning in for. It opens up at the back of your throat like a really fine cognac. Like all the herbs in this section, it's not required that you be in emotional pain to use and benefit from them!

By the way, this is also a great way to imbibe locust blossoms from the locust tree *(Robinia pseudoacacia)*. Their water too is uplifting and delightful. I learned to prepare them in this simple way from herbalist and storyteller Doug Eliot. It is perfect.

Like mimosa, the subtlety of these pea-family blossoms doesn't survive preservation quite as well in alcohol or by drying, but is perfectly extracted with simple cold, fresh water. I tincture each of these tree's flowers, too, but the infused flower waters are my favorite way to use them when they're in season. In my experience, they delight all who try them.

. . . .

I called a dear old friend of mine, and her normally joyful voice sounded odd, a little strangled. It turned out that two people she loved very much had died in recent weeks; one death had been expected, and one hadn't.

She was still in shock, and pulling her energy back into herself for healing. She'd always been giving of herself, and now needed to take time to give *to* herself. She was ready. She told me about the healing brew she put together. I named her brew:

HEAL MY HEART AND GIVE ME STRENGTH BLEND

> Dried holy basil leaves
> Dried hawthorn berries
> Dried skullcap
> Dried nettles
> Pinch of fresh spearmint
> Borage flower essence

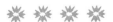

What a perfectly beautiful healing brew! I don't know exactly what proportions she used, but I'll guess it contained a tablespoon or two each of the herbs. I'm sure instinct was her guide in the moment. We shared with one another how very grateful we constantly are for these plant medicines. I was grateful that she had the wisdom to turn to them in her time of need.

Holy basil is an adaptogen that, among many other gifts, helps the spirit stay clear during or after a shock. Spearmint clears the mind and gives energy and buzz to the nervous system and spirit. Melding skullcap's deep relaxing properties with nettles' strengthening effects is a wise blending of peace and power; and hawthorn, of course, is a supreme heart-healer. Borage's name means "I bring courage," and she strengthens the adrenal glands and is particularly helpful after a sudden shock, and also when emotional energy is being depleted over time. My dear friend used borage as a flower essence.

Flower essences are vibrational remedies made by gathering flowers consciously and thankfully, steeping them in brandy (or another menstruum), energizing them in the sunlight, and then diluting them with water again and again until there is virtually nothing left of the original substance except its Spirit, strengthened by your focused intention and gratitude throughout the process. Conscious gathering, appreciative thoughts and feelings, and focused intention are the key to any harvesting and medicine-making with plants, but it tends to be more emphasized in the instructions for making flower essences.

Another herbalist I love, who had been my apprentice, told me that a young friend who was like a son to her, and who'd been greatly loved as a positive force in her community, had been mysteriously and senselessly murdered. She was in shock, and hurt down to the marrow of her bones. Everything was too painful; even looking at her own beloved children was fraught with fear and pain. She had practically forgotten that herbs existed. Then she remembered. These were the healers she turned to, drinking them and bathing in them at different times as she was inclined:

RETURN MY HEART TO LIFE (READY OR NOT) REMEDIES
- · Dandelion tea—continuity, eternality, mooring, releasing anger.
- · Motherwort tincture—mothering comfort for the heart and mind.
- · Rose baths—heart-opening; releasing grief, forgiveness.
- · Rose glycerin—for sweetening and soothing a broken heart.
- · Sassafras leaf and root infusion—joy for the spirit.

These herbs slowly and steadily helped bring her back to life, with her deeply compassionate heart opened even wider. She told me she will look for worldly justice, while spiritually opening to what is and honoring her friend with her creativity and joy.

When she first told me what happened, I felt such sorrow, and then had a distinct sense of the young man rejecting my sorrow and wanting only my joy. When I shared this with her she got quiet, and then said that when she spoke with people he'd been close to, many had felt their creativity was being stimulated (by him) in some way that truly was joyous.

A student of mine met and fell in love with a man who fell immediately in love with her too. Everything from how they met to how life seemed to have conspired to bring and keep them together felt so magical that she was on cloud nine. It was her dream come true, at last. Then he suddenly left her, just like that. She was devastated, and so angry that she knew no peace. Here is the tincture-blend recipe I made for her:

I WAS FLYING HIGH AND NOW I'VE CRASHED TINCTURE BLEND

1 part hawthorn berry tincture

1 part hawthorn flower tincture

½ part rose tincture

½ part mimosa (*Albizia julibrissin*) tincture and

1 dropper (25–30 drops) burdock root tincture

3 drops rose glycerin

7 drops cherry flower essence (*Prunus serrulata*, "Kwanzan" cultivar)

> 3 drops *flowering* cherry flower essence (These trees are so
> hybridized that I haven't been able to identify the exact
> *Prunus* species that I've been using—but any beautiful
> flowering cherry tree blossoms will work, especially if you
> feel a connection to the tree.) This is spirit medicine.

She was to take a dropper of this tincture 3 times a day in water or infusion until she finished a four-ounce bottle.

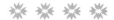

When I counseled with her, we looked at the story she was telling herself from some more enlightening and self-loving angles. I suggested two simple rituals:

Love Lost Ritual #1

First, bury the relationship: Pick an object that symbolizes the
relationship, and bury it. This is to help you see and accept that it
is dead so you can mourn it as a loss and move on.

When I suggested this, my friend responded that she'd been mourning for months, and asked if she really had to mourn more. I mention this because the answer was "Of course not!" I had assumed she was still grieving, but she wasn't. She was angry, burning mad with judgment of him and of herself. So she did "bury the relationship," but not to mourn as much as to have a concrete experience that would help her completely accept that it was over. This was a good reminder that no matter what anyone tells you as they're doing their best to be helpful, always remember that you have the final word on what you need. If she hadn't questioned me, she might have kept herself in mourning thinking that she had to, in order to do it right!

Love Lost Ritual #2

Take a bath in rose infusion to rebirth yourself as the loving,
passionate person that you are. This also acts to clear your
energy, making you available to attract the kind of person you
are looking for who is looking for someone just like you.

My apprentice used up the four ounces of tincture I sent, and did the rituals, and they helped her to trust the process and move on. As I write this, over a year later, she is in a new, healthy relationship. Hooray!

Here are some other simple yet profoundly healing recipes:

SIMPLE ROSE INFUSION

1 cup dried rose buds, blossoms, or petals

½ gallon water

Put dried, unsprayed roses into a wide mouth jar. Cover them with boiling water. Cap and let them steep for 75 minutes. Decant and squeeze out the roses. This infusion is lovely to drink or to bathe in.

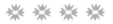

LIFT YOUR HEART OFF THE GROUND INFUSION OR BATH

1 tablespoon dried linden blossoms

1 teaspoon dried rose petals, blossoms, or buds

½ teaspoon dried lavender flowers

Cover the herbs with a cup of boiling water and steep for 15–20 minutes. For larger amounts I use 3 parts linden, 1 part rose, and ½ part lavender.

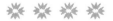

This one is lovely and soothing as an infusion or a bath. It is like a tender touch that lifts your heart when it's on the ground. (If you already feel good when you drink it, watch out—it lifts *you* off the ground!)

HEAVEN SCENT INFUSION OR BATH

1 tablespoon (or 3 parts) dried linden blossoms

1 teaspoon (or 1 part) dried rose petals, buds, or blossoms

½ teaspoon (or ½ part) dried lemon verbena leaves

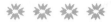

This is really another variation of the "Lift Your Heart off the Ground" recipe. Use it whenever you like, but especially when life has given you more than you think you can handle. Remember that it never does, no matter how it feels in the moment. Life is wiser than that.

CALM THOSE FRAZZLED NERVES
TINCTURE BLEND—VARIATION I

1 teaspoon (or 3 parts) violet leaf tincture

2 droppers full (or 1 part) skullcap leaf and flower tincture

1 dropper full (or ½ part) California poppy tincture

I add this tincture blend to hot water to make a soothing, sedating nervine recipe.

You can also make an overnight violet leaf infusion and add the skullcap and California poppy tinctures. Another method is to make skullcap tea (steeped for 30 minutes) and add the other two herbs as tinctures.

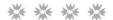

Call on this blend when your nerve endings are raw and frazzled from grieving or seething, when they've been fried and short-circuited with shock and/or anger, or you can't stop thinking and you're not sleeping well.

CALM THOSE FRAZZLED NERVES
TINCTURE BLEND—VARIATION II

1 part St. J's wort tincture

½ part skullcap tincture

¼ part California poppy tincture

Mix these tinctures into hot water. It is very effective for helping any-one frazzled. If giving it to a distressed child or an elder start with small amounts, such as 5 drops of St. J's, 2 drops of skullcap, and 1 drop of California poppy. You can always increase them. Sometimes you need to increase or decrease the amounts bit by bit to find the right dosage for yourself. The range of what is acceptable is broad. An example of a large but still safe dosage is up to a teaspoon of St. J's—roughly 125 drops—and a half-teaspoon of skullcap (though with skullcap, smaller quantities are usually more sedative than large ones), and ½ teaspoon of California poppy (here the higher quantity is potentially more sedative).

This blend will help a person to rest and sleep. It builds the nervous system even as it soothes and calms. It isn't a recipe to use forever—just for when it's truly needed. It's a lovely helper when called for.

SOOTHE ME INFUSION

> 1 cup dried violet leaves
>
> 1 cup dried oatstraw
>
> ½ cup dried hawthorn berries and/or leaves and flowers

Bring oatstraw to boil in half gallon of water and pour over the rest of the herbs. Allow this blend to steep overnight on your counter. In the morning, squeeze out the herbs and heat the infusion and put it into a stainless steel or glass insert thermos to drink throughout the day.

This is a good recipe for shock and/or grief that results in a lot of physical tension, tightness, and agitation, with or without crying. It will help relax the mind and the muscles, nourish and soothe the nerves, and aid circulation and oxygenation to help the heart.

Linden (*Tilia americana* and other species)

Linden is not only a popular wildflower for making honey, but is a "honey" of a tree. Linden opens the emotional and spiritual heart even as it improves cardiovascular circulation. If you are willing, linden helps you dance with current grief and clear out old, "stuck" grief. Linden has a divinely inspired way of opening you to the bliss of your true multidimensional nature—the larger reality we're all part of.

GRIEF-HEALING INFUSION

1 cup dried linden blossoms

1 cup dried violet leaves

½ cup dried hawthorn berries and/or flowers and leaves

Pour ½ gallon of boiled water over these herbs in a half-gallon jar. Fill it to the top, as full as possible, then cap it. Let it steep overnight, and then decant. Refrigerate, or heat and put in a thermos.

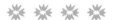

This luscious mixture is a perfect infusion to celebrate life and love when your heart is happy, or to help you heal when your heart is aching or broken, or when you've just soured on life in general. It is mood-altering, like a good glass of red wine. Taken over time, it is a transformative blend.

This tart yet sweet aromatic recipe is one you can count on to help you heal when you are grieving, even if you have turned inward, isolating yourself physically and/or emotionally and psychically. These plants have a way of helping you be with your feelings. When you allow your feelings space simply to be what they are, you can and will heal.

Taking a linden blossom bath is a particularly magical way to experience the linden tree's special medicine.

LINDEN BLOSSOM BATH

2–3 cups dried linden blossoms

Pour boiling water over the herbs in a half-gallon jar. Cap tightly and let sit 1–2 hours. Pour the liquid through a good strainer and add it to a bathtub filled with hot water.

Then pour another half-gallon of boiling water over the herbs in the jar, and let that sit overnight to drink the next day (cool or reheated). Refrigerate the remainder after that.

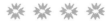

I suspect that the vast heart- and soul-opening that can sometimes occur spontaneously after a deep loss may happen because your loved one is able to share a taste of what their newly expanded state feels like.

A linden bath can help open your senses to feel your departed loved one nearby, responding to your love. Even if you are crying a river of tears, linden brings a bright, golden-light energy to touch the heaviness of sorrow over death and loss. It's as if you are dancing single-mindedly with grief, and suddenly bliss cuts in and invites you to dance in the present moment where there is no death, no separation, only awareness and love. Only joy.

Also, please remember that though these blended herb recipes are delicious and effective, the herbs are also wonderfully healing used one at a time.

· · · · ● · · · ·

Some of my favorite simple infusions for healing grief are: hawthorn berries and/or blossoms, oat straw, lavender, violet leaves, rose, linden, and nettles.

Tinctures in hot water can be wonderful as simples, too. Here my favorites are: motherwort, St. J's, oats, skullcap, borage, linden, and lavender. I also use simple tinctures of peach, evening primrose, and mullein flowers. For many years, Motherwort has usually been my first go-to herb for comforts large and small.

And then there are cherry blossoms. I often use these as flower essences. (See Some Spiritual Herbal Allies, page 27.) I infuse them in honey and vinegar and make tinctures with fresh blossoms, too. Perhaps most magical of all is the following everyday ritual. Choose a cherry tree that you can go visit every day. If you can do this barefoot, it will benefit your nervous system even more.

Cherry Blossom Ritual

Eat a pink cherry blossom every day that they are in season.
Chew it slowly and deliberately.
Experience the emotions that arise for you.
Experience the physical sensations that arise.
Taste the bitterness. Let it melt into your tongue.
Wait for the ambrosia of petal juice that follows.
Sweetness,
Nectar,
Expanding through your whole body and being.
Cherry opens a pathway to pure joy.

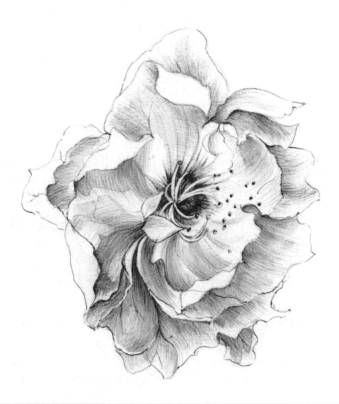

Cherry Blossom Ritual

The Respiratory System

Herbs and more for health, acute illnesses, and chronic challenges of the respiratory system; herbs to open up congestion, soften secretions, soothe inflamed sinuses and sore throats, and help bronchia and lungs to improve breathing; how to strengthen this system for less susceptibility to asthma, bronchitis, coughs, colds, flu, and other respiratory infections.

The respiratory system is divided into upper and lower sections. The upper refers to the nose, sinuses, and throat, down to the larynx. The lower respiratory system refers to the chest, the bronchia and lungs and, below them, the diaphragm.

The primary organs of the respiratory system are the lungs, which are continuously exchanging carbon dioxide for oxygen. Through the constancy of our invisible breath flowing in and out, we are invited to experience our interconnection with all that seems to be outside of us. The respiratory system is connected to the archetypal and invisible element Air (breathing and circulating movement, spaciousness and inter-being) and is related to our willingness to fully allow life in and trust its flow, moment by moment.

This system and its health, acute illnesses, and chronic challenges often offers us teachings on how to live fully in the present moment, in the same way that we can only breathe in the present moment.

Inside of the chest, the left lung is smaller than the right because it shares the space with the heart. Breath and heart are inextricably linked, both physically and spiritually. Joy and grief meet in the respiratory system. In Chinese medicine, the lungs are connected with grief, and when grieving we are emotionally living in the past, with our regrets and losses; or perhaps we are lamenting an imagined future that we won't get to experience. Grieving is a natural part of life, but when it is prolonged, when it is held onto in lieu of being fully alive in the present, it can become a damaging habit.

When illuminated with understanding and compassion, grief can be released. The respiratory system gives life to all the other systems of the body by bringing in oxygen and removing carbon dioxide. We cannot survive for more than a brief time without breathing in and out.

* * * * * * * * *

Some of my favorite respiratory allies are: pine, spruce, fir, mullein, violet, elder flowers and berries, yarrow, coltsfoot, comfrey, boneset, elecampane, chickweed, plantain, linden, usnea, sassafras, holy basil, basil, thyme, hyssop, ginger, garlic, nettles, and red clover.

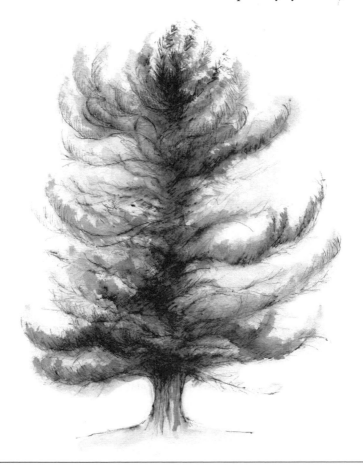

White Pine

White Pine *(Pinus strobus)*

Body: soothes, strengthens, and heals lungs and bronchia; antiseptic for lungs, skin and kidneys; eases joint pain; rich in vitamin C and tannins; resin is antiseptic for boils and wounds.

Mind: generates peace of mind, helps release perfectionist tendencies, builds inner confidence and self-esteem.

Heart: strengthens sense of unity within oneself and community; eases loneliness and sense of isolation and/or alienation.

Soul: deep peace.

White Pine

Evergreen and flowing,
Her needles packed in bundles of five,
White pine's so full of magic and grace,
Your senses come alive.

Cut the needles finely
To make a fragrant, opening tea.
It brings deep peace, reminding you that
It's enough just to be.

Take a deep healing breath,
She helps relieve a wet or dry cough,
So you expectorate more freely
Taking chest pressure off.

To create a syrup,
Steep fresh needles all day and all night,
Add in herbal honey and brandy,
Then sip to your delight.

Pine is an ancient tree,
Remaining green in the cold, dark time.
When we drink her in the winter months
The nourishment's sublime.

High in vitamin C,
Infuse the chopped needles all day long,
The healing oils are antiseptic
White pine won't lead you wrong.

A mature white pine tree is a magnificent being! Pine's healing effects on the respiratory system are due to its aromatic, resinous oils and tannins. These and more make it an important herbal medicine for the lungs that can be used on its own to good effect, as a full-strength infusion or a steam, or as cough syrup.

WHITE PINE INFUSION

2 cups fresh white pine needles

½ gallon water

Cut up 2 cups or more of fresh pine needles and the small twigs that they grow on. Use your fingernail or a knife to nick the twigs every half-inch or so, to reveal the inner bark (the green cambium layer). Put everything into a half-gallon jar. Cover with boiling water, and let the infusion steep anywhere from 12–24 hours.

This pleasant-tasting, slightly sour infusion will help relieve a cough and release tightness in the chest. It is specifically helpful for a bacterial infection and will generally support the immune system in fighting off any kind of respiratory invader. When you nick the twigs as you prepare your medicine, it will immediately release the fragrance of pine, and perhaps send you into a waking dream of walking through pine-filled woods.

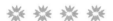

White pine is rich in tannins. These polyphenols are acid-like compounds that are highly antioxidant and scavenge the free radicals that contribute not only to respiratory infections but also to heart attacks, strokes, cancer and premature aging. Perhaps this is why, in Taoist legend, pine needle tea is an elixir of longevity.

Think of all the different pine-scented cleansers you see on grocery-store shelves, putting pine to work freshening our homes. Here, we are putting pine's refreshing qualities to work inside our bodies. This simple infusion is so antiseptic that it doesn't need to be refrigerated (though refrigeration won't harm it). In fact, if I have the time to wait, I like to let fresh white pine steep in the jar for a week when I'm preparing it as a cough syrup. (See syrup recipes on page 43.)

WHITE PINE INFUSION—QUICK METHOD

Here's another way I sometimes prepare pine needle infusion when I'm in a bit of a hurry: Put a large quantity of pine needles and the slender twigs in a soup pot, cover them with cold water, and cut it all as finely as you can with sharp scissors while bringing the water up to a boil for a few minutes. Then turn the flame way down and let the pine simmer with the lid on for about 10 minutes. Turn it off and let it continue to steep. It won't be as strong, and it will have lost more vitamin C, but it will still be very good.

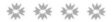

Pine softens and stimulates secretions from the bronchia too, making it a good choice for bronchitis. Sometimes I mix it with hyssop and mullein leaves or flowers. It is useful in both acute and chronic bronchial or lung infections. It is anti-inflammatory, somewhat cooling, and pain-relieving.

BYE-BYE BRONCHITIS INFUSION

1 cup fresh pine needles (or more, to taste)

½ cup dried mullein leaves (and flowers, optional)

½ cup dried hyssop *(Hyssopus officinalis)* leaves and flowers

Cut up the fresh pine needles very well and put them in a half-gallon jar. Add the mullein and hyssop. Cover with boiling water, cap, and let stand overnight, or for 8–12 hours. Then pour off the infusion, squeeze out the herbs and reheat for use. It should be refrigerated and reheated as needed, or put into a stainless-steel thermos to keep it hot throughout the day. Drink 2–4 cups a day. If you like, it can be sweetened with honey to taste.

Each herb in this blend is helpful in its own way, and could also be effective used on its own. Pine is calming and uplifting, whether or not there's an infection present. It helps clear the air passages of the respiratory system with its unique blend of astringency, antiseptic oils, and expectorant-encouraging resins.

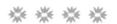

Hyssop is my oldest and foremost ally for helping people heal from bronchitis. I've found that it will safely help adults and children to expectorate even the most entrenched phlegm stuck in the bronchia and cilia of the lungs from chronic bronchitis. It is one of the first herbs that taught me that when you need something, it will taste good to you. I couldn't stand the taste of hyssop until I had acute bronchitis—then I couldn't get enough of it! I have seen this response in other people, too (to many different herbs), although some like the bitter mint hyssop anytime and find it refreshing. It is always an herb worth considering.

Finally, mullein is a reliable friend to lungs and bronchia. It will moisten, soften and melt away congested matter, and ease the dry cough that goes with it. Mullein will not stimulate coughing mucus up and out the way hyssop will. It is, instead, a good, soothing anti-inflammatory and anti-spasmodic, so it's helpful for relieving the chest pain and inflammation that can come with bronchitis and a bronchial cough.

I don't use pine just when I'm sick. I also use it as a regular tonic for maintaining good health and good spirits year-round. I use it most frequently in winter and early spring, when it's one of the only sources of fresh green plant matter around.

Pine blends well with many other herbs. I particularly like to mix fresh pine with dried sassafras leaves and either hibiscus, rose hips, elderberries, or hawthorn berries. I almost always use fresh pine for my oils, tinctures, vinegars, decoctions, syrups, elixirs, or infusions. It is, after all, an *evergreen* medicine, so why dry it? It's sweeter and stronger in spring, summer, and fall than in winter, but it's perfectly good medicine in the winter months, too. Additionally, there are usually plenty of freshly broken branches to harvest from the ground in the winter, so I can often get my medicine without any additional stress to the tree at all.

White pine is the "tree of peace" to the Native peoples of northeastern America for a number of reasons including how it encourages full, easy breathing. When you are at peace, your breathing is deep, relaxed and rhythmic. Conversely, when you are stressed, your breathing can quickly become shallow and ragged. If you are agitated, you can bring yourself to a more peaceful state of being by drinking white pine needle tea as a medicine and, if you like, as a simple ritual.

Simple Ritual of Relaxation

Pour yourself a cup of piping-hot, white pine needle infusion
and accept it as if you are giving yourself a lovely gift (because
you are). Sit in a comfortable place, perhaps looking at a view
you enjoy out the window, or sitting in a special cozy spot in your
home. Before you even drink the tea, hold the cup, close your
eyes, and imagine sitting under a great, old white pine tree. Inhale
the steam rising from your teacup and imagine it is the scent
of the tree itself after a gentle rain has fallen. Notice that your
breath will have slowed down by now or, if it hasn't, consciously
take a few easy, deep breaths. As you drink the tea, continue
to focus on steadying and deepening your breathing.
By the time you get to the bottom of the cup,
you will be more relaxed.

You will find numerous pine needle and twig recipes throughout *The Gift of Healing Herbs*. Here's one of my absolute favorites. I drink it for its deep nourishment, its medicinal properties, and to keep my spirits high, but when all is said and done the sheer deliciousness of it is compelling enough for me.

HERBAL HAPPINESS POTION

1 cup white pine needles (fresh)

1 cup dried autumn sassafras leaves (yellow, orange, red, or still partially green)

½ cup dried hawthorn berries

Put the fresh green pine needles, along with yellow sassafras leaves and red hawthorn berries, into a half-gallon jar. Cover the herbs with boiled water, filling the jar to the brim. Top it up a couple of times before capping it, as the herbs will keep absorbing and lowering the level of the water. Let it steep a minimum of 8 hours, and/or leave it 12–16 hours, for the best results.

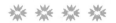

This mixture is joy-inducing. Pine brings peace, sassafras brings sweet delight, and hawthorn berries help the heart to smile. What more could we ask? And yet there is more. This brew is rich in vitamin C and iron. The hawthorn berries aid digestion. The mucilage in the sassafras is soothing to the mucous membranes, and will help relieve a dry cough, aided by pine's gifts in that area. Both sassafras and pine ease pain and inflammation in the joints, and all three herbs help clear skin. Sassafras works wonders for the lymph, kidneys and liver, and hawthorn will help the blood to circulate so that all the nutrients get to where they are needed to do the most good. What a magnificent trio!

Other evergreens—especially spruce or fir—can be used in place of white pine, and the amounts will need to be adjusted accordingly. For example, if I make the above recipe with balsam fir *(Abies balsamea)* or Fraser fir *(Abies fraseri)*, I only use ½ cup, as they are stronger and more fragrant than white pine needles. Red or black spruce can also be used, but be careful of blue spruce; it is very strong and bitter, and I don't recommend it for infusions. You can substitute elderberries for the hawthorn berries, or add ¼ cup of them, making the trio a quartet, and this will increase the antiviral, immune-supportive gifts of this recipe.

I favor herbal infusions that are red, yellow, and green like the recipe above, so you will notice a lot of those blends in this book. I find they create good remedies that work well together and taste good, too. If you're a student of chakras (the energy centers of the body), you know that these colors correspond with the root, solar plexus, and heart centers.

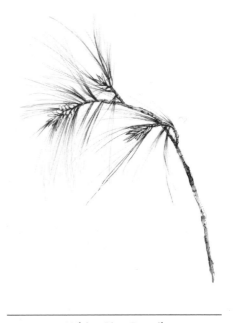

White Pine Detail

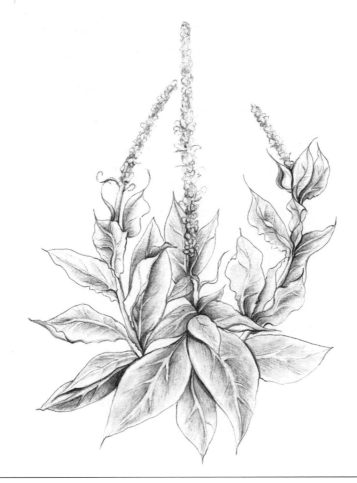

Mullein

Mullein (*Verbascum thapsus* and other species)

Body: anti-inflammatory, antibacterial, anti-spasmodic to nourish and heal lungs, bronchia, kidneys, spine, and joints.

Mind: helps open the mind to new possibilities; increases ability to see far and gain a broader overview.

Heart: softens hard-heartedness; dissolves learned toughness.

Soul: increases sense of one's body being a magical connection between below and above.

Mullein

First a rosette of leaves opens wide,
Furry leaves both scratchy and soft,
Yellow flowers arrive the next year,
Upon your tall stalk, aloft.

The rosette grows out from its center,
Your stalk shoots up straight and fine.
Open and yielding, phallic and strong,
You are a true androgyne.

Opposites are alive within you:
Your leaves are juicy and dry,
You grow low down and hug mother Earth;
You reach up and touch the sky.

You heal hurting lungs and bronchia,
Taken as syrup or tea.
And if someone with asthma can't breathe,
Your smoke helps their breath flow free

Kidneys, too, benefit from your gifts,
Again you help free-flowing.
You're also antibacterial,
Mullein, you're so worth knowing!

Leaves help slipped discs into alignment,
Your flowers, too, are divine.
Rich in mucilage and pain relief,
They are a superb nervine.

I'll end this ode to you here because,
To sum up all your powers,

And recount all the things that you do,
Would take many more hours.

Mullein is often found growing out of rocky places. Similarly, it likes to break through hard, stuck gunk in the lungs. Mullein dilates the bronchia to help breath flow in and out more easily. Growing through rocks is also a signature for a plant that can help break up bladder or kidney stones. Mullein is a gentle yet strong plant that has claimed my heart. How lucky we are that it is ubiquitous, growing in all fifty United States and beyond. I like to have it growing close to my home, so I often plant it to line my front walkway.

Mullein is a biennial plant; it lives for two years, and in its second autumn it goes to seed before it dies. New mullein babies grow from some of those seeds the following spring.

Mullein is antibacterial and antispasmodic. I use it to help people with earaches, asthma, sinus inflammation, bronchitis, dry coughs, sore lungs, and sore throats. All parts of mullein are medicinal. In the late 1980s I began to use the entire plant—root, leaves, flowers and some stalks, because a shopping center was going up where there was a beautiful field of mullein, and I harvested as much as I could before "they paved paradise and put up a parking lot" (from Joni Mitchell's "Big Yellow Taxi"). When I was about to compost the roots, the plant tugged at my consciousness, saying, "No, no, put me in the tincture, too—I will make your medicine even more effective, especially with anti-spasmodic effects for the lungs and bronchia." It was true, so I've done it that way ever since.

I've learned since then that herbalist David Winston suggests using the roots specifically for facial neuralgia, and Matthew Wood uses the roots for back pain from a slipped disc. Matthew shared a story of the wildest use of mullein leaf I've ever heard: He had someone Scotch-tape a fresh mullein leaf over a broken rib, and attested to the fact that it sped up the time it took the rib to knit together and, in the meantime, reduced the pain! Mullein is known for its effectiveness in poultices, but I'd never heard of it being used like that before. Do be careful with mullein, though, as its velvety hairs can be irritating when placed against tender skin. It's said that some Amish and Quaker women, forbidden to use rouge, would rub mullein leaves on their cheeks to make them rosy. Sounds like a good trick!

My preferred mullein medicine for asthma and coughs is to combine the above- and below-ground parts of mullein. I tincture the entire first-year plant—the roots and the rosette of leaves. I use the leaves, flowers and some of the flower stalks from the second-year plants. When I gather mullein leaves without the root, for drying or making infused oil or tincture, I gather the leaves in late spring and summer from the second year's growth because Keewaydinoquay taught me that in the first year the plants need all their leaves for themselves.

Over the years I have helped quite a few people who were reliant on inhalers for their asthma to gradually stop using them with the help of mullein, particularly by drinking mullein leaf infusion. As a general guideline, the longer you've used any pharmaceutical drug, the more your body will have become accustomed to it and depend on it, so it will be most helpful and healthful to transition off of it slowly, with care and guidance.

The first way I ever tried mullein was as a smoke. It may seem counterintuitive to smoke an herb for a cough, but it is actually a time-honored form of traditional medicine. Smoke is used ceremonially in many cultures (think of frankincense and myrrh in the Catholic church), but it is also medicinal. Mullein leaves are very fluffy when they're cut up, and need to be thoroughly dried to smoke, but they are easy to light in a pipe or dish, and will stay lit when rolled up in a rolling paper. Mullein smoke can also be directly blown into the ears to relieve ear pain. You can't do this for yourself, so you need to ask for someone's help. (Maybe this is where the sexy expression, "blow in my ear and I'll follow you anywhere" came from—maybe it began with an earache!)

In addition to drinking mullein infusions to heal the underlying condition, burning mullein can be a huge help in an acute asthma attack. I had been taught that mullein smoke could stop an attack, but when I saw it for myself the first time it made an indelible impression on me. Each time I see it work, it still amazes me. Here is how you do it:

MULLEIN SMOKE FOR AN ASTHMA ATTACK

Put the dried mullein in a fireproof dish, such as an abalone shell. If someone is having an asthma attack, or an attack is threatening, light the mullein leaves until they begin to smoke, and hold the dish so that the smoke can rise up right under the person's nose. Encourage them to focus on their exhalation, as the struggle is to inhale but usually the answer is to exhale more completely, allowing the next breath to come in more easily. The smoke will dilate the bronchia and bring comfort quickly, in less than one minute. I encourage anyone who has asthma or lives with someone with asthma to keep a pre-set dish of mullein and a lighter or matches handy for just such a need. People with asthma and other chronic breathing complaints can also smoke the mullein directly in a pipe, or rolled into paper, for short-term relief of acute symptoms of breathlessness.

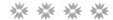

I also use mullein alone or mixed with other herbs in smoke blends to help people (including myself, quite a few years ago now) to stop using tobacco habitually. It helps with the "oral-fixation" part of the habit, and can be relaxing, too. The following blend can be used for a cough, for asthma, as part of a program to stop smoking, or simply for a ritual of relaxation and enjoyment. All the herbs must be thoroughly dried.

SOOTHING SMOKE RECIPE

6 parts dried mullein leaf

2 parts dried coltsfoot leaf

½ part dried damiana leaf

½ part dried comfrey leaf

Pinch of dried lavender flowers, to taste

Pinch of dried mugwort leaves, to taste

Blend the herbs together very well, and then put into a pipe to smoke. If you are rolling the herbs into a paper, I recommend rice papers. They are made only of rice and have no glue, but they are so thin that, when licked and sealed, they stick together without the glue. They are among the healthiest papers to use, along with cellulose papers. (See Resources, page

515.) And yes, it is true that too much of any smoke can be challenging to the lungs.

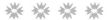

The following is an internal recipe that will be helpful if you are ready to stop smoking tobacco. It addresses both the physiological and psychological challenges of releasing this addictive and compelling habit. I say compelling because there is an ancient memory at work inside of us regarding smoke. Smoke is sacred. It is one of the oldest forms of prayer, and is still employed for prayer and ceremony in most indigenous cultures. When I stopped smoking tobacco as a daily habit, I found I could use it for ceremony in a way that felt more authentic.

Smoke is a substance that is somewhere between physical and ethereal, and has always been used as a go-between or bridge between the realms of physical and non-physical realities. Nonetheless, daily overconsumption of commercial tobacco with its hundreds of additives such as saltpeter is undeniably debilitating and harmful to one's health in myriad ways. So, all judgment aside, here is a helpful recipe to help stop smoking:

SMOKE-RELEASE TINCTURE BLEND

½ part mullein tincture

½ part oat-top tincture

¼ part lobelia tincture

¼ part burdock tincture

Combine tinctures in a dropper bottle. Shake the bottle and take ½ teaspoon or less of the mixture in water, tea, or juice, 3–5 times daily. You can also take 1–3 drops directly under your tongue now and then as needed. Alternately, put one or more droppers of the blend into a water bottle and sip throughout the day and evening.

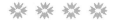

This tincture is helpful in numerous ways. It is good in acute craving. It will help in relieving the difficult emotional responses that can come with withdrawal from tobacco. The oat tops are soothing and calming, and the Lobelia *(Lobelia inflata)*, nicknamed "Indian tobacco," helps satisfy the physical craving for nicotine by providing lobeline and isolobeline, chemicals that are received at the nicotine-receptor sites in the body as if they were nicotine. While lobelia is sedating to the nervous system, oats are strengthening. The tops are considered by some herbalists to be the crème-de-la-crème of the oat plant. If you squeeze the fresh, unripe tops, they will exude drops of milky liquid. This is a perfect metaphor for a "mothering" plant that offers you comfort in times of need. I tincture the oat tops, yet most often prefer the whole plant, tops and straw all together, for infusions. Oat infusion acts as a long-term sustainability tonic. The tincture is a bit more anti-depressant, while the infusion is most nourishing.

In a lecture I attended at a conference, herbalist (and now MD) Tieraona Klar Low Dog spoke of using oat tops to help people going through withdrawal from heroin or morphine in the clinic she'd once had in New Mexico. She also said that quitting smoking can be harder than letting go of heroin, and many addicts back this up, so the oats and/or other strengthening relaxants are definitely needed. What most impressed me was the benefit and wisdom in using something as simple as oats in such a serious situation. (Read more about oats and releasing addictions, pages 193–195.)

The burdock in this mixture will support your commitment and confidence as it helps your body more easily and completely release the tar and nicotine that are tobacco's waste products, clearing your blood and lymph. It will also help you stay strong and grounded during the challenging process of letting go. Oats and burdock can both help with the tendency to put on weight after stopping smoking. Each of these herbs is deeply nutritive and therefore satisfying, and helps adjust and balance blood sugar. Infusions will be most helpful for that, and it would also help to eat burdock root and oatmeal as foods.

Finally, the mullein in the mix will help your lungs with the process of self-repair that begins as soon as you stop smoking commercial tobacco.

MULLEIN EAR OIL

I make and use infused oil of mullein flowers for one of its classic uses—ear pain. If there is an infection, mix 1 drop of mullein flower oil with 1 drop of garlic infused oil, warm them, and put a drop in each ear. These days, mullein-garlic oil can be purchased as a pre-made mix for ear infections. Do take an anti-infective or immune-supportive herb such as echinacea internally as well. (See a list of immune-strengthening allies, beginning on page 108.) When you can help yourself from both the inside and the outside, do it!

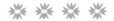

If mullein flower oil is not available, you can use infused oil of St. J's wort. (This is what I call St. John's wort. That plant is sometimes called St. *Joan's* wort, which makes students wonder if it is two different plants. "St. J's" is my solution to the confusion. It is all the same plant, *Hypericum perforatum*). This oil or evening primrose oil *(Oenothera biennis)* can be used for ear pain.

I particularly love mullein flowers, not only for earaches and lung challenges, but also for the nervous system. I find tincture of mullein blossoms to be a reliable relaxant and soother of nervous tension. When you are jumping from one thing to another (in Ayurveda this is called having too much *vata*, or wind, in your system), and you are anxious about everything but nothing you can put your finger on, mullein flowers are indicated. When I went through menopause and often felt irritably hot and cranky, I found mullein flower tincture invaluable. (My mate was quite pleased with me taking it, too!) When it wasn't mullein flower tincture that I wanted, it was evening primrose. Sometimes I mixed them together, which was lovely too. (See more menopause recipes, page 329.)

I love mullein flowers for inflamed sinuses, both as an internal tincture and as infused oil for external use. I recommend taking the oil with you when traveling by plane, or for a long train or bus ride, especially if you wear contact lenses; but all of us are prone to dry and potentially irritated nasal passages when we have to sit for a length of time in artificial, re-circulated air. Come to think of it, with more and more office buildings being built without windows, you may want to take the mullein flower oil to work, too. You can put the oil in your nostrils with a Q-tip, a tissue, or your pinky. Massage the oil externally over your sinuses, too, above your eyebrows and just above your cheekbones out to your ears. It's also very useful if you live at a high altitude with a dry climate.

As I said earlier, breath and heart are inextricably linked. A nurse and herbalist named Mary who was my apprentice called me from the hospital one afternoon. Her elderly aunt was suffering from congestive heart failure and taking oxygen. My student called to ask if there was anything she could give her aunt to make her more comfortable. I said it was unlikely to help much in such a dire situation, but I suggested mullein to help with the excess fluid that was collecting within and outside of her lungs (characteristic symptoms of congestive heart failure). It may sound as if I'm making this up, but after she drank a cup of mullein tea the woman took off her oxygen mask, flung it across the room, and said she felt the best she'd felt in ages. My student called me back, ecstatic. I told her it couldn't hurt to start her aunt on a mixture of hawthorn berries and mullein leaves!

Famed French herbalist and healer Maurice Mességué used mullein leaves and flowers made into syrup with glycerin and blackstrap molasses, to be taken by the tablespoon twice a day for angina, palpitations, and other coronary disorders.

Gail Faith Edwards writes that the Ojibwa people use the inner bark of mullein roots to stimulate the heart, and that ancient Greek healers used mullein for both physical and emotional matters of the heart.

Mullein syrup is a great remedy for winter coughs and congestion. I have made many variations.

Here's one that combines mullein leaves and flowers.

MULLEIN LEAF AND FLOWER SYRUP

2½ cups mullein leaves

½ cup mullein flowers

1 ounce mullein flower tincture

Vegetable glycerin or dark honey to taste (vegan options are maple syrup, agave, or blackstrap molasses)

Put mullein leaves and flowers into a half-gallon jar. Cover with boiling water and leave to steep overnight. In the morning, pour the infusion into a saucepan, squeezing every bit of infusion you can out of the herbs. Compost the spent plant material. Simmer the infusion in an open pan on a very low flame, being careful not to boil it. When half the volume of liquid has been reduced, you have made a decoction. To turn the decoction into a syrup, remove from heat and stir in the alcohol and the honey or glycerin.

This syrup will keep in the refrigerator for several months. If there is no alcohol in it, it may last for a shorter time, about 4–6 weeks. Label it and use it straight by the tablespoon several times daily, or add it to healing teas when you need to benefit from the gifts of the marvelous mullein plant.

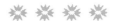

A few other ways I like to enjoy mullein are in the following infusions:

Mullein leaf/sassafras leaf/elderberry: A deluxe recipe for respiratory- and lymph-system strengthening, support for the urinary system, help with bacterial and viral infections, and a tasty way to start the day.

Mullein leaf/sassafras leaf/red clover blossom: Yum! Lymph nourishment as well as support for a healthy musculoskeletal system.

Mullein leaf/sassafras leaf/sassafras root infusion and/or syrup: The addition of a very small amount of root (⅛ part) adds a delicious medicinal bonus to this infusion when you turn it into a syrup.

Lobelia *(Lobelia inflata)*

Let's talk about lobelia, a plant of decidedly mixed reputation. From reading alone, I was frightened of this plant and didn't use it at all for years. Now I really love lobelia. This Native American plant is slender and grows only about a foot tall, but she has a big presence and takes on powerful challenges in an assertive way. Lobelia is both stimulating and relaxing, depending on dosage, and definitely doesn't fall into the realm of gentle-yet-potent herbs that I use most frequently. Lobelia is potent, but not gentle; her nicknames "pukeweed" and "gagweed" attest to that! You can taste a bit of pepper on your tongue when you taste either fresh lobelia or a fresh lobelia tincture.

Lobelia is frequently used in small amounts in recipes for asthma and bronchitis, and is effective at quelling painful spasms and uncontrollable coughs. As the nicknames suggest, lobelia can be nauseating, so the dosage needs to be carefully chosen. It is also used as an intentional emetic in cases of poisoning, or in cases of such thickened bronchial secretions that an emetic is needed to provoke vomiting out the congested matter. I have only read of that kind of heroic approach, and never practice it myself. I use lobelia internally when it's needed, in respiratory remedies, pain-relief blends, and in the smoke-release recipe above, but I use it far more frequently in external preparations.

The following recipe provides a helpful liniment for topical use that I can confidently recommend as effective and completely safe for breaking up painful tightness and congestion in the lungs.

LOOSEN-IT-UP LOBELIA LINIMENT

3½–4 cups fresh lobelia leaves, stalks, flowers, and seed pods (or 2 cups dried lobelia)

1 quart apple cider vinegar

Cut up the fresh herb. Put the lobelia and then the vinegar into a non-aluminum saucepan. Bring it to a boil, then turn it down and simmer it on the lowest possible heat for about an hour. You can use it immediately, but it will get better if allowed to stand and infuse. I usually put the whole mixture into a bottle and let it stand for 6 weeks or more. If you don't have time to wait, let your mixture stand overnight in the saucepan; then strain it, squeeze out the herbs, and bottle it. When you put the label on your jar, besides writing "Lobelia Liniment" and the date, please mark your bottle "for external use only." This vinegar is *not* one you want to put on your salads.

This liniment can be applied freely, front and back, on the skin over the bronchia and lungs.

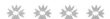

Cooking and infusing lobelia in vinegar brings out its anti-spasmodic benefits, and they are felt immediately. There will be less constriction throughout the chest, and a decrease in pain. The smell of vinegar is strong at first, but completely dissipates in a short while. It should generally be used along with internal herbs to remedy the underlying situation.

Let's Talk about Colds

What does your cold feel like? Do you feel hot and dry, stuffed up and separated from everything and everyone by thick mucus clogging your nose and limiting your sight and hearing? Or is your nose running copiously while you feel chilled and shivery? Treat yourself accordingly by taking care in choosing whether you want more or less warming, cooling, moistening, and/or drying.

For example, if you are cold and have chest congestion with a wet, productive cough, you might want to use an infusion of ginger root because it's warming and drying. If your cough is harsh and dry, and it feels like mucus is stuck deep in your lungs, you might use an infusion of cooling, moistening sweet blue violet leaves, or bronchial-easing mullein leaves and flowers; or if that cold and congestion is accompanied by fever and you feel hot and parched, perhaps a tincture of saponin-rich, juicy-stemmed, cooling chickweed would be just the thing. Matching the "energetics" of your symptoms (hot, cold, wet, dry) to the herbs can help you choose the herb or herbs that will be most healing for you.

All of the above herbs have anti-inflammatory and immune-building properties specific to the respiratory system, as does anti-infective, expectorant elecampane root tincture *(Inula helenium)* or lung-healing, cough-soothing plantain leaves (*Plantago* species) used as tea or tincture, or even a familiar spice herb like basil (*Ocimum* species). Basil is antiviral and can be helpful for any type of cold when taken as a simple tea, tincture or infusion. Antibacterial thyme *(Thymus vulgaris)* can be brewed as a tea and also used for a steam. It is one of the best warming herbs for healing a chilly cold with a bad cough.

You have options, so if you have one herb available and not another, don't worry; just use the best herb(s) available to you. Last but not least, which taste is most appealing to you at that moment? I've found that to be a surprisingly reliable way to choose the most effective herbs for the person who needs them.

When it comes to sinuses, yarrow flowers or combined flowers, leaves and stalks are one of my "go-to" herbs, both internally as infusions and tinctures and externally as steams. The white flowers with tiny yellow centers are best gathered when the oils that give yarrow its characteristic complex aroma are at their peak. That's when the medicine is most potent. I value yarrow highly in my herbal medicine chest (see Wound and Bruise Healing, page 471), so each year I grow and also wildcraft yarrow (gather it from the wild) to use medicinally.

I will turn to yarrow when the situation is chronic or when I want to warm the person, and sometimes if they have fever. Yarrow is a powerful healing plant with a contractive effect. I use tissue-toning, astringent yarrow when I want to stem a flowing tide of mucus from the sinuses, or when there is deep, compacted congestion leading to ongoing inflammation and painful sinus headaches. It's also helpful if there is any tendency to nosebleeds. "Nosebleed plant" is one of yarrow's old nicknames.

Yarrow is most helpful with the additional properties of strengthening the liver and improving inadequate functioning of the whole digestive tract, which is often a causative factor in chronic sinusitis. Yarrow helps through an array of bitter volatile oils, resins and other chemical constituents, and can often relieve the most terrible sinus headaches. When it doesn't bring complete relief, at least it usually makes a person comfortable enough to sleep and heal. Many chronic sinus infections are fungal, and this is one reason these infections often return when treated with conventional antibiotic treatment, or even herbal antibiotics that target bacteria rather than fungus. Yarrow also has antifungal properties.

I don't usually use elder and yarrow flowers together, preferring to alternate them, but you certainly can. Mixed together with mint, they are actually a time-honored cold remedy. My partner likes to use yarrow and elder blossom tinctures together to help him when he gets sinus infections. I will often suggest adding echinacea and elderberry. Or we'll add homemade tincture of usnea lichen, as it's an excellent antifungal for the respiratory system.

The recipe below is a tincture blend, but it could be made as an infusion with dried roots, flowers and berries and would be just as effective if not more so.

SINUS INFECTION RELIEF TINCTURE BLEND

3 droppers echinacea root tincture (about ½ teaspoon)

2 droppers elder blossom tincture

1–2 droppers yarrow flower tincture (also use the leaves and
stalks if making your own tincture)

3 droppers (about ½ teaspoon) elderberries (or use a tea
spoon of Elderberry Elixir, page 153)

This is a strong tincture blend. Mix tinctures into a mug of boiled or very
hot water. Sip and enjoy. Sleep and heal. This mixture, along with steams
and infusions, has helped my partner get through some very difficult sinus
infections. How much herbal medicine people need varies greatly based on
their general state of health, on how rested or exhausted they are, and on
the quality of the herbs being used. You could start by using this recipe 3
times daily; or put the herbs into a thermos and simply sip from it all day
and perhaps sip another thermos all evening.

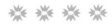

WILDLY DELICIOUS COLD AND
SINUS RELIEF INFUSION

1 cup fresh pine needles

1 cup dried autumn sassafras leaves (If you use fresh leaves, only
use ½ cup, or your brew could get too gooey. You want
to extract that wonderful soothing mucilage, but not overdo it.)

¼ cup dried rose hips

¼ cup dried elderberries (or more, to taste)

Cut up the pine needles and break up the sassafras leaves. I crush the rose
hips in a mortar and pestle to draw out more of their properties, and leave
the elderberries alone, as they will yield their gifts easily to boiling water.
Put the herbs into a half-gallon jar. Cover with boiling water and let steep
overnight (8–12 hours).

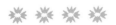

I named this tangy mixture "wildly delicious" the first time I made it because I had gathered all the ingredients from the wild, and though I hadn't tasted it yet I knew it would be superb. I was right!

This is a great recipe when a cold is lingering and you are feeling a bit blue about it, as well as tired and perhaps cranky. The high concentrations of vitamin C in the pine, rose, and elder will help your immune system to heal you. The pine will help you breathe easier, and its antiseptic oils will prove very beneficial if there is any infection present in your lungs. Pine also soothes and calms the spirit, helping you to be more easily at peace with what is. And sassafras—ahhh, sassafras!—lifts your spirits as she puts a sparkle back in your eye, and a lilt in your walk. She helps your lymph, skin, kidneys, liver, and lungs—all the main filtration systems in the body.

Sassafras softens what she touches, whether it's inflamed lung tissue, raw mucous membranes, irritated skin, or anger. Sassafras will even help the irritations that tend to form under and around the nose after frequent sneezing, blowing, and wiping. Please do *not* use tissues with "soothing" additives. The chemicals used are extremely irritating, and potentially toxic!

COMMON-COLD TEA

½ cup dried comfrey or alfalfa leaves (Since there is ongoing debate about whether comfrey is safe to take internally, I offer alfalfa as an acceptable substitute in this recipe.)

¼–½ cup dried rose hips or elderberries

¼ cup dried elder or yarrow flowers

Put the herbs into a saucepan with one quart of water. Bring everything to a boil and then allow it to steep or simmer for 30 minutes or longer.

Rest and drink the hot tea throughout the day, with or without honey. This recipe can also be made as a slow infusion by putting the herbs into a quart jar (doubling the quantities if making a half-gallon). Let everything steep overnight, as usual, and then strain, squeeze the herbs into the infusion, compost them, and gently reheat the infusion, storing it in a thermos to drink it hot all day. The remaining amount should be refrigerated.

❋ ❋ ❋ ❋

If you can supplement this recipe with a hot, immune-strengthening vegetable, beef, or chicken soup made with onions, garlic, carrots, mushrooms, and astragalus, so much the better. (See Everything Is Medicine, page 383.)

A cold will still have to run its course, and we usually "catch" a cold—or "get caught" by one—when we are run-down and need permission or an excuse to rest. However, the severity and duration of the symptoms will be lessened with the help of the herbs.

MORE COLD REMEDIES

Here's the promised recipe for elderberry syrup:

EASY ELDERBERRY SYRUP

> 1 cup dried elderberries
>
> 1 vanilla bean
>
> Honey, to taste
>
> ½ gallon water
>
> 4 ounces brandy or, better yet, herbal infused brandy
> (optional)

Cut off both tips of the vanilla bean, and cut it in half lengthwise. Scrape out all the seeds with a knife or small spoon, and then cut up the rest of the pod into approximately ¼-inch pieces. Put all parts of the vanilla bean and the elderberries into a half-gallon glass jar. Pour boiling water over the herbs. Fill the jar to the top and then wait a minute or so, then top it up 1–2 more times until it is as full as possible. Then cap the jar so it is airtight.

Let this brew infuse on your counter for 12–18 hours. Next, pour the liquid into a stainless-steel or enamel saucepan, and squeeze the berries and vanilla bean pieces until you can't get anymore liquid out of them.

Put the strained infusion over a very low flame until steam rises off the top of the liquid. Keep it steaming, just below a simmer. You have to keep an eye on this kind of preparation. It is definitely not the sort of thing where you want to go and check your email or get involved in a movie or conversation. Trust the voice of experience: You will burn pots and lose wonderful medicines if you distract yourself while preparing herbal syrup on an open flame.

When the liquid is reduced to half, you have made your simple decoction and it is almost done. I use a chopstick to measure the original brew, scratching a little mark into the chopstick to mark the original depth and then periodically dipping it until the liquid is reduced to the desired level, halfway from the mark to the bottom of the chopstick.

When the decoction is ready, take the saucepan off the stove and stir in honey to preserve it, make it even more delicious, and add the natural anti-bacterial gifts of honey. The more honey you add, the better preserved your syrup will be. In general, I like about 1 tablespoon per cup of liquid, but add more or less to please your own palate. The darker the honey, the more nourishing and medicinal it will be.

I store my syrups in the refrigerator, labeled, and they last 1–3 months. If you choose to add brandy, it adds anti-spasmodic and relaxant qualities and increases the stability of your syrup. It can last for 6 months or more with alcohol in it.

This simple recipe is a great base from which to be creative. Some ingredients to try adding in are: cinnamon sticks, elder flowers, ginger root, cloves, rose petals, spruce, pine, or balsam fir needles, coltsfoot flowers, and more!

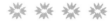

This is one of my all-time favorite syrups for colds and flu. The vanilla bean adds a delicious flavor and brings its calming presence to the potion. When you are ill, take a tablespoon or more of this syrup every couple of hours throughout the day as an immune-vitalizing, antiviral tonic that's rich in antioxidants, iron, and circulation-enhancing bioflavonoids. You can also add this syrup to a cup of infusion. Or, if you aren't ill, put it on ice cream or yogurt!

Warning: This recipe is so delicious that you may have friends coming by pretending to be sick to get you to share your elderberry syrup!

A great thing about syrups is that you can have them prepared ahead of time and not have to fuss with making something when you are feeling awful. If you are well and looking to stay that way, you can use a tablespoon a day of this syrup as an immune-strengthening tonic.

And here are a few more recipes:

STUFFY-HEAD INFUSION I
(plus bonus facial)

2 cups dried rose hips

Elder blossom tincture

Echinacea root tincture

Infuse rose hips in a half-gallon jar of boiled water for 8–16 hours. Decant the infusion, squeeze out the rose hips well, and set them aside. Reheat the rose hip infusion, and before drinking it add 1–3 droppers (25–75 drops) of elder blossom tincture, plus half your body weight in drops of Echinacea tincture, per serving.

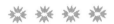

BONUS ROSE HIP FACIAL

When you decant the rose hips, you may want to take a brief sidetrack and give yourself a gentle facial. The steeped and squeezed rose hips will now have a gelatinous consistency. Massage them into your skin in gentle circular motions, and leave the rose hip gel on your face for as long as you like before rinsing it off. Rose hip's oils are quite healing to skin, and help smooth out wrinkles.

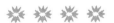

This simple and excellent remedy is for colds, especially if they are threatening to get a lot worse before they get better, possibly because you are run down and in need of deep rest. There is an abundant supply of vitamins C and E in the rose hips as long as they are gathered after a frost and don't have their seeds removed. And echinacea is famous for generally nourishing the immune system back to optimum functioning.

The herbs can be combined and used in different forms. Here are two examples:

STUFFY-HEAD INFUSION II

1 cup dried elder blossoms

½ teaspoon rose hip tincture

½ teaspoon echinacea root tincture

Steep the elder blossoms in a half-gallon jar for 2 hours, and add ½ teaspoon each of rose hips and echinacea root to each cup of hot infusion. I also like to tincture rose hips in vegetable glycerin, which results in a sweet/tart flavor. You could also add rose petal honey (see page 466).

STUFFY-HEAD INFUSION III

2 cups dried echinacea root

1–3 droppers rose hip tincture

1–3 droppers elder blossom tincture

Pour boiling water over 2 cups of echinacea root in a half-gallon jar. Cover and steep for 8–12 hours. Then decant it, reheat it gently, and add 1–3 droppers each of the rose hip and elder blossom tinctures, to every cup of infusion.

Drink about half a cup of this infusion, warm-to-hot, 4 times daily.

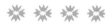

Echinacea root infusion is underused as a healing preparation. When you pour the boiling water over the dried root to steep it rather than boiling the root itself, it may help preserve some of the more delicate polysaccharides (healing sugars) present in the root. People tend to imagine that tinctures are more potent than infusions. Perhaps tinctures look (and taste!) more like "real medicine" than a cup of infusion does. However, over the years I've found that when echinacea tincture is not working the way I'd hoped it would, echinacea infusion is often the ticket-to-ride back to health and re-energized well-being.

Colds can often be brought on by feeling overwhelmed or overburdened, as when you get run down from lack of sleep, overwork, and/or not eating well. In other words, a cold is often brought on through lack of attention to self-care. It can be your body's way of calling attention to itself and its need for care and consideration, and *its* need is *your* need.

A HEALING STORY—COLD AND COUGH

A couple of friends of mine called me on a Sunday morning when they had bad colds that were getting worse. Her head felt heavy and was hurting badly. She was very congested, and concerned that it might turn into pneumonia, as had happened to her the year before. He was feeling weak and sick, and coughing a lot, which made his chest hurt. They'd been sick for a day or two at that point, and had been "trying everything" as people so often do. "Simplify," I suggested.

They already had echinacea tincture, so I came over that night and brought them elderberries and yarrow flowers. I knew they weren't up to doing much themselves, so I gave them the simplest instructions I could.

SIMPLE COLD AND COUGH RECIPE

1–2 teaspoons dried elderberries

1–2 teaspoons dried yarrow flowers

Pour 2 cups of boiled water over the combined herbs, and steep them on a very low flame for about 20 minutes.

Drink the tea warm-to-hot, with or without honey, at least 3 times daily.

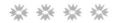

For the first day or so, they were each to take 2–3 droppers of echinacea tincture every few hours in hot water or tea. After that, they could take it 3–4 times daily as they continued with their tea, as needed. When I talked to them two nights later, they had both been resting (not something they do a lot of) and taking the herbs, and were amazed at how quickly they were feeling so much better!

We sometimes act as if we really aren't fond of ourselves at all. I don't think that's what we mean to do—but if we are honest, it sure looks that way a lot of the time! I call this dis-ease "SCDD"—Self-Care Deficit Disorder—and the cure is tending to yourself as you would tend to someone you *truly* love and care about. Let that person be *you*!

Everyone is different, with unique needs and their own variation on common needs, but self-care is a universal recommendation.

Some of the Most Important Things You Can Do for Vibrant Health

Spending time with yourself ... taking time for friends, fun, pleasure, play, singing and dancing (Have you heard the expression, "If you can talk, you can sing; if you can walk, you can dance"? I would like to add, "If you can't talk or walk, you can sing and dance with your spirit.") ...

Staying warm enough in cold weather and cool enough in hot weather ... exercising, or any regular physical activity ... engaging in thinking that challenges and stretches your mind ...

Managing energy by spending and conserving it as consciously as possible ... being outdoors regularly ... being in a natural, wild environment at least sometimes ...putting your bare feet on the earth ... touching trees ...

Doing something that feels valuable to a larger community, ideally as part of a community ... working with and freeing blocked energy through a practice such as yoga or *chi kung* ... meditating daily ...

Eating healthy cooked and raw foods,including high-quality fats ... drinking daily herbal infusions ...taking relaxing baths ... resting ... getting enough sleep consistently ...

Learning to trust your own senses ... circulating sexual energy through your body and experiencing sexual fulfillment (whether on your own or with another) ... being generally happy and content ... laughing and crying freely ... expressing your truth ...

And, most importantly, having good, respectful relationships, and at least one true friend who helps you feel loved and cared-for.

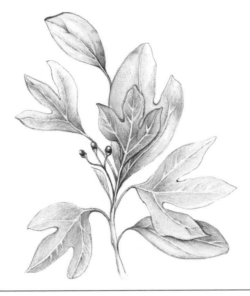

Sassafras

Sassafras *(Sassafras albidum)*

> Sassafras makes me happy.
> Sassafras makes me whole.
> Sassafras teaches
> Wholeness and uniqueness.
> Sassafras makes me whole.
> —song by Judith Berger, author of *Healing Rituals*

Body: soothes mucous membranes, clears skin, increases flow through lymph and urinary systems, supports liver, and relieves dry coughs.

Mind: breaks through dark, brooding thoughts, relieves depression, clears mental fog, dark clouds and gloom, brightens outlook.

Heart: brings happiness and joy, melts psychic armor that has out lived its usefulness, offers an alternative to melancholia.

Soul: dispels inner torment, uplifts the spirit, brings light, delight, and enlightenment.

Sassafras

Sparkling with golden energy,
She lifts the clouds away.
Famous for her mitten leaves,
She brightens up my day.

Sassafras is such an imp,
She won't let you stay sad.
No matter what is going on,
She says, "It's not that bad."

Her spicy taste is famous—
You've had it in root beer.
She helps lymph fluids get flowing,
And makes skin smooth and clear.

Sassafras in fall and spring
Is a fine a physician
For kidneys, lungs, and to help with
Seasonal transitions.

She's so mucilaginous
And soothing to your throat.
I use the yellow leaves the most
And barely touch the root.

A little goes a long way
In so many recipes.
In winter months she lights me up
To joy she holds the keys.

"Sassafras teaches wholeness and uniqueness" in the song above refers to the three different-shaped leaves on most sassafras trees, which are entire, mitten-shaped, and three-fingered. It's almost uncanny how people fill with delight when they're standing under these trees. I've taken people to groves in Central Park, and contagious and irrepressible smiles break out, especially when they smell the leaves and bark. I like to nibble a few sweet, spicy yellow flowers just a bit in the spring, like a young deer.

Sassafras is native to North America. It is a local tree where I live, and I enjoy having an abundance of these trees in the forest nearby, and along the small road on which I live. I start to gather the green leaves for infusions every summer, and continue through the late autumn as the leaves turn orange and yellow and begin to dance down from the trees. Sassafras is an urban tree too. I used to gather the falling leaves to dry for tea every autumn when I lived in New York City. When they feel moist and supple, like skin, they're still good to gather. When they get thin, dry, and crepe-papery, they're no longer viable for medicinal infusions.

Sassafras lifts my spirits and makes me happy. Sassafras leaf tea is a delicious and uplifting drink that is used, along with root tea, as a medicine in many parts of the world to clear skin and lymph, to help a dry cough, and as a folk remedy for a variety of cancers. Her dried, powdered leaves are well known as the base of the Louisiana spice filé gumbo. Even the pith inside the twigs and branches is used as a demulcent remedy for inflamed eyes and to sooth a cough.

Sassafras makes one of the best spirit-lifting infusions. I prefer the term "spirit-lifting" to "antidepressant." I've often used sassafras leaves in recipes for people who are weaning themselves off pharmaceutical anti-depressants and/or tobacco. Sassafras loves to help. Though traditional write-ups and modern studies are most often focused on the root bark of sassafras, I find the leaves gentler and more to my liking. I get very little argument from people who taste sassafras leaf infusion—it's delicious!

Sassafras root tea is traditionally taken as a spring tonic, especially in the southern United States, where it's known as a blood cleanser. It's native to eastern North America, growing as far north as Maine and Ontario, but is a larger tree down South both in size and in lore.

Sassafras Mountain, in the Blue Ridge range, is the highest point in South Carolina.

In the United States sassafras root has been labeled as carcinogenic, but I don't believe it. I don't think former FDA official and esteemed botanist James Duke believes it either; he notes that the safrole oil in sassafras root beer, now banned in the United States, is one-fourteenth as carcinogenic as the ethanol in regular beer. The suspect is the safrole oil in the root. This volatile aromatic oil is what gives sassafras its spicy smell. The roots are more intensely aromatic than the leaves, which also contain far less safrole oil. The leaves, in fact, legally sold as filé gumbo, are designated "GRAS" (generally regarded as safe) by the FDA.

Plants suggest to us by their intensity how much to use them. Just as you wouldn't sit down to a meal of cinnamon, you wouldn't consume sassafras root in as great quantities as you might consume an herb like basil or dandelion greens. Something else to consider is the difference between a chemical constituent of a plant and the whole plant itself. Isolating plant chemicals and then finding them potentially or even actually harmful is not the same thing as proving that a whole plant, leaf, or root is harmful.

Plants are complex, synergistic, living beings. When a chemical is isolated and lifted out of its living matrix, or "re-created" by being chemically synthesized, as is often the case, it is no longer the same. This seems like common sense, and yet it's still the standard way to "scientifically study" herbal medicines, rather than studying them in their natural state or in ways that they're actually used.

Plants with strong, potentially poisonous chemicals usually (though not always) contain their own natural buffers to those harsher compounds, making them safe to use. In other instances, fear arises from certain attributes of plants being misunderstood, as when plant sterols are confused with actual hormones and discussed as if using those plants will produce the same effects as taking hormones, or when chemicals are mistaken for one another, as when common cyanogenic glycosides in plants are confused with cyanide. They're not the same thing—and even if they were, that chemical is actually found in many popular foods and herbs, including apples, cherries and peaches, and is rendered inert by boiling water. It can be recognized in the subtle smell of almonds and in the almond smell of anisette, or in the scraped bark of a wild black cherry tree twig.

A more detailed discussion of plant chemistry is beyond the scope of this herbalist or this book, but for those who want to research it further, there are reliable resources such as herbalist Lisa Ganora's book *The Phytochemistry of Herbs.* Additional information, including helpful publications and websites, can be found in the Resources list at the end of the book (page 507).

Back to sassafras: This tree provides a tonic medicine to be used repeatedly and rhythmically when the seasons are changing, perhaps for two weeks or a month at a time. Different rhythms will work for different people.

I find sassafras very helpful for making it through the first, sometimes dreary, stages of spring in the Northeast. It's still cold and wet, and people want it to already be warmer and more comfortable. Sassafras leaf (or, traditionally, the root) gets your blood and lymph stirring, waking up, ready for more warmth and activity to come.

I also like sassafras in the late fall to help the kidneys, lungs, lymph, and liver function optimally, to keep the body healthy and strong through the upcoming winter. Sassafras infusions drunk at this time can help prevent the colds and coughs that typically knock people down as the seasons change.

WHAT'S IN A NAME?

In winter, I drink sassafras to chase the blues away. It can be used to good effect for people who say they have SAD (Seasonal Affective Disorder). It brings the feeling of honeyed sunlight in every sip! I'd like to note that—although I understand the power of a name and the sense of control that comes with having a name for something that's happening to you—I try to use the names less and less, especially for mental challenges and chronic conditions. I've found that when you say, "I have (SAD, arthritis, cancer, migraines, etc.)" it invites you to be attached to that condition, which gives more power to the symptoms associated with that condition.

Within thirty minutes of having her cancer diagnosis confirmed, I watched my mother's pain level increase exponentially, never to decrease again. And she is not alone in this. Her belief about what was supposed to happen influenced how she was experiencing what was happening. This is human nature, unexamined.

Whatever "it" is, you think you have it—it is yours. This is one of the first ways we become attached to a story about our health and illness. When you say, "I have a bad (back, knee, shoulder, etc.)" this "bad part" becomes part of your identity, how you see yourself, and who you are or are becoming.

By holding a condition firmly in your mind, you actually help the condition become more entrenched in your body. I can say, for example, "I have arthritis in my fingers." If I say, instead, "My fingers are sore and swollen," I have not frozen them into that state by "having arthritis" in my mind as well as in my body. When a condition lodges in the mind in this way, it is harder to heal. When you let go of it in your mind, even a bit, it frees the condition to be absolutely true in the present moment and only the present moment, assuming nothing about the future.

Investigate this for yourself. It goes far beyond positive thinking; in fact, it has nothing to do with positive thinking. Describing the realities rather than labeling your maladies can be a valuable key to healing everyday challenges, acute injuries, chronic problems, and degenerative or life-threatening conditions.

Time and again, I have seen this conscious mental shift help people with chronic, degenerative diseases open to the herbs and facilitate their own healing to a surprising degree. I have experienced it myself. I have deep respect for herbalists I know, or whose work I have read, who understand diseases and the workings of the body far better than I do. I am not trying to take anything away from the brilliance of their knowledge. I simply believe we all stand to benefit if we hold our learned ideas and book knowledge, and even our experientially gained knowledge, a bit more lightly in regards to the inevitability of any particular dis-ease or diet or situation's effects.

We are all powerful cocreators of reality, living in a time when our species is evolving and consciousness is growing. We do best when we create unprecedented spaciousness for healing possibilities that we may never before have conceived of, for ourselves and our clients.

MORE ON SASSAFRAS

I've used sassafras to help people with skin and respiratory challenges, and for what used to be called the blues. I've happily brewed and drunk sassafras leaf infusions for breaking the ice in difficult situations, such as when I've held classes at battered-women's shelters or homeless shelters. It's helpful to serve sassafras when you want to help people lighten up and relax in a tense situation. It's a great infusion to serve at a party, perhaps at dinner when you are introducing your beloved to your family for the first time, or any similar potentially nail-biting scenario.

Mostly I use sassafras as a seasonal tonic to promote wellness. It is one of the most beloved ingredients in my regular wellness tonics. It's one of the herbs that I make absolutely *sure* to harvest a big bag of every fall when the leaves are changing color and beginning to fall to the ground. I gather some green leaves in the summer, too, to mix in with the yellow and orange/red ones. You can also drink sassafras leaf tea fresh, but be careful not to make it too strong or it will come out goopy. (I like "goopy" as a technical term, better than "mucilaginous.")

I often drink sassafras as a simple, but I also like to make tasty, healing blends with one or two additional herbs (see below). I figure I'm taking care of all my body systems with the variety of herbs that I rotate and drink on a daily basis, in addition to specific herbal medicines I drink when I get sick or for chronic conditions. Sometimes I choose the simple (single herb) or blend with specific and clear intent; at other times I'm intent on making it taste good and on general systemic nourishment. I trust my mood when I'm choosing my infusions. If I'm not sick, I seem to make what I need when I give myself time to look at, touch, and smell the different dried herbs I have stored in paper bags.

Here are a few blends that I enjoy and suggest as full-strength infusions to receive the maximum benefits of the dried herbs. You'll notice they are often red, green, and orange (or golden-yellow) because the sassafras leaves are mainly gathered in the autumn.

RARIN'-TO-GO INFUSION

½ cup dried elderberries

¾ cup dried nettle leaves

1¼ cup dried sassafras leaves

This infusion is best steeped at least 8 hours, but even better steeped 12–16 hours.

This blend brings joy as well as great strength. It's rich in many factors that nourish the immune and respiratory systems. It offers replenishment and will have us "rarin' to go" by strengthening our adrenal glands if we have become depleted or exhausted.

Elderberries are well-known for their antiviral properties, immune-nourishing vitamins A and C, and good supply of easy-to-assimilate iron. Nettles are used to prevent exhaustion, and contain an abundant supply of minerals such as chlorophyll, iron, and calcium. All three of these plants are helpful for keeping the joints flexible, and help us breathe easier too.

RESTORATIVE INFUSION

1 cup dried sassafras leaves

½ cup dried red clover blossoms

½ cup dried nettle leaves

These amounts make a half-gallon of infusion. Covered in boiled water and steeped overnight, then decanted, this restorative recipe tastes light and delicious, is nourishing to the nervous system, and makes a good lymphatic-system tonic. It will rev up the immune system and can help with allergies, coughs, and colds. It makes a good kidney tonic too. Sumach berry honey, or goldenrod honey, can be added to your cup to make this mixture even more restorative for the kidneys.

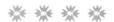

THREE-TREE TEA

1 cup dried sassafras leaves

1 cup dried spicebush leaves

3 cinnamon sticks

Break up the leaves and cinnamon sticks. Put them into a half-gallon jar and cover with boiled water. Cap tightly and wait overnight if possible. It will be delicious within the hour, but more medicinal if left to steep longer.

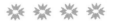

I call this fragrantly spicy, aromatic blend "Three-Tree Tea"—but don't try to say that three times fast! The spicebush tree *(Lindera benzoin)* is our Native American version of the herb allspice, and is often found growing near sassafras trees. They like to work together.

I always think of both of them as friendly trees, and recently learned from Native American herbalist Jody Noé, ND, that spicebush has traditionally been used at gatherings to help people feel more friendly toward one another.

Spicebush is often found along the edges of flowing bodies of water, especially streams meandering through the woods. This suggests its connection with one or more of the fluid systems in the body. It will, in fact, help improve blood circulation, being a warming spice like cinnamon. The above blend is also helpful for your digestion and for stabilizing blood sugar. It can help with mild queasiness or nausea. I often use cinnamon alone for severe nausea and vomiting, especially if caused by an intestinal bug.

RESPIRATORY RELIEF INFUSION I

1 cup dried mullein leaves

1 cup dried sassafras leaves

Cover equal parts of the herbs with boiling water to fill a half-gallon jar, and steep overnight. This infusion is specific as a fall tonic and a moistening respiratory blend. It is best when drunk hot; raw or herb-infused honey can be added if desired.

Both mullein and sassafras moisten the lungs and soften hardened, congested mucus in the lungs, making it easier to get it out. A stronger expectorant such as elecampane or hyssop tincture can be added if a person is too weak or run-down to cough the mucus up and out on their own. This infusion can also be decocted (boiled) down and sweetened to make a great syrup for soothing inflamed bronchia or lungs.

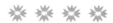

RESPIRATORY RELIEF INFUSION II

1 dried cup mullein

1 dried cup sassafras

½ cup dried elderberries

Steep this brew for at least 8 hours, preferably 10–12. Then reheat it gently in a pot on the stove so you can drink it hot.

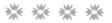

The elderberry makes this an even stronger immune-nourishing, antiviral brew for colds or flu. At the risk of repeating myself, it also makes it even tastier! This blend can also be made into an effective lung and bronchia healing syrup to be used as needed, or daily by the spoonful as a preventative medicine.

OOH-LA-LA INFUSION

1 cup dried sassafras leaf

½ cup linden blossoms

¼ cup rose buds or blossoms

Steep the sassafras and linden in a quart jar overnight. Steep the roses in another quart jar for about 75 minutes. When both infusions are done, decant and combine them. When ready to use, gently reheat in a saucepan on the stove. You can store what you don't drink immediately in a thermos or in the refrigerator.

Ooh-la-la! This blend of dried herbs is sensuous and delicious. It will lift your spirits like the day you were eight years old and woke up to find you had an unexpected snow day off from school! Some people may find this recipe more soothing than that experience, but it's just as pleasurable.

It is also a lovely medicine to use for a cold when you are sniffling, congested, and too hot, perhaps with a low-grade fever. If you can't sleep because you're agitated, this could be a good blend to take in the early evening to help you sleep later. If you're feeling sad with the blues or the blahs, please try it—I think you'll like it. And if you're having a party, this blend will bring out the best in your guests!

And please remember that Sassafras can be enjoyed all by itself as a simple infusion for the multitude of benefits it offers. The best way to get to know any herb is to experiment with it on its own, just as you get to know a person differently when the two of you get together on your own rather than in a group.

Of course, getting out to meet and spend time with the trees themselves is vitally important for getting to know sassafras, as for any plant you use as herbal medicine. Whenever possible, do that first. You can help that happen by learning to use the plants and trees that grow close to where you live. It's also meaningful to take food and medicine made of plants that grow where your ancestors came from, if that's different from what you currently call "home."

Try sassafras leaf infusion (with or without a bit of root in it—about 1 part root to 8 parts leaf). It's good hot or cold, and has a tendency to provoke joy no matter how you use it, and no matter what you are using it for.

Sassafras says, "Have fun! Enjoy!"

12

Skin—The Integument System

Herbs and more for health, acute illnesses, and chronic challenges of the integument system; healing herbs for first aid, itchy rashes, blisters, boils, infections, burns, wounds, acne, eczema, and psoriasis.

The living tissue that comprises your skin is made of layers of varying thickness that progress from the most exterior layers (epidermis) to the most interior layers (dermis). This system is magical: It is nearly waterproof and acutely sensitive to pleasure, pain, and temperature changes; and the inner layers contain connective tissue, lymphatic vessels, nerves, sweat glands, hair follicles, veins, and arteries.

The skin is the largest organ of the body, and contains what you generally think of as "you" within it, safely tucked inside. Enveloping you, the skin creates a boundary that separates your insides from everything outside. Still, your "outer shell" is soft and constantly being sloughed off (up to nine pounds of skin each year), and your pores provide multiple openings to and from the outside world.

This system is connected to the element Air, related to breathing and circulating movement, spaciousness and inter-being. Skin is an extension of your respiration.

Skin is part of your innate immune system, too, providing you with protection via an acidic mantle that covers the skin and traps and prohibits intruders from entering. This acidic layer of protection becomes depleted through overuse of soap and water. Washing with soap removes the acid layer, turning the skin alkaline. This makes skin more vulnerable to infections, including those that enter the body through the skin. Using a natural soap like Castile is good for your skin, and for our land and water. And moderation is a good thing, including when washing yourself.

The skin system's health, acute illnesses, and chronic challenges often offer you teachings and challenges around a healthy sense of self, of knowing where you end and another begins. Challenges that manifest through the skin, whether bacterial, viral or fungal infections, rashes or even continuous insect bites, often have to do with strengthening your personal boundaries. This can involve learning how to say no to others and developing your ability to know who you are and what you need, and being willing to ask for it as well as open to receive it. This doesn't mean there isn't a physical cause such as a need for a change in diet, or an allergic reaction, but whether you choose to address it immediately or not, there will always be a spiritual core within the physical problem that will first "request" and then ultimately require your loving and compassionate attention, reconnection, and healing.

· · · · ● · · · ·

Some of my favorite herbal allies for the skin are: oats, chickweed, plantain, calendula, lavender, rose, birch, elder blossoms, nettles, red clover, burdock, and sassafras.

Plantain

Body: healing to skin, respiratory, digestive, urinary and immune systems. Leaves are astringent and demulcent, antiseptic, antiinflammatory, mucilage-rich and soothing, styptic, drawing, wound-healing, and itch- and pain-relieving. Leaves are nourishing raw or cooked, useful for an eyewash, specific for anemia and "failure to thrive" in infants; roots are used, too, especially for venomous bites. Seeds are a mucilaginous, bulk-forming laxative, and are used in the treatment of parasites.

Mind: refreshes and renews a tired, jaded, or cynical mind.
Heart: uplifts the heart by connecting it with the joy and
abundance of simple treasures that are underfoot.
Soul: relieves deep pain in the soul in a quiet, unassuming way.

Plantain

Little plantain
Has big healing powers
And a rosette of leaves,
With tiny white flowers.

Close to the Earth,
Plantain's a humble weed
Who heals rashes and cuts
So they won't itch or bleed.

Wounds get cleaned out;
Infections are stopped, too.
Plantain's leaves draw out stuff
That is no good for you.

In the body
Lungs, kidneys and guts,
Are all toned by plantain,
With no ifs, ands, or buts.

Her seeds heal, too
As a bulk laxative
They're gel-like and tasty.
She's got so much to give.

If there's one herb
That I would not be without,

It is soothing plantain
About that there's no doubt.

She heals so much
As a poultice or tea,
Yet never causes harm—
What a great way to be.

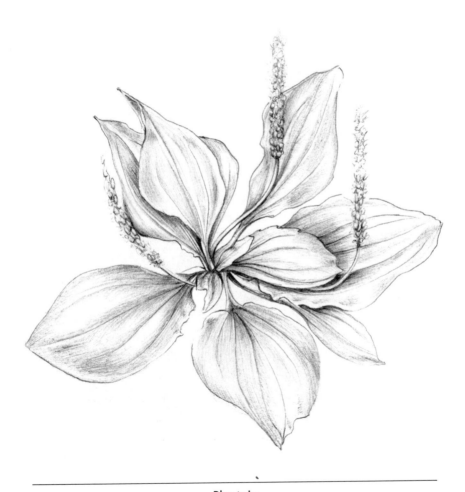

Plantain

I have often said that if I had to choose only one plant for medicine—one plant that I would never want to be without—it would most likely be plantain. Fortunately that isn't a choice I need to make, but I say this because of a casual conversation I had with herbalist Ed Smith one day at an herbal conference. He shared his definition of the three qualities he looks for and most values in any herb, and plantain matched them all: It is ubiquitous, does an astonishing variety of things for us, and is completely benign, doing no harm.

A PLANTAIN STORY

I had moved into my new home in the winter, so come spring I was outside digging up my front lawn by hand to create gardens. My friend and student Deb was working as my gardener, so she was out there helping me. I wanted a peaceful vibration in my gardens that didn't involve working the earth with power tools.

I asked Deb to transplant a bunch of narrow-leaf and broad-leaf plantain plants into their own bed. Plantain is too important to me not to have a good supply of it right outside my front door. (Never mind that I transplanted it from a very short distance away!) She created a lovely half-moon plantain garden right next to my front walkway. But she was quietly indignant, spluttering and muttering now and then—I guess you are not supposed to plant an inconspicuous weed in such a prime showcase spot!

Deb found this a very annoying use of her gardening skills and wondered what on Earth was wrong with me. She told me this sheepishly because of what happened to her the next day when she was in line to pay for groceries at the supermarket. The woman behind her wasn't paying attention, and whammed her cart right into the back of poor Deb's ankles. Deb was furious, but at least she knew what to do. She went outside and gathered up some plantain, chewed it up and sighed with relief as the pain and small lacerations were immediately soothed. She decided that she owed plantain and me an apology, and also made a bottle of plantain oil for herself that very day.

Legend has it that Native people of the North American continent gave plantain the nickname "White Man's Foot" and said that everywhere the white man walked, this plant appeared. Well, it is good to know that Europeans did at least one marvelous thing for Native Americans, even if unintentionally! It wasn't easy to decide which section of *The Gift of Healing Herbs* to put plantain in—skin, respiration, digestion, immunity, or wound and bruise healing, as it could go in any of them. The power of plantain leaf often surprises people because it's such a common weed (the Russian name for it translates as "plant by the side of the road") but this humble plant is actually an international star.

I frequently use plantain for first aid. It is chewed up and plastered over a mosquito bite to stop itching and swelling. It can also be chewed up and applied over a fresh cut to help staunch bleeding. It will relieve pain and bring down swelling or bruising. Additionally, it acts as an anti-infective. If you chew it, a potent antitoxin in the plantain called aucubin mixes with an enzyme in your saliva and turns into an even more anti-bacterial substance called aucubigenin. If you are hesitant about chewing it, you can use boiled water over a fresh leaf, or open it with a mortar and pestle, and it will still work. If you are using dried leaves, boiling water is best for opening up the cell walls of the plant. Plantain is also helpful for relieving the itch of poison-ivy rash.

I dry and powder the leaves of plantain, and store the powder in a little jar or tin. It can be sprinkled on an open wound when fresh plantain isn't available. This is a great item for a first-aid or travel kit. It can be used alone or mixed with other wound herbs like yarrow or witch hazel to be make it more blood-staunching and bruise-healing. When there is an open wound, whether you use the leaves or leaf powder, plantain's anti-infective, immune-strengthening qualities are most helpful. In addition to cleaning the wound and helping it stop bleeding, plantain leaves will also begin the process of skin healing; the leaves stimulate the growth of new granulation cells that will form new skin.

Plantain is effective at drawing out a thorn, splinter, or piece of glass embedded in the skin when used as a "green band-aid," chewing up a leaf and sticking it on. These are also called "spit poultices." This kind of poultice can be taped on, or held in place with a piece of cloth if needed.

ANOTHER (KIND OF FUNNY) PLANTAIN STORY

I walked into Central Park with my apprentices one afternoon. When we'd last been together the week before, I'd been teaching them about plantain. One of the women said, "I wish I would get hurt so I could use plantain and see for myself how it works." I immediately cautioned her, "Be careful what you wish for!"

It wasn't five minutes before she suddenly shrieked in pain and bounced up and down on one foot. "Ouch!" she said. "I don't know what could have happened!"

"Looks like you got your wish," the other women chided her. She was wearing very thin-soled shoes, and a thorn had gone right through them and pierced the tender flesh on the bottom of her foot. It had broken, too, embedding the point in there. So we set to work.

She sat on the ground and gathered some plantain leaves, and everyone else picked some too. She mashed them up with her teeth, mixing her saliva into the leaves well to increase their anti-infective properties. She put a nice thick wad of them up against the sore, red spot, and then we waited with her. The pain eased presently, and then she replaced the spit poultice with a fresh, smaller one. After that one was removed, it had pulled out the last bits of the thorn that had splintered in her foot and we went on our way.

A MORE DRAMATIC PLANTAIN STORY

I was gathering yellow dock and plantain leaves in Central Park in New York City. I planned to blanch and freeze them so I could have wild greens to eat in the winter. After I'd been gathering from one hillside for a little while, a man joined me who didn't look very healthy. I was intrigued that he was also busily picking weeds in Central Park, and kept watching him out of the corner of my eye.

We were both going up and down the hill; I was picking plantain leaves, and he was digging up the whole plants. I had never heard of using the roots before, and I finally asked what he was doing. But he didn't speak English, and I didn't speak Spanish. What to do? We used sign language, with my little bits of Spanish and his little bits of English until he helped me understand that he had a terrible rash that had gotten dirty and infected and led to blood poisoning. He'd been dismissed from the hospital because he didn't have insurance. He gestured to indicate that he'd had a red streak going up his leg. He had heard that this plant, *llantén* in Spanish (pronounced "yan-tain"), could help him. He was using it, and was getting better. He showed me his leg, and I could see that it was in the process of healing.

He indicated that he had been putting the plants on his leg as well as drinking the tea. I showed him that drinking an infusion made from the bitter yellow dock root could also be helpful to him, and he gratefully gathered some of that, too.

Since then, I have heard of several other people who used plantain internally and externally for blood poisoning, along with echinacea root tea or tincture internally, when they had no other options—usually because they didn't have money for medical care in this confused culture we live in. The good thing about our confused cultural values is that they are, ironically, prodding us to return to our good green Earth for our medicine.

AN EVEN MORE DRAMATIC PLANTAIN STORY

I will always remember Anishinabeg herbalist Keewaydinoquay telling the story of how three women, two of them her students, were in a desert garden somewhere out west and were bitten by an unknown type of spider. Two of them, remembering Kee's teachings about plantain, put the chewed-up leaves on the spider bites. The third woman didn't do that. All three had to go to the hospital later that night with serious adverse reactions to the bites. The women who used the plantain were eventually okay, but the woman who had refused to use the plantain wound up dying from the bite!

I have successfully used plantain leaves combined with osha root (*Ligusticum porteri*) tincture, externally and internally, to help people bitten by poisonous spiders.

In more everyday uses, plantain oil is a staple in my herbal medicine chest. I make a fresh batch of oil and ointment every year to have on hand when the plant is out of season. It is useful for all kinds of everyday boo-boos as well as diaper rash, shaving cuts, and even acne. It can be dabbed onto pimples, and helps reduce them even though it is in an oil base. Plantain is effective for wounds, ulcers, eczema, psoriasis, boils, burns, sores, and more. It soothes and shrinks hemorrhoids, and quickly eases the pain of bee or wasp stings. Eating the fresh leaves and/or drinking fresh leaf tincture (or tea made with dry leaves) will help from the inside too.

Dry the leaves for teas and infusions to give you a boost of vitamins and minerals (especially iron), as well as to soothe the digestive and uri-nary tracts, to ease bowel movements and urinary flow, and to calm a dry, tickling cough. Plantain infusion can also be used as a skin or eye wash.

Plantain works beautifully as a simple, or it can be combined well with other herbs. I mix it with calendula for rashes, yarrow for wounds, and thyme for coughs. I've used it in conjunction with slippery elm to help the bowels, and with corn silk for the urinary tract.

Here's another skin-healing story about plantain: Three dermatologists and a podiatrist (I know, it sounds like the beginning of a bad joke) were completely baffled by my client's poor feet. They were deeply cracked all along the bottom and sides, and the fissures were dry in some areas and oozing in others. She was in a lot of pain, and nothing was helping her even though they gave her ointments and internal medicines, and sent her from one professional to the other searching for "the answer."

When they couldn't find it, it was decided that she should take an exceedingly powerful antibiotic. She called me at that point, scared about following this regimen of strong drugs when they didn't even know what the problem was. Their guesses ranged wildly from a previously unknown bacteria or virus to a reaction to a sexually transmitted disease (which she didn't have).

When in doubt, turn to plantain!

We had this woman soak her feet every night in an infusion made from the dried leaves of garden sage *(Salvia officinalis)* and plantain. Sage is helpful in foot soaks, and here its antiseptic, drying qualities were a welcome boost to the soothing, anti-infective plantain, especially since I wasn't sure what I was dealing with beyond what I could see.

She also massaged her feet with plantain oil each night, and drank burdock root tincture in water several times daily. The final piece of her plan was to warm castor oil at night, dip pieces of flannel or cheesecloth in the oil, wrap her feet in the cloths, and then cover them with plastic wrap and put a sock over that to keep everything in place while she slept. She didn't heal overnight, but she did heal. It took a few months, and she did the night wraps not every night but as frequently as she could. In between, she just massaged her feet with plantain oil.

When she went back to her podiatrist a year later (for a different problem), he was amazed at how beautifully her feet had healed. Her skin was perfect. That was years ago, and I checked in with her recently to ask permission to use this story; she told me that her feet are still "beautiful" and she's never had a problem since.

She's done a lot of healing with herbs, but considers this one of her most amazing herbal healing stories. I have to agree! She deserves a lot of credit, because she followed through in caring for herself, working with the herbs to help her healing happen. Also, being the wise woman that she is, she asked for help to look into her own issues around "standing on her own two feet" and all that that meant to her. So she not only healed her feet but also resolved some old emotional pain and let go of limiting beliefs that were being played out in her body in order to bring her awareness there so that she could heal fully.

White birch *(Betula alba/pendula* and *papyrifera)* and Black Birch *(Betula lenta)*

The different varieties of birch (and there are many more than black and white) are so beautiful that I sometimes swoon with pleasure simply to see them. So I'm not claiming objectivity here. Birch, especially white birch, is a tree of the north with many legends surrounding it. Most of my physical ancestors come from the northern part of the world, from Russia and Poland, where birch is revered. Birch even grows in the Arctic Circle. It is also a tree much used by Native Americans, often for healing, but its best-known use was for making boats, so it is also known as canoe tree or canoe birch.

White birch is represented in the first letter of the Celtic tree alphabet (called the Ogham), and it symbolizes the magic of beginnings. White birches tend to grow in faery circles, and sometimes they're planted that way, too. They draw faery magic to them in the summer months, and strong Nature spirits year-round. They form the most natural and gently powerful sacred circles, most often in clearings in the midst of the woods, but also in meadows and fields.

While at a conference at Skidmore College, I discovered my personal birch circle outside one of the dorms. There I learned much about birch's gentle and creative healing spirit as I walked inside the circle from tree to tree, feeling soft, green moss under my feet, tasting and reveling in the sweet tartness of the young leaves and the whispering messages of the winds moving through them, and doing rituals both alone and with others within their magical circle of roots, trunks, smooth tooth-edged leaves (with slight fuzz underneath), and golden catkin flowers.

I first became aware of white birch as a medicinal ally when a student sent me a New York Times article in the 1990s that reported studies had shown successful correlations between white birch preparations and skin-cancer healing. The article ended with "don't try this at home." In 1994, scientists at the University of North Carolina reported that chemicals found in white birch bark slowed the growth of HIV. The following year, a researcher at the University of Illinois reported that betulinic acid (from birch) killed melanoma cells in mice. (See Notes, page 519.)

According to the American Cancer Society website:

> Betulinic acid has not been studied in humans, but several laboratory studies have looked at its effects when it is added to cancer cells growing in laboratory dishes. These studies, using the pure chemical betulinic acid rather than birch bark, have been published in peer-reviewed medical journals and suggest that betulinic acid holds some promise for patients with melanoma, certain nervous system tumors, and other forms of cancer. Three German studies concluded that betulinic acid showed antitumor activity against cells from certain types of nervous system cancers in children. Two laboratory studies conducted at the University of Illinois indicated that betulinic acid might prove useful as an antitumor drug.[1]

Birch trees have a long history of use in folk medicine. Everywhere it grows, it's leaves, twigs and bark are universally used for skin problems such as boils, rashes, and eczema. I've begun experimenting with using black birch topically as an infused oil, tea wash, or tincture to see if it might help rouse the body's life-force to heal basal-cell carcinomas. Whether or not that proves to be a good use for black birch, the betulinic acid in white birch has indeed been shown to be helpful against systemic skin cancer, specifically the much more severe melanoma.

Recent studies, such as those conducted in 2006 by Brij Saxena, PhD, who works in reproductive endocrinology at Cornell University's Weill Medical College, demonstrated that in mice with induced prostate cancer, the ones injected with betulinic acid had slower tumor growth, and greater cancer-cell death, suggesting that white birch may be helpful for men with prostate cancer.

I don't personally think it's desirable or ethical to do medical experiments on animals. It's been demonstrated in both test tube *(in vitro)* and animal *(in vivo)* studies that betulinic acid helps induce apoptosis (cell death) of cancer cells. Betulin is the powdery white substance that comes off on your fingers if you gently rub white birch bark. This betulin converts into betulinic acid, which is also concentrated into mushrooms that grow on birch trees, such as chaga mushrooms or birch polypores. These mushrooms, especially chaga, are now recognized as powerful immunomodulators that also have specific resonance for helping people healing from cancer. However, no plant or tree is simply a sum of constituents. It has a spirit, and is part of the unity of consciousness like everything else.

White Birch Bark Ritual

Gather some white birch bark from a fallen tree or branch. Let it dry thoroughly. White birch bark peels off the tree in strips and represents shedding what is no longer needed—what you've outgrown yet may still be clinging to. It is often used in rituals related to death and rebirth. Never peel the bark off all the way around a living tree trunk, because that can seriously harm or even kill the tree.

When you want to initiate a change in your life, meditate and ask for guidance to see how you are holding yourself back from being your whole, true self. Ask to be shown what you could choose to release in order to live more fully and with less fear. It may be a familiar theme that you are being asked to take to a deeper level; or something you've never looked at before may reveal itself to you.

Write a phrase or word, or draw an image that symbolizes whatever it is that you want to let go. This could be any physical habit, habit of mind, or old belief that is no longer serving you. Make sure that it is something for you to do, or stop doing—not some way in which you want someone else to change. Whenever we think that getting someone else to change is the key to our happiness, we are not seeing the truth. We can only be responsible for our choices, not someone else's.

Writing what you are letting go, on this bark "paper" that represents beginnings, symbolizes how endings are always followed by new beginnings. Rebirth follows death as spring follows winter. Release whatever you have written on the birch paper into a ritual fire. When you burn the bark, say aloud what you are releasing, or say it silently to yourself. Either way, you have powerfully initiated a change, and now the day-to-day work begins. It is spiritual-growth work you've chosen for yourself, so persevere and it will be worthwhile.

Many witches do this ritual on Halloween night (our new year), but I have introduced this ritual at New Year's Eve parties and found it well-received then too. Everyone enjoyed doing something meaningful as one year ended and the new one began. If there's a need for this ritual in your personal life at any time, though, then that's when you do it.

Among the various birch species, the one I know best is the black birch, also known as cherry birch or sweet birch. It's easy to mix up actual black cherry trees with cherry (black) birch trees because the leaf shapes are not that different at first look, and the bark of each has a relatively smooth, dark appearance that gleams with a red undertone. Both species have horizontal lenticels, small vents or breathing pores, all along their trunks. However, though you may easily confuse these trees by sight, you won't forget how birch smells when you learn to "scratch and sniff" the twigs, and black birch's unmistakable, delicious fragrance reveals itself. The distinctive aroma comes from methyl salicylate, or wintergreen oil. This is one of the constituents that make black birch as medicinal as it is delicious—it is rich in salicylic acid, making it pain-relieving and useful for sprains, aches, and arthritic pains.

It is one of the first fresh plants I harvest for infusions every spring and these infusions are almost universally loved. Fresh birch twig tea gets vital energy flowing through the body, akin to the way sap begins to flow through the tree again as the light and warmth revive its circulation, calling it back to an active phase of growth after its winter's rest.

BLACK BIRCH SPRING DELIGHT INFUSION

2 cups fresh black birch twigs

½ gallon water

Harvest small twigs from a black birch tree, ideally before it has leaves. (If you use twigs from a tree that already has leaves on it, you can put a few leaves into your infusion and dry the rest for a different infusion. Leaves are beneficial to the kidneys, but I leave them out of this infusion to get the maximum taste of wintergreen.)

Nick the outer bark every half-inch or so to reveal the green cambium layer underneath and help release the fragrant oils. Then cut the twigs into approximately half-inch pieces. Put them in the jar. Cover with boiled water. Cap and let steep overnight.

Enjoy!

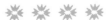

One day I was out in the woods and found myself drawn to a silvery-gray birch tree. I wrapped my arms around it and heard a female voice say, "I'm called Lady of the Woods, or you can call me Moon Birch." The first question that rose in my mind was, as always, "Did I make that up?" The first answer I gave myself, as usual, was, "Does it matter?" I've found that if I'm making it up, that means my imagination is finding a way to translate a truth into a story of some kind. More often, upon researching, I find that there is recorded history that verifies my intuitive experience, as in this case. Silver birch has long been known in the British Isles and Scandinavia as "the lady of the woods."

When I or one of my students intuitively "pick up" a piece of healing information, sometimes science has not yet discovered it. I've learned not to disregard these intuitive, magical experiences with the green ones, even when there is not yet any corroborating evidence, which often comes later.

My personal experience with black birch mostly involves using the tree's twigs as tea, tincture, and infused oil for healing skin conditions, especially eczema. Recently a friend was required to take blood thinners after surgery, and his back broke out almost immediately in a terrible rash (a known side effect of his medication). His girlfriend, who is allied with the black birch tree, used her homemade tincture on his rash, which immediately began improving as the tincture dried and soothed it. I suggested she also give him some tincture internally. Whenever possible, help skin heal by using herbs both inside and outside the body.

Birch is also frequently used to stimulate healing of the liver and lymph system, and the leaves are used to bring anti-inflammatory and other healing energies to the kidneys. Black birch bark and leaves help things flow generally, and can be beneficial for benign prostate gland enlargement (BPH).

Herbalist Ananda Wilson has written of her love affair with black birch. She has some creative suggestions such as:

Birch baths are excellent for the flu. They help dispel the fever, soothe retching, and relieve the aches. After soaking, oil the chest, lymph areas, and feet with birch infused oil, and wrap up nice and warm. Birch baths are also excellent for athletes after sports.

Here are some recipes for skin that include black birch, which I've used successfully with clients, family, and friends:

SKIN BLEND

¼ cup dried burdock root

¼ cup dried black birch twigs

½ cup dried sassafras leaves

1 tablespoon dried sassafras root

Put the herbs into a quart jar and cover with boiling water. Let steep for about 8 hours, and then decant and refrigerate, or heat and put into a stainless-steel or glass-insert thermos for drinking.

For a chronic or acute skin challenge, drink 1–2 cups daily for about six weeks, and then take a break. This allows you to shift to other herbs that you might want to drink, and also gives your body a chance to work on its own after having received this optimum herbal nourishment consistently for a time. You can always repeat a cycle of use after a break of two or more weeks. If you are using the herbs simply as a tonic without a specific need for it, then you might choose to drink it for two weeks or so, 3–4 times a year. In the spring it is also a nice wake-up tonic blend to drink after the cold winter.

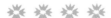

This blend of common herbs creates a delicious and powerful infusion for skin-clearing. It will deeply nourish and tone the liver, lymph system, and kidneys, helping them do their jobs so that the skin isn't overburdened as a filtration system. In Matt Wood's book, *The Earthwise Herbal,* he writes of burdock:

> With low absorption of lipids there is a shortage of these substances around the body. Burdock is thus associated with dry, scaly skin conditions and dry skin in general. Sometimes the sebaceous glands get blocked, due to a lack of oil moving through them, resulting in inflammation—hence the association of burdock with acne and boils.

The following is another skin-clearing recipe that helped a young man who had had a dramatic case of eczema on his face, hands, back, arms, and legs for about ten years. It had recently become year-round rather than "only" a winter manifestation, and it would "drive him crazy" with itching and peeling skin. His filtration systems had also been seriously taxed by eight years of psychotropic medications for his diagnosed schizo-affective disorder.

ECZEMA RELIEF INFUSION

2 parts dried red clover blossoms

1 part dried burdock root

1 part dried sarsaparilla root

½ part dried sassafras root

Fill a quart jar with the herbs, which should equal about one cup when combined. Cover with boiling water. Cap and steep the herbs overnight.

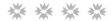

This combination of herbs to help the young man's skin also worked to strengthen his lymph, liver, and kidneys, similarly to the Skin Blend recipe above. In addition, the red clover helped to strengthen his nervous system and stabilize his mental state, while the burdock provided him with the deep grounding that he needed in order to heal on deeper levels. I have found that burdock can help someone know and accept that "you have a place in this world." He enjoyed drinking this infusion, and soon he no longer had to use the steroidal creams he'd been using for years.

We were also able to shift his diet from his staple white rice to brown rice, and to more whole foods, fruits, vegetables, wild foods, and other common herbs (such as dandelion and plantain) to help him reconnect with himself and his true nature. He went back to college, and graduated. He was able to work with his psychiatrist to slowly wean himself off of his psychotropic medication, and eventually was able to discontinue it altogether. He also began to garden in numerous gardens, working with me in the medicinal garden we were creating for our town.

Getting his hands in the earth on a regular basis brought him greater peace inside himself. It helped him know that, in addition to his intellectual pursuits, working with the earth was what he loved to do. In fact, he got in touch with me recently to let me know that he is feeling happy and healthy and is traveling around the country. He is having fun with friends, and doing meaningful, environmental work that gives him a sense of purpose.

Herbs for Burns

Nearly everyone is familiar with using fresh aloe leaf gel for a burn. Unless you live in a tropical climate where it's growing wild everywhere, it's smart to keep one or more aloe plants in your home for that purpose. In the kitchen, if you burn yourself on the stove, take a deep breath, thank your plant, gently pick a leaf, slit it open, and then spread some gel on the burn to help bring relief. It also helps if you've gotten sunburn. The aloe may sting at first, but then it soothes. Aloe gel is also nice as a skin conditioner—just apply it to your face at night before bed.

I often turn to lavender tea for burns (see below). Drinking it and washing the area with it soothes the pain and begins the healing process. People also use essential oil of lavender for healing burns. That works, too, and is convenient to carry with you. I make infused fresh-lavender oil, and this can be spread, or sprayed from a spray bottle, onto a burn. Lavender honey is marvelous to enjoy in tea or on toast, but it is a great healer for simple burns, too. Lavender honey will help prevent infection when used externally on a fresh burn.

The following skin-healing recipe is amazing and reliable. The amounts are approximate.

RELIEVE-THE-BURN-WITH-FLOWERS RECIPE

½ cup dried calendula blossoms

¼ cup dried rose blossoms

⅛ cup dried lavender flowers

Combine the flowers in a quart jar. Cover them with boiling water. Cap and let them steep for 20–30 minutes, no more than an hour. Strain out the herbs and let the tea cool down. Once it has cooled, dip a soft cloth into the tea and apply it as a cool fomentation, gently washing the burned skin for both immediate relief and skin-healing.

For whole body burns, add 1–2 quarts of the strained tea into a cool bath and soak for 20–30 minutes. Repeat often, until no longer needed.

Another good way to make this recipe is to put the calendula and rose into a pot, bring them just to a boil, and immediately turn the flame down as low as possible. After a minute or so, turn the heat off. Add the lavender into the pot and cover. Let the mixture stand, then strain the herbs out after 20–30 minutes.

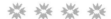

This blend, prepared either way, soothes burns so quickly that it has become one of my favorite recipes. This mixture is good to drink for skin- and nerve-healing, too, so you might want to put up an extra jar. I like to make the infusion a little lighter and drink some, too. It also helps the skin cells to repair in record time, especially with the calendula in it. The calendula marigold is a classic vulnerary or wound healer and a bad burn is a kind of injury to the skin and nerves within.

One of my former apprentices, herbalist Rossana Rossi, told me that she decided to try this blend for a client with a very bad case of itchy eczema, and it worked beautifully for that too. For maximum benefit, remember to drink it as well as put it on your skin.

Apple cider vinegar that has been infused for a month or so with either roses or elder blossoms is a fine medicine to relieve sunburns. These preparations are good to make ahead and keep on hand in case of need. Drinking elder blossom or rose teas, separately or together, nourishes the skin and the capillaries just below it, improves your circulation, and nourishes your skin to keep it fresh, smooth, and glowing with health.

Lemongrass infusion, once it's cooled down, is also helpful for healing burns. Lemongrass is often called "fever grass" in the tropics. Here, it grows in our gardens. In the tropics, it grows widely like the wild weed that it is.

St. J's Wort (*Hypericum perforatum* and other species) is another important herb to help the skin heal. I use it for burns of all sorts, but especially sunburn. I prefer to use it preventatively, so I slather the oil on myself to prevent sunburn. When I have the option I use the ointment because of the little bit of extra thickness that the beeswax layer provides.

ST. J'S WORT OINTMENT

1 ounce St. J's wort oil

1 tablespoon grated beeswax

Begin by making homemade St. J's wort oil. Steep flowers for at least 6 weeks in olive oil before squeezing them out and pouring the oil off. This oil should be a rich red color. (You can also buy St. J's wort oil; see Resources, page 509.)

Pour the oil into a shallow saucepan, and stir in beeswax. Keep stirring while you warm it over a very low flame, until the wax is completely melted and there are no lumps left in the oil.

Pour the warm oil-wax mixture into a jar, and cover it. It will solidify from the bottom up. Ointment is easier to carry than oil, so you can take this with you everywhere. It doesn't need to be refrigerated.

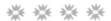

I have fair skin and used to sunburn badly, ever since I was a child. Then, starting in the mid-1980s when changes in the environment were escalating, I began to get fever blisters around my mouth every time I went out in the sun. They were painful, and it was pretty rough to deal with—I'd be leading weed walks with fresh leaves plastered over the sores! I've always felt a bit like the canary in the coal mine, with my body so very sensitive in response to my environment—an accurate predictor of reactions that would become more common among more people in the near future.

I've observed that St. J's isn't really a sunscreen. It is protective, but more as an adaptogen for the skin. In the past twenty-five years of using this herb for sun "screen" it has helped my skin adjust to the changing environment, specifically to the depletion of our planet's protective ozone layer. My skin is not as vulnerable as it always was to burning, and I don't get those fever blisters anymore. I've asked others who use this herb for skin protection what they've noticed about their skin, and many have reported similar responses.

I theorize that the plants are adjusting to the changes, and are helping us adjust, too, even though the process of natural evolution is usually much slower. Alarmingly, even people with beautiful ebony skin are suffering from burns these days, so it's wise to protect your skin even if you never used to need protection before. When you're out in the hot sun, or in the water, reapply it frequently. Also, if you must undergo radiation treatment, St. J's wort oil is a good herbal ally to protect your skin from radiation burns.

I use St. J's oil for viral infections that show up on the skin, such as chicken pox and herpes. St. J's oil will be absorbed through the skin into the nerve endings to help bring relief and soothe the pain. It will also hasten the healing of the condition. It is a specific for relieving the pain of shingles, and for herpes sores on the mouth or genitals. I like to combine or alternate it with essential oil of camphor for mouth sores, so as to supplement St. J's moistening, soothing, healing effects with camphor oil's drying properties to speed up the closing of the painful sore.

Oats are well known for being restorative to the skin, and can be turned to anytime there is a red, itchy rash or other skin inflammation.

It is used both internally as an infusion and externally in washes, baths, scrubs, and soaps.

SIMPLE OAT STRAW SCRUB

Loosely grind rolled oats in an electric grinder (or a mortar and pestle). Put these into a glass jar in your bathroom and combine with warm water for a gentle exfoliant, to stimulate healthy skin on your face and body.

This recipe is easy, inexpensive, and effective, and my favorite way to use it, but it also combines beautifully with a small amount of other herbs such as rose or lavender.

Another lovely addition is ground almonds, though that mix may be more likely to spoil without refrigeration. Make small batches to be sure it's fresh, and also so you can try different recipes and see what works best for your skin.

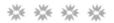

Here is a nice astringent, tonic recipe that's helpful to reduce and remove small bumps on any part of the skin.

BUMPS-BE-GONE SKIN INFUSION

¼ cup dried yarrow flowers

¼ cup dried chamomile flowers

Pour boiling water over the dried flowers in a pint jar. Cover and let them steep for 30 minutes.

Strain very well. This infusion must be kept refrigerated, though a small usage bottle can be left out for a day or two if it's not too humid or hot. If it is too hot to leave it out, the refrigerated herbs will feel great on your skin!

Splash it on the affected area with your hands or apply it with a washcloth twice a day.

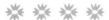

This recipe originated when a woman came to me who had tried everything (of course) over the counter, prescribed, and herbal, to help her with an annoying and slightly embarrassing problem. She said, "I always have little tiny bumps on my butt that never really go away. They don't hurt, but sometimes they itch and are uncomfortable, and I really don't want them there. Can any herbs help?" I figured they were probably some kind of heat rash.

These herbs helped like nothing else had, and she was happy with her baby-soft bottom. Meanwhile, I asked some men to try it for shaving bumps, and they liked it too. I find it to be a cooling astringent, particularly nice on my face in the summer after a day out in the sun. It smells good, and yarrow is a pretty good insect repellent, too.

Chickweed *(Stellaria media)*

This plant, which Susun Weed sweetly calls, "the little white star-flower plant," is a wild and delicious edible, so diverse in her healing gifts that her healing capabilities are out of all proportion to her size (to paraphrase Juliette de Bairacli Levy, referring to petite *Veronica officinalis*).

Chickweed likes brisk weather, and grows abundantly in spring and fall. If you are lucky enough to find her in the summer, it will always be in wet, shaded places. She doesn't enjoy the hot sun shining directly on her, and similarly discourages excess dry heat inside our bodies.

I remember my first herbal healing class and weed walk in New York City in the 1980s. It was very early spring, and had been snowing on and off for days. I took the students for a stroll around my urban block, starting on 14th Street and 6th Avenue. On 15th Street, in a sheltered doorway, I used a discarded paper cup to shovel away five inches of fresh snow, revealing a vibrant patch of chickweed in full flower. Everyone ooohed and aaahed at this miracle! This is one *cool* herb.

I primarily use fresh chickweed, whether I'm eating it in salad or mashing it up with saliva, in a mortar and pestle, or in boiled water to apply as a poultice. I use it secondarily as a dried herb for teas, fomentations, and poultices. When it's not available fresh, I also use it as a fresh-plant tincture or as infused oil or ointment. The last two preparations are tricky to store because of the natural moisture in the plant, but it can be done. Recipes for all three follow the chickweed stories below.

I love chickweed for skin—especially for hot, dry, itchy skin—as chickweed epitomizes cool, moist juiciness. Chickweed is helpful internally and externally for bacterial and viral infections manifesting through the skin, such as chicken pox or measles, and for dissolving hard or fluid-filled cystic lumps that are pulling the skin taut as they grow. Chickweed is also great for drawing foreign objects such as splinters or glass shards out of the body.

One of my former apprentices (Donna Reynolds of Willow Moon Herbals) had been trying unsuccessfully to interest her brother in using herbal medicine after he'd injured his hand in a carpentry incident. He had been able to extract a large wood splinter, but his hand remained swollen and painful even after a full round of antibiotics. Next he had gone to the local medical center, where they shone strong lights through his hand, determined that the wood pieces were all out, and couldn't figure out why he still had that "ghost" pain. It became a red-hot burning pain, and his index finger swelled and began to fester. As so often happens, the help of herbs is finally accepted when conventional medicine has nothing else to offer and the person feels they have nothing to lose in trying herbs.

Donna gave him some fresh chickweed tincture, with instructions to apply a bandage soaked in it. Within 2–3 days of applying fresh, chickweed-soaked bandages, a wedge-shaped piece of wood approximately an inch long, which had originally lodged in the palm of his hand, emerged from just under the first joint where the index finger meets the palm. This piece had been in his hand for a month, causing him severe pain and ongoing infection, until her homemade chickweed tincture cooled everything off and pulled it right out!

My best girlfriend had a large, hard cyst protruding from her right cheek. The skin was pulled taut, and looked like it was straining to cover the round lump. Surgery was scheduled. Before the surgery date, we met in New Mexico for some needed time together. I brought some home-made chickweed ointment for her, explaining that if she used it consistently it would help soften and dissolve the cyst, potentially saving her a surgical procedure.

During our road trip (I was mostly the passenger) I noticed that she wasn't remembering to use it often enough, so I took the ointment back. While we were driving, or in our apartment—or anytime I thought of it—I applied it to her cheek myself, perhaps 6–8 times a day. When she returned home a week later, the cyst was gone. Surgery cancelled. No recurrence. I don't recall if I had her drink chickweed tincture in water as well, but that would have been a wise choice. Whenever it's possible to approach healing from both inside and out, do it! You need to have chickweed oil to make the ointment from. So we'll start with that:

SIMPLE CHICKWEED OIL

Fresh, never-washed chickweed stalks, leaves, and flowers

Olive oil

Cut up the chickweed and completely fill a glass jar. Cover with olive oil. Cap and label the jar. Set it on a saucer, out of direct sunlight.

For the first week or two, top up with oil as needed, and continue to poke any chickweed down under the oil to discourage mold.

Decant after exactly 6 weeks for maximum strength without spoilage. Let the decanted oil sit for 24 hours, and then pour it off one more time, carefully leaving behind any water sitting on the bottom. That tiny bit of watery oil can be discarded, or would be fine for immediate use within a couple of days.

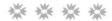

CHICKWEED OINTMENT

1 ounce chickweed oil (see above)

1 teaspoon–1 tablespoon beeswax

Gently heat the decanted oil. Stir in grated beeswax to achieve desired firmness. Pour the mixture into a jar when all the beeswax has melted, and cap it. It will be ready for use in about 15–30 minutes, depending on how much you are making at once.

Remember to use a wide enough jar to get your finger into even when the ointment is almost gone.

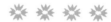

SIMPLE CHICKWEED TINCTURE

Aerial parts of fresh chickweed, preferably in flower

100-proof vodka

Follow the same procedure described for making the infused oil (above).

Use 100-proof vodka as the menstruum instead of olive oil. With vodka, there isn't the same concern regarding mold, so you can let it sit longer than 6 weeks. Still, do top up the tincture with vodka for the first week or two. Tincture faeries *love* to sip chickweed.

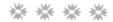

Fresh, mashed chickweed makes a soothing poultice for eyes, too. I use it for tired or dry eyes, for people who wear contact lenses, and/or after spending a lot of time staring at screens. I especially value chickweed poultices for infections such as pinkeye (conjunctivitis). They are very effective. A poultice that you use to moisten dryness or soothe fatigue can be reused if necessary, but never reuse a poultice for drawing out infected matter, because you can all too easily reintroduce the infection that way.

I love the salty, green taste of fresh chickweed. Her high vitamin and mineral content aids the body as a nutritious wild vegetable that can be eaten raw or lightly cooked. Chickweed, rich in saponins, helps cellular membranes become more permeable, so they can better receive nutrients and release wastes, thus benefiting every system in the body.

I value chickweed as a tonic for the glandular/endocrine system, too. I have a client with chemical sensitivities and Sjögren's syndrome who is benefitting from daily use of chickweed tincture. I turn to chickweed for reliable help in dissolving ovarian cysts, even unusual ones, such as dermoid cysts. It is of value in helping to nourish and tone the thyroid (especially when low-functioning), and aids healthy metabolism.

Chickweed's saponins also emulsify fat. These tonic and emulsifying properties have helped chickweed gain a well-deserved reputation as an herb that's helpful for releasing excess weight. Chickweed's wet, cooling nature is healing for dry coughs, and generally will help activate and move the lymph along when there is a feverish infection in skin, lungs, or intestines. I combine chickweed with oats and nettles internally (and externally in baths) for infectious, itchy skin conditions as well as for the endocrine system. I have used it with mullein leaf infusion or tincture for dry coughs.

I have seen it work effectively with dandelion root for supporting good elimination. We need digestive fire for assimilating our food, but if we lack enough moisture in the intestines, elimination can become hard, causing dry stools and constipation. This can also lead to bleeding in the rectum. I have used chickweed successfully (often in combination with slippery elm powder and yogurt) for blood in the stools originating from constipation that ended up causing bleeding hemorrhoids. I have also used it for anal fissures and for raw, bleeding tissue caused by poor diet, bacterial infections, or unknown reasons that needed to be explored further after the symptom had been resolved. I have found chickweed infallible. It can also be applied as oil or ointment, or made into a suppository. It combines happily with witch hazel, plantain, yarrow, and/or calendula oils for this purpose. Internally, 1–2 droppers of tincture added into water or tea is used 3–4 times daily.

ONE MORE CHICKWEED STORY

My friend Tommy was excited to be the best man at his older brother's wedding. Those of us in the wedding party gathered at the family home a few days before the wedding. The first morning, Tommy awoke with a large swelling on his otherwise handsome chin. He was unhappy about the prospect of sporting a lump the size of an oversized marble on his chin throughout the wedding and in all the pictures. But he shrugged his shoulders and accepted it as something that couldn't be changed. After all, the wedding was in three days.

Herbs to the rescue! I went out to the lawn and found chickweed growing there. "Perfect!" I said to myself, grateful to so easily find just what he needed. I called him outside and explained that chickweed excels at dissolving cysts and other lumps and bumps, especially hot, fluid-filled ones. It can help infected cuts and rashes too. He looked at me doubtfully, and said this had happened from an ingrown hair.

"No problem," I replied. "It will help your body deal with it, by drawing out the hair or helping your body reabsorb it, and it will take the redness and heat out too. It looks like it is getting infected. Does it hurt?" He affirmed that it did. "This will help. It will get the swelling down substantially, if not all the way," I added confidently.

Tommy agreed that there was nothing to lose, and though he gave me a strange look when I said that either he or I should chew up the small handful of chickweed I was holding and then press it to his chin for about ten minutes, he did it. About ten seconds passed before he said, a little suspiciously, "It took the pain away. Did it numb it out?"

"No, it cooled it off. And it's drawing out the inflammation that's your body's natural immune response to an 'invader'—in this case, the ingrown hair."

"Wow," he said, with a new degree of respect and appreciation in his voice. I left him holding the poultice against his chin while I gathered about two more cups of chickweed from the lawn to store in a ziplock bag in the refrigerator. We repeated the poultice twice more that day and three times the next, each time using enough chickweed to cover the area liberally. The bump got smaller, softer, and cooler to the touch each time.

On the last day, I mashed up the fresh chickweed a bit with a mortar and pestle, and then poured a cup of boiled water over it to make tea and a poultice. After it steeped for about fifteen minutes, Tommy used the herbs for his poultice and drank the tea. Since this was the final day before the wedding, I wanted to help his healing from the inside out too.

By the next morning there was no lump—just a tiny swelling without pain or redness. Tommy's comfort and vanity were soothed, and he could enjoy the day fully!

We can all celebrate chickweed's great healing powers. Her smooth stalks have tiny hairs that spiral around them, indicating chickweed's helpfulness for all parts of the body that have hair on them, such as lungs, intestines, and skin. Her leaves end in sharp points, indicating her ability to help with cuts and wounds. She is juicy, indicating her ability to moisten anything she touches, helping inflamed joints, dry bronchia, lungs, or intestines. Finally, chickweed is vibrantly green, indicating the deep nourishment that she offers us.

Women's Sexual/ Reproductive System

Herbs and more for health, acute illnesses, and chronic challenges of the female reproductive system; hormonal support and optimum nourishment for life-long vitality and joy through menstrual, mothering, and menopausal life-cycles and beyond.

The proximity of the urinary system to the sexual/reproductive organs brings the health of the kidneys and bladder into play when we look at the health of this system, and that information is equally relevant to men's health, as is much of the herbal and spiritual healing information in this chapter.

This complex system, mostly Water and Earth, but incorporating *all* of the elements, is comprised of the connections between our psyches and our nervous, hormonal/reproductive and endocrine systems. It is a rhythmic system that pulses through our bodies, changing them continuously and cyclically throughout our lives.

Our bellies and breasts wax and wane again and again, like the moon guiding the tides of the sea to rise and fall. Lymph fluid flows through our breasts, and milk flows out of them. The health of our liver and digestive system is reflected in the health or illness found in our ovaries, cervixes, and wombs, and in the nutrient-rich lifeblood that builds up and releases during our menstrual cycles and forms and nourishes our babies' bodies during pregnancy.

Nourishing the workings of the digestive, cardiovascular, and musculoskeletal systems, as well as the skin, often takes center stage for keeping this system healthy during our menopausal years. The menopausal years can be as confusing in some ways as puberty and adolescence, but they also offer us a rite of passage with a more mature focus, a passage that calls for intense self-care and reflection, a time of going within that allows for shedding of old skins and growth into what we are becoming. At best, this culminates in stepping more fully into one's changing role in the world as a complete and confident woman of power who can now use her love and energy in devotion to the health of the larger community.

That then launches us into the final chapters of our lives when we grow into being elders. The more nourishment and care we've provided ourselves during the years leading up to this, the stronger and healthier we will be in our post-menopausal years, and the more ready we are to take on the mantle of our personal power.

This system and its health, acute illnesses and chronic challenges often offer us teachings around enhancing the quality of our relationship with our bodies/ourselves (Earth), and deepening our self-acceptance and self-love (Water). Illuminating the quality and nature of our relationships with others is key, too, in this most intimate system (Fire and Air, passion and joy, spaciousness, and inter-being). All of our past and present relationships can impact our sexual/reproductive health, starting with our relationships with our mother and father, whose relationship and shared sexuality brought us into being in the first place, incarnating us here in form.

Many challenges center around how we view our bodies and our femaleness within the matrix of the culture we live in. We are taught that our primary value is in how well we fit into standardized images of false beauty. Women are also taught that sexuality is the foremost measure of our worth, and at the same time that expressing our own sexual pleasure and bliss is not acceptable, and certainly not spiritual, and that our sexuality puts us at risk of harm. And if we are harmed, it is our own fault for being too sexual.

These confusing and dangerous messages from our adolescent, patriarchal culture can often wreak havoc in women's bodies and psyches. It literally makes women (and men) sick.

Women's bodies are very responsive to our emotional states of being, and we take a lot of our unprocessed emotional "stuff" into our breasts, wombs, and ovaries. I remember Rosemary Gladstar once joking that a woman could have a fight with her lover and five minutes later have a vaginal infection. I've seen it happen. It can also be a way of saying "No" to being sexually active (just not the healthiest way).

And though I've looked at sexual health mainly through the lens of women's health and female bodies, I see the same and other disempowering internal and external messages affect men who stuff their feelings into their bodies too (even though false power—power over women—is offered instead).

There are also external, health-disrupting factors such as processed food, excessive electromagnetic frequencies, endocrine disrupters and exogenous estrogens in our environment. Sexual health, like all areas of our health and all things related to living a satisfying, creative, healthy life, is not only a personal, physical issue but a societal one.

The good news is that our bodies respond really well to love and attention, time spent in nature, regular movement, and to whole foods and the right herbs. Herbs love people, and bring much healing to anyone who will give themselves the time and attention and herbs they need to heal. That's been my experience far more often than not. And it's never too late to start taking time to care and tend to you. You're worth it!

· · · ● · · ·

Some of my favorite women's sexual/reproductive-system allies are: artemisia, motherwort, red clover, red raspberry, lady's mantle, skullcap, chaste berry, dandelion, violet, peach, lemon balm, chickweed, and wild carrot.

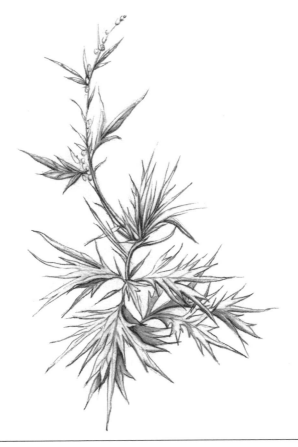

Mugwort

Mugwort/Cronewort (*Artemisia vulgaris* and other species)

Body: steadies nerves and strengthens digestion; minerals
nourish bones and joints; hormonal regulator and tonic for
ovaries and uterus.

Mind: sharpens intuition and perception; strengthens memory.

Heart: reawakens the heart's truest desires; strengthens the courage
of one's convictions; awakens wild and free nature.

Soul: reawakens awareness and embodiment of divine, fierce female
energy and your deepest dreams; opens you to guidance from
night dreams.

Mugwort/Cronewort

I am Artemisia—
I'm bitter and green.
I tone liver and stomach
And keep your mind keen.

I have vitamins galore
And minerals, too.
They've called me eldest of worts—
You know it is true.

I keep harmful bugs out of
Your belly within,
And I help with removing
Rashes from your skin.

And not only that,
You can put me in a drawer
And wool-eating moths
Won't bother you anymore.

What I really love
Is to tonify your nerves
So that you are strong
Even when life throws you curves.

I balance hormones,
Increase your menstrual flow,
Help you with cramping
And PMS, too, you know.

I help you to dream,
To envision what you need,

To journey within
So your true passions you'll heed.

Drink me and you may reclaim
Your Self, free and true.
Eat me and I'll help you dance
And howl moonward, too.

For men I am Pan;
For women, I'm Artemis.
I am eldest of worts.
Medicine is part of us.

This sacred wild herb, this prolific weed, has leaves that are green on top and silvery gray underneath. In the early spring when the leaves are tiny, they are dainty, bright green and innocent-looking. The hair underneath is subtly white and feels like felt, not yet woolly and silver with age. Over the course of the growing season, the shape of the leaves changes utterly, from a multi-lobed leaf to a spear-shaped one, and the green grows into a deeper olive color.

Artemisia is a wise being and wants you to be one, too—to acknowledge and use your wisdom. The Anglo-Saxons called her "the eldest of worts" and consider her one of their nine sacred herbs. This is a moon or lunar-energy plant, a woman's medicine that helps with regulating menstrual cycles, relieving cramps, generally easing symptoms of premenstrual and menopausal challenges through abundant nourishment and tonic effects on the liver.

She isn't for women only, however, as artemisia is a systemic tonic with effects throughout the body. This plant offers green medicine that strengthens nerves, digestion, kidneys, lungs, and the musculoskeletal system. I turn to artemisia tincture, vinegar or tea when there is simple indigestion or heartburn after a meal. Not much is needed—between 1 teaspoon and 1 tablespoon of mugwort vinegar in water or tea, or 25–30 drops of tincture, or one cup of tea. It can be used similarly half an hour before a meal, as preventative medicine. Artemisia vulgaris is a bitter aromatic tonic for the digestive system. Regular use of this herb will lessen the symptomatic need for a curative remedy. She is also a mineral-rich tonic for the central nervous system, and thus nourishes the brain and improves memory.

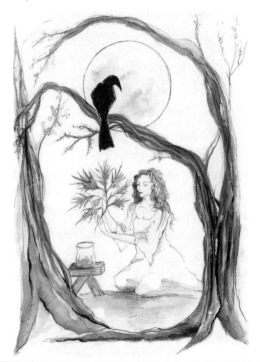

Full Moon Tincture

MAGICAL MOON-BATH/ *ARTEMISIA VULGARIS* TINCTURE

Fresh *Artemisia vulgaris* leaves and upper stalks

100-proof vodka in glass bottle

Gather artemisia under the light of the full moon, nearest Summer Solstice in June (December if you're in the Southern Hemisphere). Sit outside, bathing in the moonlight as you make an artemisia leaf-and-stalk full-moon tincture. (You can also gather the artemisia at dusk for another especially magical tincture.)

Tear or cut up your artemisia plant parts very well and put them into a glass jar, filled ½–1 inch from the top, neither jammed in nor loosely packed. Cover the plant material with vodka, pouring it in slowly to see that all the plant material gets saturated. You can poke through the plant material in the bottle with a chopstick or twig to help. Make sure the plant material is not sticking up out of the liquid. Fill the bottle as full as possible with the vodka. This helps the plant's properties to be more fully extracted into the menstruum.

Wait about 6 weeks for your full-moon tincture to be ready. That will be around the time of a dark, new moon, and this is a great time to carefully decant your magical mugwort tincture into another jar or into a spouted pitcher.

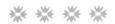

Another beautiful and magical preparation can be made by gathering artemisia's yellow and red flowers just as they open—late summer into early fall—and tincturing them on their own. Herbal guidebooks call these and other wee flowers "inconspicuous." That depends on how closely you're looking, so look closely and they will be conspicuous to you. If you don't have a local teacher yet, spend time outdoors, walking slowly, and stop often to observe the plants and trees that live around you.

These flowers don't need to be cut up at all, just put into your jar. This makes a divine and delicious tincture for visioning.

Speaking of vision, smoke dried artemisia leaves and flowers in a pipe or rolled in rice paper to strengthen your intuitive wisdom and inner vision. I call this plant *the intoxicant that helps you to remember.* Remember what? Whatever it is you need to remember, including who you truly are and what your purpose is here. Artemisia helps you access the truest dreams of your heart and soul. Like a wise grandmother, she will guide you and help you to access your own questions and answers. *Listening* to your inner wisdom, however, is up to you. It is your choice. She will, if asked, strengthen you for your journey of life and help you have the courage to live it authentically.

Artemisia, whether drunk, smoked, eaten, or bathed in, strengthens a woman and encourages her in claiming her independence and self-esteem, the kind of belief in herself that needs no external validation. The goddess Artemis is known for teaching women to be physically strong and vital, to stake claim to their own bodies and minds. Artemis, also known as Diana, the huntress, is a virgin goddess—"virgin" in the original meaning of a woman who is whole unto herself and owned by no one.

Artemisia can also help men reclaim their belief in themselves and the wisdom of the divine feminine. This helps them not only to respect and value the women in their lives, but also to connect to their own healthy, natural sexuality through freeing their minds from culturally programmed self-definitions. Male sexuality has been subverted, packaged and sold in Western culture to the detriment of men, women, children, and our planet. Men, like women, have been largely brainwashed and programmed. After drinking a cup of tea made with flowering artemisia, a man in class said, "This plant sharpens me. It makes me keen." Yes, it offers an intriguing combination of sharpening both internal vision and external perceptions as well as helping us to soften our vision and go within and dream—quite a talented plant!

Though artemisia is undeniably a plant that opens a direct link with the divine feminine and the intertwined web of life, this plant has profound physical medicine to offer us. Herbalist Susun Weed recommends artemisia steams for rapid relief of bronchial congestion, and the tea or tincture for children's fevers.

Artemisia vulgaris is not only an herbal medicine, but an integral part of the cuisine in Japan, and is also eaten in China, Korea, and Germany. Artemisia vulgaris is rich in trace minerals that nourish the nervous system, as well as nutritive vitamins such as ascorbic acid (vitamin C), beta-carotene (vitamin A), and the B complex. To benefit from the nutritive gifts of artemisia, eat the young spring leaves in salads, and the fresh growing tops in summer. The older leaves can be cut into small pieces and added to cooking. Putting the plant up in vinegar is viable at any time of the year and is one of the best ways to extract her nerve- and bone-strengthening minerals. Experiment with making vinegars in spring, summer, and fall when she is in different stages of growth. Young artemisia vinegar has a lighter, aromatic bittersweet taste while artemisia's bitter taste and digestive-tonic qualities increase with age.

ARTEMISIA VINEGAR

Fresh young *Artemisia vulgaris* leaves and stalks (or mature leaves)

Apple cider vinegar

Wide-mouthed pint (or larger) jar

Gather and rip or cut up enough fresh mugwort/cronewort to fill the jar. Cover it with apple cider vinegar and fill to the top. As with any vinegar preparation, put a piece of unbleached parchment paper under a metal lid to prevent rusting, or use a plastic lid or a cork. In six or more weeks you can decant your vinegar by pouring off the liquid and squeezing out the leaves.

Use the vinegar for cooking or for salad dressings and in sauces as a tasty, nourishing tonic, or take a tablespoon of the infused vinegar in water half an hour before or after a meal as a digestive medicine. It can also be used daily by the spoonful, taken alone or with an equal amount of raw honey in a glass of water, to ease the stiffness of arthritis.

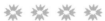

Artemisia helps uterine and ovarian pain when taken as a tea or tincture, so I use it for menstrual cramps, menopausal discomforts, and the pain of ovarian cysts. Artemisia moves energy in the uterus and can be especially helpful for women with clots. Be aware, however, that it may increase the menstrual flow as it does this.

For cramps it can also be mixed with aromatic, antispasmodic herbs like chamomile flowers or catnip leaves (flowers optional), which will also soften the strong taste. Add about one tablespoon of the chamomile flowers or catnip leaves to a quarter-cup of artemisia herb per quart jar. This works better than sweetening it with honey because shifting the bitter taste too much will diminish artemisia's ability to tone and strengthen the liver, improve bile production, and aid digestion. These additional herbs are not necessary, but will add to the pain-relieving qualities and help ease the digestive distress that accompanies menstruation for many women, too.

I was a fledgling herbalist the first time a client came to me who had gone to doctors for almost ten years looking for both the cause and the answer to her horrible menstrual cramps. She had tried drugs, and couldn't tolerate the side effects. She had tried therapy, and found it irrelevant. She was simply tired of losing so much time each month to severe pain, and found it distressing that there was nothing to be done about it. She told me that she couldn't even believe she had come to see me because, honestly, what was the point?

We discussed some dietary changes she might make, and some alternate approaches to stresses in her life. As we talked, she shared with me that she loved being a woman and didn't have mixed feelings about her body. As I listened to her, I heard the truth in her words and realized that she carried less shame and baggage than most women discover we've been carrying when we take the time to investigate.

Her only problem was that she had come to hate and fear her monthly menstrual cycle and that was, of course, a big problem. I have since heard variations of this story thousands of times—usually with much more self-judgment issues connected with the physical distresses, but not always.

I had had problems with severe cramps all my life too, and could fully relate to what she was telling me. I told her that I had found enormous relief from reconnecting with and learning to love the ever-changing roundness of my belly, and with delving into the intuitive and psychic magic that was part of becoming a more conscious menstruating woman. I shared stories with her about the healing I was experiencing by taking time for myself during my moon time, and that two herbs had helped me more than any others that I'd tried. I suggested that we start her with those. I'm not exaggerating when I tell you that she laughed so hard that she fell off my living-room couch! She could not believe that anything so simple as taking two herbs would help her at all. "Well, they won't hurt you," I gently persuaded her, handing her two tincture bottles, "and I made these myself, so would you like to try them?"

Within one month of using motherwort tincture *(Leonurus cardiaca)* several times during the daytime, and mugwort tincture or tea, and sometimes baths, during the evening and night, her cramps had decreased considerably. She told me this in utter disbelief.

Sometimes there is a dramatic response to herbs right away, as if the body is saying, *Thank you, I needed that!*—and then the dramatic healing response decreases as the adjustment and assimilation process goes on. It is as if the herb is giving you a taste of what's possible, but the body and psyche need time to adjust. Then slow, gradual change begins, which will be more sustainable. In this young woman's case, her monthly experience changed from intolerable to tolerable to healthy. She stayed in touch with me for another four or five years and actually came to love her monthly cycle. She also shared the simple, yet profound medicine of mugwort and motherwort with many of her friends and the women in her family. I imagine her now and wonder if perhaps she's teaching her own daughters how to love and support their bodies' natural rhythms as they enter into their own moon-times.

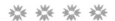

Another way I like to use artemisia is in a bath for both physical and spiritual healing.

ARTEMISIA BATH PREPARATION

2 cups dried artemisia leaves and stalks (up to 4 cups if fresh)

½ gallon water

Pour boiling water over the herbs in the jar. Cap and let the herbs steep for 2–4 hours. Pour through a fine strainer after the tub has been filled with water, and swirl it into the bath water.

This bath will ease pain, stimulate dreams and intuition, help resolve fungal skin infections, calm your nerves and inspire you to continue to practice self-care. Soak for at least 20 minutes for maximum benefit.

❋ ❋ ❋ ❋

RITUAL ARTEMISIA BATH PREPARATION I

You can also prepare artemisia as a ritual bath. A ritual bath is a bath that has a specific intention connected with it, such as to release something that's been troubling you, or to ask for guidance about a particular issue.

Use stalks gathered when in flower to make the infusion for this bath. If that's not possible, prepare it as above, with conscious intention, and ritually add 13 drops of flower tincture to the bath before you enter it.

After you've soaked for some time, pour the water over yourself with a gourd (or special cup) to complete your spiritual bathing. Allow yourself to air-dry naturally when you get out of the tub.

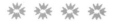

RITUAL ARTEMISIA BATH PREPARATION II

If you are doing this ritual outdoors somewhere, and are not getting into a tub, gather together a bundle of 1–3 foot long fresh stems of artemisia.

You can simply hold them together or tie them. Dip the bundle tips into cool or tepid artemisia tea and then tap them on different areas of your body, effectively sprinkling and spraying the infusion all over you.

Make sure that when you are done, you leave the plants you used and any leftover tea outside on the ground as an offering. Do not reuse these plants.

This last version is actually lovely to do with and for others, especially in a wild setting, though it could be done in a suburban back yard or living room as well. I first experienced this kind of spiritual bathing with a *curandera* in Mexico. Ecuadorean wise woman Rocío Alarcón reintroduced me to its gentle power, for which I'm grateful. It is perfect for a releasing ritual.

You may choose to mix other herbs into the bath or bundles to suit your physical and/or spiritual purposes, but please don't underestimate the power of simples either. Each herb is complex—really about as "simple" as any human being!

Artemisia is a metaphysical ally, a woman's herb that's also beneficial to men. It is also a strengthening food and, like the majority of plants written about in *The Gift of Healing Herbs,* can be enjoyed in many beneficial ways whether you are ill or not.

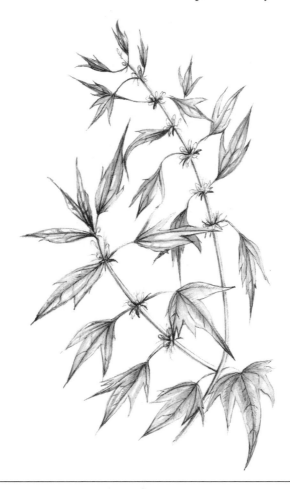

Motherwort

Motherwort *(Leonurus cardiaca)*

Body: relaxes womb, helps female hormonal imbalances, steadies
a fast or irregular heartbeat, calms an over-active thyroid, relieves
constipation.

Mind: induces calmness, eases anxiety.

Heart: soothes emotions—turmoil, anger, frustration, grief,
resentment, heartache.

Soul: invokes openness, acceptance, and peace.

Motherwort

Oh motherwort, dearest motherwort,
You are more precious than gold.
We call you the lion-hearted one;
It's time your story was told.

You are complex, bitter to our taste
Yet sweet of spirit and heart,
When anyone asks you for comfort,
You're willing to do your part.

I've seen you support stressed new mothers;
Of course you calm fathers, too.
Even kids benefit from your gifts.
You help us all shine like new.

You bring peace and soothe anxiety
afflicting heart, mind, or womb,
And fill us with determination
So we won't give in to gloom.

It's said you bring immortality,
And whether or not that's true
You help me feel so much happier,
I will always live with you.

Motherwort's lower leaves are maple-like, and her upper leaves become thinner and thinner until they are like little spears. Her flowers are glorious, orchid-like pink blossoms that are nestled inside of spiky whorls at the junctures of the leaves and central stalks. Her thick stalks are perfectly square (an indication she belongs to the mint family) and grow deeply red over time, reflecting motherwort's relationship to the blood and her resonant power to regulate the rhythms of the heart and womb.

I was taught that many plants helpful to the womb also help the heart. Motherwort's botanical name, *Leonurus cardiaca,* means "the lion-hearted one" and motherwort, also known as the mother's weed, does benefit the heart both physically and emotionally. When someone has palpitations or an irregular heartbeat, motherwort is a great remedy. I have seen it resolve palpitations quickly and completely. It is also helpful in cases of angina.

This beautiful bitter herb brings profound relaxation to the womb. Motherwort is anti-spasmodic, and thus helpful for relieving menstrual cramps. Think of a tightly clenched fist relaxing into an open hand to appreciate motherwort's action on the uterus.

If you are a woman with a very heavy menstrual flow, proceed with common-sense caution and use small doses of 5–10 drops of tincture in water to check out how the plant works with your body, since motherwort can increase menstrual bleeding for some women. I used to have heavy menses, and motherwort never increased my bleeding no matter how much I used. I relied on it every month for relief. Motherwort can also be helpful for a woman with amenorrhea, or lack of menstruation. This is not a plant for frequent use by women with fibroids or endometriosis, though occasional use is not contraindicated unless your inner sense or body wisdom tells you otherwise.

Motherwort is a hormonal and nerve tonic, and as such is a fantastic herb to use for that irritable time of pent-up emotion or heightened sensitivity that many women experience right before menstruation begins. She nourishes the nerves with assimilable calcium. She also prevents menstrual cramping by helping relax the stomach and intestines, easing the digestive distress and belly tension that can accompany menses.

Motherwort is not a laxative but a relaxant, so when digestive distress, especially constipation, is due to nervous tension, motherwort is an excellent ally taken as a bitter tea or as a tincture. Additionally, if you get tense having to move your bowels in unfamiliar surroundings and suffer from constipation when traveling, motherwort is a good ally to take along with you. Motherwort is underrated as a digestive bitter to promote healthy bowel movements. It should be taken unsweetened for the best digestive effect.

It is especially valuable in any condition where nervous tension or anxiety is the root of the problem, because motherwort is deeply calming to the nerves and helpful for congestive states in general, including emotional congestion.

MOTHERWORT FOR MENSTRUAL CRAMPS

Rina Nissim, who runs the Dispensaire des Femmes in Switzerland and is the author of *Natural Gynecology for Women,* writes that three cups a day of motherwort decoction will help with painful periods and anemia. I like to nibble motherwort leaves, but they are so bitter that most people don't choose to join me when I indulge in it. I like motherwort but still can't imagine drinking three cups of decoction a day. Many herbalists, myself included, recommend and most often use motherwort as a tincture because of the taste. I have always found the tincture effective.

No matter how you take it, motherwort is unexcelled for relieving cramps of a congestive, tense nature, and it nourishes the hormonal system at the same time. It can be used on a continuum of tiny to large doses depending on the woman and her situation. There were some months when all I wanted to do was sit near the plant, and other months where I needed frequent doses of tincture to alleviate my menstrual cramps.

MOTHERWORT TINCTURE

Fresh motherwort (above-ground parts in flower)
100-proof vodka

Tear up the plant into small pieces. Fill a jar with it. Cover the plant material and fill the jar completely with vodka. Wait 6 weeks or more before decanting it.

Put 10–13 drops or more (up to a huge dose of 1 teaspoon) in any amount of room temperature-to-hot water or tea. Warm or hot liquids tend to be more helpful for opening up congestive conditions. Drink your motherwort and take some deep breaths to help your womb soften. If you can apply a hot-water bottle to your belly, do that too. That can be a great help for easing menstrual cramps, and is nice to sleep with. If your cramps are not relieved in 10–15 minutes, repeat the tincture dose every

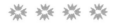

10 minutes until relief is felt. Repeat as needed. You could also put 25–50 drops in your water bottle and sip it throughout the day.

This is my favorite simple remedy for menstrual cramps. When I had an IUD as a young woman, I didn't realize that the awful menstrual cramps I experienced were my body's way of protesting that unnatural foreign object implanted in my womb. I thought the intense cramps were normal. Motherwort would have been a great help in those years too, had I known to use it. As I educated myself about the potential side effects of the IUD, I had it removed and felt lucky that nothing worse than terrible cramps had ever happened because of it.

When I began to learn about herbs I bought motherwort tincture for the first few years, until I learned how easy it is to make my own. And when I was first using herbs "back in the day," the quality that was available for purchase was so poor that I wouldn't even use those herbs now. But in a testament to the power of herbal medicine, even those poorly made preparations helped me!

When you're gathering your own motherwort, harvest the above-ground parts of the plant early in the flowering season before the calyx that surrounds the petals gets spiky and sharp to the touch. You can gather motherwort anytime she's in flower, but this makes it a lot easier to handle, both at the beginning and the end of the tincture-making process. The resource section at the end of *The Gift of Healing Herbs* includes herbal companies that will ship fresh herbs in season, if you are ready and willing to make your own medicine but don't have motherwort growing near you, or don't yet know how to identify the plant "in person." (See Resources, page 509.)

Another lovely thing you can do for yourself when you have cramps—or even when you don't—is to massage your womb/belly with infused motherwort oil. Motherwort oil is a great ally. Using it externally can help relax your belly, and as your belly relaxes so does your whole body and being.

I love motherwort and know that she loves me, too. She's come to live all over my land. She's a very loving plant to everyone, and helps us to remain calm or to find calmness, even serenity, in the face of life's challenges. I feel she wants to help us learn to accept that life's bitter experiences are an intrinsic and natural part of life.

Grief is a natural response, but ultimately loss needs to be accepted. But numbness, refusal to believe or accept what has happened, or ongoing angry protest over the apparent unfairness of life, won't change the situation. And if you're burnt-out from working to change some aspect of "the system," trying to help everyone by addressing one of the many injustices we live with, motherwort is the balm you need—the balm we all need. Motherwort will help you find your equanimity without giving away your aliveness, your emotional responsiveness. She is bitter, but so kind-hearted and restorative.

I sometimes think that maybe it's this quality that's behind motherwort's ancient reputation for bestowing long life. She helps our hearts to stay healthy, but perhaps there is more to it than that. In both Chinese and Japanese lore, this beloved herb is seen as a longevity herb, and in some stories motherwort is considered an herb of immortality!

When we are emotionally at peace with life and not anxious, furious, resentful, or frustrated so often, we tend to live longer. It certainly would make most people want to live longer! Motherwort helps us to live more joyfully and peacefully.

I wish I'd known about motherwort when I was a hurting, self-conscious teenager. This plant often comes to my mind when I'm with teens that are lashing out at themselves or others in hormonally charged confusion and anger. When I have the chance to offer some drops of tincture in a glass of water, the results have always been positive and surprising to the teenager. (Come to think of it, the parents of the teens could use some motherwort love, too!) The Chinese name for motherwort is *yi mu cao,* which translates to "benefits-mother herb." This is generally understood to refer to the benefits of using motherwort in early labor or after delivery, though not if there is heavy bleeding. But again, "benefits mother" may have wider implications!

Herbalist/MD Aviva Romm, who has spent her professional life supporting women and their families as a midwife and an herbalist, suggests motherwort not only as a uterine tonic for menstrual and post-partum challenges, but also for menopausal symptoms ranging from insomnia to night sweats, to anxiety, depression, and heart palpitations. This matches my herbal experience with motherwort.

One of the other special things about motherwort is her ability to relax all three types of muscles in our bodies—smooth, skeletal, and cardiac. The smooth muscles line many of our internal organs such as stomach, intestines, uterus, esophagus, veins and arteries, and are part of the involuntary nervous system. The skeletal muscles are what we use to move different parts of our body. These muscles are striated (striped) and are under the control of the voluntary nervous system, meaning that we consciously direct these movements.

All muscles in the body are stimulated by electrical impulses between nerves and muscles, but smooth muscle is also stimulated to contract (often rhythmically) by hormones. Think of the action of the heart and the uterus, the muscular organs that expand and contract, rhythmically and repeatedly. Cardiac muscle is generally considered to be a third type of muscle, but it can also be seen as a synthesis of the two types— striped like skeletal muscles but controlled by the involuntary (autonomic) nervous system like smooth muscle.

Noting the powerful relaxant effects of motherwort on smooth and cardiac muscles when used internally made me decide to infuse motherwort in oil. That proved to be so effective and relaxing as a belly and womb rub that I next experimented with it on skeletal muscles. It has turned out to be effective here, too, though more subtly. Motherwort's anti-spasmodic effects are drawn out very effectively by infusing the fresh flowering tops in olive oil. I use the leaves, flowers and stalks, and let them sit infusing in the oil for two months or longer. I have come to love fresh motherwort oil for pain relief. I haven't found the dried plant oil as helpful, but it's possible that cooking it rather than infusing it would be better at drawing out its healing properties. It's worth a try if that's all you have.

The quality of the herbs you start with makes a difference in how effective the medicine is. If you're going to try infusing oil with dried motherwort, for example, you ideally want it dried that season, not three years earlier. Always use the best-quality herbal medicine available, and whatever you are using, thank it and bless it for its help. Your energy goes into your preparations and genuinely makes a difference in their quality.

Applying motherwort externally engenders its famous relaxation response. There isn't much written about using motherwort externally, but I can definitely recommend topical applications (along with internal use) for helping to ease cramps, constipation, tension and digestive headaches, neck tension, anxiety, menopausal mood swings, hot flashes, premenstrual irritability, insomnia and more.

One of my apprentices gave a friend her homemade motherwort oil to use after surgery. It eased the pain and sped up the time it took for her bruises to heal, so noticeably that her doctors commented on it. I was pleased but surprised by this when she told me about it, and tried to understand what might be at work. Here's an educated guess: Since smooth muscle also lines our veins and arteries, perhaps motherwort's tonic effect on the blood vessels had helped. The hormone-balancing properties of this extraordinary yet ordinary weed, which help bring a steady rhythm to smooth muscle contractions, may have played a part in how the plant reduced her pain. *Leonurus* is also said to "enliven the flow of blood," so that too could have helped speed the healing of her bruises.

SOME USES FOR MOTHERWORT AS A SIMPLE

Her bitter taste is important, so I don't sweeten this herb. Begin with 10–13 drops of tincture in any amount of water. Increase dosage as necessary.

Try using a fresh tincture of motherwort when you feel overwhelmed with too many responsibilities and not enough time or help to keep up with them.

Motherwort is a gentle yet powerfully effective soother when you feel frazzled and emotionally overwrought, as if the slightest thing could set you off.

Motherwort is great for "simple anxiety" such as you might feel before a job interview or an audition, or when you have a big project to complete. Motherwort is an invaluable ally to take before having a conversation or confrontation that is emotionally challenging for you.

Motherwort is an herb you can turn to for help if you suffer from constipation that strikes when you are traveling.

Another way to use this plant to nourish the nervous system is to infuse the fresh plant in apple cider vinegar to extract her abundant minerals. Motherwort is loaded with calcium and tastes good prepared this way.

I discussed alternating Motherwort and Mugwort/Cronewort in the section on Mugwort/Cronewort. (See page 311.) Motherwort can also be alternated with the following herbs, or they can be blended together.

Here are some motherwort blend recipes:

MOTHERWORT-PEACH BITTERSWEET BLEND

1 part flowering tops of motherwort

1 part peach pits, leaves, twigs, or flowers

This "bittersweet blend" is for bittersweet times in life, and can be used as tinctures or infusions or in any combination. To make 1 quart of infusion, use 10 dried pits; cover them with boiled water and steep for 2–3 hours.

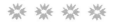

Bittersweet Blend can be helpful during menopause, for example, when the person you have known yourself to be no longer feels relevant and you're doing your best to discover who you are becoming.

Use this recipe for any transition times when feelings of bitterness and crankiness may be alternating with loving feelings, or with feelings of hope and excitement about the unknown future.

Perhaps you've instigated a break-up after a long relationship, and you've gotten what you wanted but still resent the past and are frightened of the future.

Peach helps calm your nerves by reducing heat and irritability and adds her sweet, cooling moistness to the blend, while motherwort continues to nourish the hormonal, reproductive, and nervous systems, lending a soothing, strengthening hand to guide you and relieve your growing pains.

MOTHERWORT-MELISSA BLEND

1 part motherwort

2 parts *Melissa* (lemon balm)

Here again we have two very different flavors and energies working together. This recipe is mostly a calming yet uplifting digestive aid. I particularly like this recipe as vinegar, though it can be taken as teas and tinctures, again combined however you like. You could use motherwort tincture in lemon balm tea, or use both plants as tinctures, or whatever other combination you might like to try. (See pages 41, 53, and 47 for general directions on making herb teas, vinegars and tinctures.)

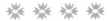

This mixture is good for lifting depression and relieving nervous anxiety. It can help to aid digestion that is slowed down due to emotional blocks and resistance to letting-go. I haven't yet used it to help someone who is weaning from anti-depressant or anti-anxiety medication, but imagine that this blend could be helpful in that situation.

MOTHERWORT-SKULLCAP TINCTURE RECIPE

2 parts motherwort

1 part skullcap

I have been grateful to this blend in the past, and usually use both herbs as tinctures. This mix is good for shock and trauma. (See page 47 for general directions on making tinctures.)

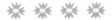

I used it once when I was almost run off the road. I took the motherwort as soon as I pulled over, and it definitely helped. But when I took the skullcap shortly thereafter it increased the calming effect of the motherwort, and vice-versa.

This beautiful blend will help you to release trauma both physically and emotionally so that you can shake it off without having to deal with unnecessary aftereffects.

Motherwort helps the emotional and mental release, and skullcap supports physical release; then both plants work together on every level, supporting your full recovery whether something has actually happened, almost happened, or happened nearby and left you feeling fearful and physically vulnerable. These plants work together to quickly dissipate the residual effects of shock and trauma. Using them as soon as possible after an event will speed the recovery time, but it is never too late to address and bring healing to post-traumatic stress.

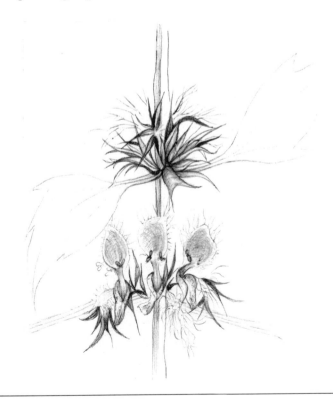

Motherwort detail

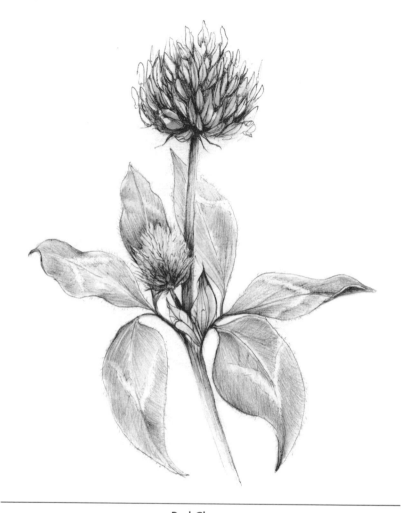

Red Clover

Red Clover *(Trifolium pratense)*

Body: alkalinizes blood, clears skin, strengthens lymph,
supports hormonal, nerve, bone, and joint health, digestion,
and respiration.

Mind: stabilizes the mind.

Heart: calms and soothes the emotions.

Soul: opens the connection between body and soul.

Red Clover

Oh, darling Red Clover,
Who doesn't like you?
You're gorgeous and tasty
And lymph-clearing too.

When it comes to hormones
That have gone astray,
I'd turn to Red Clover
On any old day.

She'll contain breast tumors
And not them let them spread,
And soothe dry hacking coughs
That hurt your poor head.

Her flowers are sexy—
Look at them up close.
They're sexual organs,
And help yours the most.

So rich in minerals
And vitamins too,
Infusing this plant is
A smart thing to do.

Gently thinning to blood,
And softening to skin,
And it strengthens your skeleton;
How can you not win?

If you haven't chosen
Red clover to drink,

Then eat the fresh blossoms,
You'll like them, I think.

Red clover soothes your nerves
And your digestion.
Keep the blossoms nearby—
That's my suggestion!

The next wonderful weed I'd like to talk about is one that positively affects so many body systems it's hard to know where to place her in the book. I decided that since there was no wrong place, I'd put her in this section because she's such an important herb for women to know about and make part of their daily lives. I use her for men and children, though, just as frequently.

Trifolium pratense is the botanical name of red clover, and refers to what she looks like and where she lives. Red clover has sets of three leaves *(tri-folium)* and is found in meadows *(pratense)*.

Red clover is the national flower of Denmark and the state flower of Vermont. Though I've never yet gathered her blossoms in Denmark, without question the most beautiful red clover I've ever gathered was in Vermont with my first apprentice, Martha. Please read on to meet red clover so that you can discover that she's not really red, and a whole lot more.

Red clover is a beautiful member of the legume family, gentle and strong, with glistening pink-to-purple hairy blossoms, exquisitely patterned sepals, and white chevrons on the leaves. She grows abundantly in open fields, and blossoms in the early part of the summer. Found in healthy meadows and also in disturbed soils, red clover is a valuable medicine. Red clover benefits the whole body, especially the lymphatic, digestive, female reproductive, musculoskeletal, nervous, and integument systems (skin). This is a classic "alterative," a plant known to reliably improve long-standing chronic conditions over time.

This special plant is rich in all of the standard amino acids that form the building blocks of protein, which are the building blocks of life. Protein is found in all of our cells and is second only to water as the most essential nutrient for the human body. Red clover provides an easily digestible, complete protein that can help a person who is convalescing from a long illness and having trouble eating enough food to maintain their health and strength. It can also be a blessing when someone near the end of life has lost interest in food.

The first time I saw this was when a friend of mine was dying from an AIDS-related illness. He asked me to stop bringing him anything except red-clover infusions. They soothed him mentally and physically, and he had no trouble drinking them even after his desire for other food and drink was gone. The amino acids in red clover also provide our bodies with the material to create neurotransmitters, such as serotonin and dopamine, to help maintain a healthy, stable state of mind. Red clover provides optimum nourishment, providing vitamin B complex, vitamin C, calcium, chromium, magnesium, manganese, niacin, phosphorus, and potassium.

I use red clover to help balance the acid/alkaline levels in the body. This is useful for challenges including chronic heartburn, arthritis, and both acute and chronic skin rashes. It is a gentle and safe herb for children with eczema. Red clover is also helpful for hormonal health, reversing premature menopause, for example, and easing menstrual cramps and other discomforts. It is one of the herbs that a woman can call on to help dissolve cystic breast lumps. Red clover is a supremely nourishing tonic that improves both physical form (blood, tissue and bones) and function (assimilation, elimination and filtering through the digestive system, skin, lymph, and lungs).

As stated earlier, red clover has long been considered an alterative. What exactly is an alterative? Herbalist James Green says that alteratives are blood cleansers that help us assimilate nutrients, eliminate metabolic wastes, restore proper functioning, and build health generally. Herbalist Amanda McQuade Crawford says, "Alteratives alter a longstanding condition by aiding the elimination of metabolic toxins."

Here "toxins" can be understood to include seemingly benign substances such as white-flour products like white bread and pasta that your body can't assimilate and excrete easily or, in other words, can't metabolize in a healthy way. As another example, red clover can be used to help children who have had bad reactions to standard vaccinations causing unforeseen side effects. It can also be used preventatively. Red clover is indeed a superb alterative.

Red clover is also an adaptogenic nervine, nourishing the nervous system slowly yet definitively. Regular use of red-clover infusion will help a person alter how they respond to stress. It builds inner strength and promotes calmness through nourishing the nervous system with an abundance of vitamins and especially minerals. Red clover supports the health of our endocrine system, including our adrenal glands.

This beautiful plant is commonly available and abundant, except in years when it's very wet. In 2009, when it was very rainy in the northeastern United States, there was a severe shortage of red clover, and prices went sky high. I've been very impressed with red clover for many years and would sorely miss this multi-talented healing herb if it were not available to me. This is another reason it's so important to grow plants in your own garden and to get to know them in the wild.

I use red clover quite regularly as an infusion to nourish, strengthen and soothe my nervous system, keep my skin clear, and support my immune and hormonal health. I use the flower heads and include the first set of upper leaves, well-dried, except when eating just the blossoms fresh in salads. I delight in eating the fresh blossoms in my salads when they're in season, usually in June. The delicately sweet, pink-to-purple fresh blossoms make any dish more beautiful. Pull off the individual flowerets from the flower head, and add them atop salads and sandwiches for a visual, edible treat. You may remember pulling apart the flower heads as a child and sucking the sweet nectar out of the individual flowerets. If you haven't done that in a long time, I recommend that you do it again. In this way, red clover can also keep you young at heart!

Red clover excels at alkalinizing the blood, benefiting the digestive and musculoskeletal systems, particularly the joints. I was in my twenties and teaching my earliest classes when I first suggested daily red-clover infusions to an elderly student to help forestall her scheduled hip replacement. She made some helpful dietary changes, and drank two cups of red-clover infusion daily. Though she was already well into her seventies at the time, she told me she felt so encouraged by the improvement that she had cancelled her hip-replacement surgery. I was as excited and encouraged by the power of herbs as she was! One year later, she was still feeling so much better that she still hadn't needed the surgery.

Red clover is high in antioxidant, immune-supportive isoflavones such as genistein, and is known to inhibit the spread of cancer. But there is some confusion about red clover. I often read misinformation about it, especially on the web, such as the following completely erroneous statement: "This herb has been recently questioned because it adds artificial hormones to the organism. By doing this, it can produce side effects like breast cancer." This is completely irresponsible "reporting," and outrageously inaccurate. No plant whatsoever can add artificial hormones into our bodies since plants don't actually have hormones (and if they did they could hardly be called artificial). Plants such as red clover have phytosterols that are building blocks for hormones, helping the body to create a healthy hormonal environment within.

We have different pathways that hormones such as estradiol (one of the forms of estrogen that has been linked to breast and other cancers) can travel as they move through the body. There are short and long paths. Unnatural estrogens take the long path, which is more dangerous to us, whereas natural estrogen that is supported by legume-family plants in general (lentils, for example), and red clover in particular, moves through the body via the shorter, safer pathways.

Another way to understand the gift of phytosterols is that the body in its natural wisdom will always choose the best quality of a substance that is offered to it. If the hormonal receptors are busy with what red clover provides them, they are not available to take up exogenous estrogen from outside sources, such as plastic leached from microwave-cooking containers. Red clover has also been shown to cause cancerous cells to be replaced with healthy ones, and to help prevent cancerous cells from metastasizing. Red clover improves lymph circulation, boosting the strength and effectiveness of the immune system. The book *Breast Cancer? Breast Health!* by Susun Weed is an excellent resource on this subject, as is Lisa Ganora's herbal-chemistry website (see page 513) for more scientifically minded readers.

I have come to think of red clover more often than not as a perfect medicine when a woman comes to me with hormonal imbalances that may have led to infertility, breast tenderness, breast lumps, irregular menstrual cycles, painful menstruation, or menopausal difficulties.

Herbalist Deb Soule wrote that, "Each floweret looks like tiny wings that resemble the flowery opening of a woman's vagina." It is true! Look at a single blossom with a magnifier. It is made up of many individual flowerets, and you will be astounded at its beauty. Here is a snippet excerpted from writing I did after a plant meditation with red clover: "Beauty, sweet-pea family, female, many blossoms joined as one, community gathered together; vulvas, ovaries, breasts, vaginas, alkalinizing everywhere except where it needs to be acidic. Female genitalia. Red-clover blossoms are circles of women buzzing with community, alive with life in the wild fields and meadows."

Herbal wise woman Gail Faith Edwards writes that red clover was sacred to the Celts, who "believed it helped get them in touch with their eternal soul."

HEALING FOR A WOMAN WITH A LARGE BREAST LUMP

Here is a healing story that highlights the physical and spiritual gifts and attributes of red clover.

One of my apprentices discovered a lump in her right breast and began to drink about one quart of red-clover infusion a day. The lump began to dissolve soon thereafter, and disappeared completely after about two months.

Then, the following year, a hot painful lump appeared in her left breast. It kept growing in spite of the fact that she'd embarked upon an intense multiple-herb regimen. The lump became so large it changed the shape of her breast and was even visibly poking out under her blouse. It was radiating intense heat throughout her breast and armpit and down her arm. She came to see me as a client after about six months of using different herbal formulas in her own attempt to dissolve the lump. She had such great faith in herbs that it had to get that bad before she heeded her husband, who had been pleading with her to get help.

Asking for help and receiving guidance is often a vital step in someone's healing process. I know that when I'm ill it's true for me, too.

It was time to help her get back to a more simple, loving approach to healing. When we are frightened we tend to assault our bodies with herbs rather than breathing deeply to center ourselves, and then seeing what we need to do to nourish the body systems within that are designed by nature to help us heal. In this case the systems we wanted to nourish were both lymphatic and hormonal. We also needed to address her fear. Finally, we needed to start from the wisdom that where there is illness there is an opportunity to bring healing not only to our beloved bodies but to our whole selves. I often say that our bodies love us enough to get sick for us, if that's necessary to bring us into a greater experience of our wholeness—of who we truly are.

This woman said she hadn't been drinking red clover for quite some time. The first thing I suggested was to put the red clover infusions back into her mix. She also made infused red-clover oil and started using red clover poultices, daily at first, then a few times a week. (The oil and poultice recipes follow, below.) Then she gradually decreased the frequency of the poultices, using only the oil for her external treatments until her healing was complete. The whole process took time, but the lump itself began to shrink as soon as she simplified her herbal blend and changed her diet.

Upon questioning, it turned out that she had started a popular weight-loss plan and the food she was eating every day was highly processed and had lots of unfermented soy in it. She began to see good results almost immediately when she stopped that diet, even though she had stopped it reluctantly because she really wanted to lose the weight. The lump itself was fully dissolved in six months. More than that happened, though.

She also got in touch, through guided meditation, with the fact that she'd been holding onto a traumatic event that had occurred five years earlier. She saw that she held herself partially to blame for it, and had never let it go. She further realized she had put on the weight after that experience in order to hide, and had never been the same since, not even being willing to ever share her beautiful smile for a photograph.

Over the course of her healing process, as I helped her to look at the past situation through new eyes—the eyes of self love—she reconnected with her true self and was able to free herself from those limitations. She is now a shining and radiant woman, confident in her beauty and abilities, and creating her own work as a healer, which is actually a continuation of her family's multi-generational herbal tradition. And yes, she also lost the weight. Knowing that this kind of lymph congestion is one of the ways her body expresses itself, she takes care to nourish her lymphatic and hormonal systems regularly with red clover, and other lymphatic helpers like dandelion roots and flowers, cleavers, red root, and violet leaves. (See the chapter on the immune-lymphatic system, page 101.) Now she freely beams her gorgeous smile when she is photographed, too.

RED CLOVER POULTICE

> ½ cup or more dried red clover blossoms, depending on the size of the area to be covered
>
> Water—just enough to cover the blossoms
>
> Washcloth, or piece of flannel or muslin

Put the red clover blossoms in a shallow bowl or saucepan. Use enough blossoms to generously cover the area you are making the poultice for. Boil the water and pour it over the blossoms. Steep them for about 15 minutes, then strain the blossoms and squeeze them to get out any excess liquid.

Use the steeped blossoms as a poultice over the affected area. It's fine if it covers the surrounding skin, too. You can place your hands over the herbs to hold them in place, and/or take a washcloth or soft piece of flannel, and place it over the herbs that are lying against your skin covering the lump. (I don't actually use the word "lump," though. I call it a "bump" instead, as this word doesn't have the same fear associated with it and even sounds a bit humorous.) The client in the story above was happy to experiment with using a different word to create a different vibration, and even the suggestion made her smile, releasing some tightly wound tension.

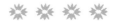

One of the things I suggest in using any poultice for breast healing is to apply the poultice to the nipple as well as to the area being treated. Nipples are designed to allow milk to flow out, and thus are helpful portals when drawing out a breast infection. I learned about this from a student. We were taking a class together when she spoke up to share a success story. It featured the Mediterranean tradition of cutting open and warming up fresh figs, then applying them to nipples for breast infections no matter where in the breast the infection has shown up. I thought this was brilliant, as did our teacher, Keewaydinoquay. One important caution: Do not reuse these herbs. Make a fresh poultice each time.

RED CLOVER BLOSSOM OIL —VARIATION I

1 part fresh red clover blossoms

1 part olive oil

Gather enough vibrant red clover blossoms to almost fill whatever size jar you are using. Do *not* wash the blossoms. Pull apart the whole blossoms and fill the jar with the flowerets, optionally including the top set of leaves that are just under each flower head. Cover with olive oil and fill to the rim of the jar, poking out the air bubbles with a chopstick.

Let this preparation sit for about 6 weeks, periodically opening the jar, poking out air bubbles, and topping up the oil if needed, and then pour off the oil. Squeeze out the herbs as fully as possible, adding the oil to your medicine jar and composting the spent flowers. After about 24 hours, watery liquid will have collected underneath the oil. Slowly, carefully, pour the oil out into a fresh, dry jar, and let go of the watery residue, or use that part right away. Your medicinal oil is now ready to use.

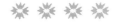

RED CLOVER BLOSSOM OIL —VARIATION II

½ part fresh red clover blossoms

½ part dried red clover blossoms

1 part olive oil

Follow the same directions as above except in this variation, fill the jar half full with the fresh blossoms, and then finish filling the jar (nearly) to the top with dried blossoms. The dried blossoms can be left whole or pulled apart.

Red clover is so high in protein that the infused oil is prone to mold and must be watched rather carefully while it is infusing. This method (Variation II) of preparing the oil discourages mold from forming, as there is less natural moisture to begin with. I got this tip from Gretchen Gould, herbalist and owner of Herb Hill (see Resources, page 509).

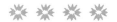

RED CLOVER BLOSSOM OIL
—VARIATION III

1 part freshly dried red clover blossoms

2 parts olive oil

If you don't have fresh flowers, or if you're in need of the oil right away and don't have time to wait, you can make your herbal oil using dried blossoms.

Combine the ingredients into a saucepan, and gently and slowly heat on a very low flame. You can use a double-boiler if you like. Simmer the oil very gently for around an hour, being careful not to let it bubble and boil, and then turn off the flame and let it sit, steeping. This process can be repeated 2–3 more times over the course of a day. Then strain the herbs, squeeze them out and bottle the oil.

If you have the time, pour the cooked herbs and oil into a jar together and let them steep for up to 6 weeks before you decant them. This oil can be massaged on in between poultice treatments to help dissolve breast lumps (bumps).

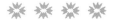

I don't like to use a crockpot to cook my herbs, especially for breast medicine, since electromagnetic frequencies (EMFs) are implicated in breast cancer. It simply doesn't make sense to me to use oil made with electricity on my breasts if I have a choice. This is true whether I'm doing breast massage for lymphatic circulation to support breast health, or using an herbal oil to heal an existing problem.

Violet leaf oil (*Viola odorata* and other species) can be mixed with, or alternated with, the red clover oil. Violets, too, have an affinity for breast health and will help strengthen lymphatic circulation. Violets have long been used in folk medicine for the treatment of breast and other cancers and, as a simple, Violet is one of my favorite oils for regular breast massages. (See Violet leaf- and Dandelion Flower-Infused Breast-Massage Oil, page 336.)

HEALING FOR A MENOPAUSAL WOMAN WITH AN OVARIAN CYST

I had a client who made an appointment for help with an ovarian cyst. But it's never really just one thing, is it?

Her stated goals were to feel relaxed and more energized, happier and better connected to life. She wanted to dissolve a complicated cyst on her right ovary and a few smaller ones on her cervix, and continue building and strengthening her immune system. She had been diagnosed with Lyme disease and a co-infection from another tick-borne bacteria two years before I met her. She was still struggling with fatigue, some achiness, and mental fogginess. Her relationship to her health, marriage, children, and career were all in a state of flux. She was receptive to any help that herbs could provide her in easing the way through all the transitions she was going through.

At some point in our conversation, I nearly always ask a client to consider what is the best they can imagine coming out of our work together. Her answers were profound. The best she could imagine was that she would trust her inner wisdom and nature's wisdom, feel the infinite love, let go and surrender to the flow … "anchor my connection, move with grace through this health/life challenge with clearer vision, and better understand my purpose." Now clearly here is someone in touch with a larger perception of her own evolution!

This thin, wiry woman was in the early stages of her menopausal years, commonly called perimenopausal; but that implies a clear-cut "before, during and after" bleeding, as if our menstrual and ovulatory years finished neatly all at once rather than in the natural, gradual progression that takes place over years. She had a lot of nervous energy, dry skin, and was physically running very hot. She was also "hot" in the sense of feeling irritable and annoyed with everything. She was having ongoing pelvic pain that had recently gotten worse, which was what had motivated her to seek medical advice.

She brought me her sonogram results. They showed a four-centimeter septated cyst (septated means segmented, divided into separate compartments by walls of tissue of various thicknesses). It was on her right ovary, filled with both fluid and semi-solid matter. This is considered a potentially dangerous kind of cyst. She also had multiple, harmless nabothian cysts on her cervix. When she said she didn't want surgery or medication, the recommendation of the doctors was to do a follow-up ultrasound in three months. The assumption was that the cyst would continue to grow larger, and then they would operate to relieve her pain, removing the cyst and possibly also the ovary.

Her diet was superb. She was doing everything she could to support herself with food and lots of physical activity. She had been able to recover from the worst symptoms of her double-whammy of tick-borne infections, though she was still chronically exhausted. Her tension level was currently very high, along with dissatisfaction with her life in general. Through all that, though, she trusted in the process of life and healing that she was engaged in, and was wholeheartedly open to using herbs to continue her process of healing, including dissolving those cysts. She'd been trying this, that, and the other thing, as people often do, so I worked with her to simplify her herbal recipes to give her confidence in the herbs that were chosen, and to benefit more fully by taking them consistently and rhythmically.

We agreed upon the following recipes for an infusion, tincture, bath, and poultice.

NERVE- AND WOMB-STRENGTHENING INFUSION

    ½ cup dried nettles
    ½ cup dried red raspberry
    ½ cup dried oat straw
    ¼ cup dried skullcap

Put the herbs into a half-gallon jar. Pour boiling water over them and cap tightly. Let them steep for about 8 hours, or overnight. Decant and drink 2–4 cups daily, hot or cold.

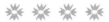

This blend was strengthening to this woman's immune and nervous systems through the multitude of vitamins and minerals in all four herbs. Nettle is one of my favorite herbs for exhaustion and adrenal depletion. Red raspberry brings healing medicine and energy to the whole reproductive system, and is a specific healer for the womb. Oat straw was a must for her—soothing, cooling, and inducing more grace and flexibility both mentally and physically. It also helps counter the astringency of nettles and red raspberry with its moistness. Skullcap adds a deeply relaxing quality to the whole blend, and a nice minty flavor, too. These herbs are commonly available and were familiar to her, like old friends. I took her out to meet each of them in my planted and wild gardens.

CYST-DISSOLVING TINCTURE BLEND

13 drops chickweed tincture

5–10 drops motherwort tincture

10 drops peach pit tincture

Add these to hot or cold water for a "tincture tea," or put the drops into another tea or infusion. Each tincture can be used separately in order to be precise with the dosage, or to allow you to make adjustments in the amount of each herb used, as needed. Or, just to make it easier, a one-ounce bottle can be filled with the pre-mixed tinctures and then shaken well. Then add a single dropper (about 25–30 drops) of this blend into the water, tea, or infusion.

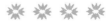

My client took this mixture three times daily. One of the interesting things about this recipe is that it blends together several very different tastes. The chickweed is salty and soapy, the motherwort is a bitter mint, and the peach pits are sweet.

Chickweed *(Stellaria media)* is an excellent dissolvent herb for ovarian and other cysts. It was a good choice for her because it is moistening and cooling. Chickweed, rich in hormone-like, frothy saponins, helps cells absorb nutrients and release wastes. It is also mineral-rich, and strengthens the nervous system. Chickweed is a gentle yet potent immune-supportive herb through its array of antibacterial and antiviral components. Herbalist Susun Weed calls chickweed "maidenwort" and the "little white-star flower lady." This young lady packs a powerful healing punch!

Motherwort *(Leonurus cardiaca)* is a mint plant that helps both nervous and reproductive systems come into a more harmonious working order. It brings calm to the mind and emotions. Its bitterness felt like a good match for this client considering the difficult challenges she was experiencing all at once.

It seemed important to include peach *(Prunus persica)* in her recipe to bring back the possibility of sweetness at a time that felt so bitter to her.

Peach *(Prunus persica)* and Other Soothers

Peach

I'm sweet, juicy, cooling, and moist,
Relaxing nerves and tissue.
I help you when you're not content
In fact, I like to kiss you!

I allay severe nausea—
That is one of my great gifts,
Especially in pregnancy—
Use my flowers, leaves, or pits.

I am such a beautiful tree,
And I support your liver.
My fuzzy fruit's round and luscious;
Your life flows like a river.

Peach, the tree of immortality in China, has a good humor about it. It is very soothing to the nerves, to moisten and cool off my client in the story above, mentally and physically. Peach is also a very sensual plant medicine, and since that woman relates to life very much through her senses, peach seemed like a good match for her on every level. I found it helpful in my own menopausal journey to cool me off when every little thing seemed irritating. It's almost as if I could hear peach giggling at me and saying, "What are you so hot under the collar about?"

SWEETHEART LEAF POULTICE

Fresh or dried violet leaves *(Viola odorata)*

Water

Use enough violet leaves to generously cover the area. If you are using fresh leaves, tear, pound, or cut them up into small pieces. Pour boiling water over the dried or fresh leaves, using just enough water to cover them. Let them sit for 5–10 minutes, then remove the leaves, squeeze them out, and apply them directly over the area being treated—in this case, the ovary and womb. Fresh leaves can also simply be macerated (chewed) and applied directly. If you have plenty of leaves, you can place them over the whole lower belly, covering both ovaries and the womb. Relax and imagine cysts getting smaller and smaller. Visualize the entire area sparkling with good, vibrant health.

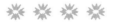

Violet is another herb that is effective for dissolving cysts. It, too, is cooling and moistening. It can be used internally as infusion or tincture, but in this case I chose to have her use it externally to complement her internal herbal medicines. Whenever it's possible for hands-on healing to be part of a person's journey, I encourage it because it makes it very personal. In the case of a woman bringing healing to her reproductive area or breasts, I consider it almost essential. This is working on two different levels—first, to put plant medicine directly over the area that needs healing, to be absorbed through the skin, and secondly to bring your own loving touch to your body.

SWEET AND SOOTHING HERBAL BATH

1½ cups dried oat straw

¼ cup dried lavender flowers

Put oat straw into a half-gallon or more of cold water in a soup pot. Bring it to a boil, and then turn it down to keep it on the lowest possible flame for about 30 minutes. Turn it off and stir in the lavender. Cover the pot and wait another 30–60 minutes. Squeeze out the herbs and pour the strained tea into a full bath of hot water. Soak for 20 minutes or more. Light an unscented palm-oil (sustainably harvested, please) or beeswax candle if you want to create an even more relaxing experience for yourself.

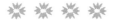

This is my "go-to" bath recipe, the first one I think of when I want to help someone move through stress and anxiety. I use other bath recipes, too, but this remains one of my favorites for soothing. It brings immediate relief of physical and emotional distress and pain. The more often you do this for yourself, the more benefits you will retain. Sometimes when someone is rude or cranky with me I want to throw her or him into a bath like this! (That reaction shows me I haven't been taking enough oat/lavender baths myself!)

She was diligent in her follow-through; she took her herbs and did her poultices, sending love into her body as she did them, and enjoyed soaking in her healing baths a couple of times a week. Her pains began to subside, she felt calmer and clearer, and she began to make even more healthy decisions for herself.

When she returned to the doctor for her follow-up several months later, all her cysts had completely dissolved.

She also went on to split up with her husband, leave her steady employment of many years that had become unsatisfying, and try her best to work things out with her son. She is rebirthing herself, emerging slowly and surely out of her old shell into a moister, juicier, happier version of her beautiful self. I am so inspired by her!

Sparkling Seeds

Women are sowing the sparkling seeds of the rebirth of our world,
And to do our job,
To lead the way for all,
We need to fan the flames of joy and delight.
What are you doing to fan the flames of your own joy?
To reclaim your right to pleasure and delight?
Please … say YES to yourself, and YES to life!
This is what's being asked of us.
I call it "eve-olution"!

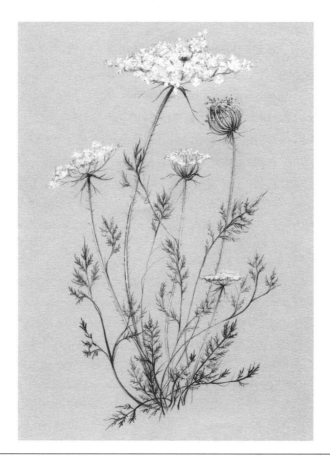

Wild Carrot

Wild Carrot *(Daucus carota)*

Body: urinary system tonic; aids conscious contraception; may support conception; thyroid and pituitary stimulant; dissolves gravel and stones in bladder and kidneys; aids digestion; increases breast milk; carminative.

Mind: stimulates clear thinking, insight, and perception of beauty.

Heart: encourages playfulness, community, and laughter.

Soul: teacher of shape-shifting; awakens third-eye consciousness; increases awareness of energy, oneness.

Wild Carrot

Shape-shifter,
White lacy light,
Orange mandala,
Shining at night.

Red-dot blood
In the center;
Wild carrot is a
Sexy mentor.

Flower heads
Spread wide open,
And then they contract,
Seed heads hoping,

Pulling in,
Becoming womb,
Expanding outward.
Open to moon.

Orgasms
Express delight.
She does this again,
Night after night.

Whether wild or domestic, carrot is a member of the huge Apiaceae family, sometimes called the parsley family. She is a relative of familiar plants such as anise, caraway, fennel, and of course parsley. Every part of carrot, from root to seed, has value as food, and the entire plant has also been used as medicine.

Wild carrot is the ancestor of our domesticated orange carrot, and this is one of the rare instances when I think the domesticated version of the plant tastes better than the wild plant. Interestingly, if you put wild carrot in your garden it will never become a domesticated carrot, but if you let a domesticated carrot go to seed, it will go wild! Hmm ... I think there's a human analogy that can be made here, but I will continue, undistracted for now, to talk about wild carrot.

Wild carrot's root is a whitish color, and a bit bitter. If you are going to eat it, raw or cooked, it is important to know that carrot is a biennial, and therefore you want the first-year, not the second-year, root of this herb. My favorite way to eat this plant is to make an infused vinegar with the first-year roots and leaves. (See directions for Herbal Vinegars, page 53.) Like most biennials, carrot will have pulled all the juiciness out of the root the second year in order to have energy and nourishment available for the hairy green stalks that grow two to five feet tall the second summer, then come alive with flowers and seeds for several months. The root is no longer needed much after that, so what is left is a woody, stick-like growth under the ground, instead of the vibrant, living root it once was.

Wild carrot, also known as Queen Anne's lace, is fiery—a lover of full sunlight—and yet moves airily. She is a dancer, moving and swaying her many arms in the breeze while her main stalk is strong and stable. Her flowers are lacy-white, tinged with subtle and sometimes not-so-subtle pink, and they have a dark blossom right in the center that can range from light to deep red to magenta-purple, to not being there at all! Carrot is expansive, spreading out her flower blossoms wide, and yet also contractive, closing them up, over and over again until they mature into fertile seeds. She then opens and closes some more until she closes up her seed heads into cup-like "bird's nests" (one of her most common nicknames) and then finally opens them wide, wider, widest, to disperse the seeds freely. Wild carrot is wild, not tame, and she just won't be pinned down.

Wild carrot supports conscious contraception. I have written about this extensively online and in my booklet, *Wild Carrot: A Plant for Natural Contraception.* The following information is gleaned from two small grass-roots studies and anecdotal information collected from women and their partners who use wild carrot as a natural contraceptive, and from other herbalists.

Wild carrot is a most magical plant. As an example I offer the following anecdote: I was interviewed by herbalist Karyn Sanders on her Pacifica radio program *(Herbal Highway)* about using wild carrot for contraception. Karyn had been living on the same land for seven years without wild carrot anywhere on it, and yet, a few weeks after our radio talk, a very young plant popped up on her land in a noticeable location. Her students asked her about it. When it grew large enough for her to identify, she saw it was wild carrot!

It's clear that Ms. Carrot loves the attention that we give her—but she has a contradictory nature.

Herbal literature suggests that wild carrot also supports healthy conception. I and thousands of other women would love to understand how best to use wild carrot to achieve these very different outcomes. Of course there are no guarantees. I have been studying wild carrot in this regard for over twenty years, and will do my best to summarize what I have learned here.

When I have sat in meditation with this plant she has told me that she knows everything about both holding and releasing. This immediately made me think of her dual gifts of supporting contraception and conception.

One evening I looked at wild carrot and asked her for some insight that I could share with other women thirsty for knowledge, for ways to be in deeper relationship with their own fertility. I saw a powerful woman rise up out of the wild carrot plant with a ball of orange light and energy swirling in her womb center. She said, "I hold the powers of life and death. It is up to you to choose. "I can help you hold a pregnancy. I can help you release a potential pregnancy. The choice is yours."

She is an herbal ally who supports the commitment a woman makes, consciously or unconsciously, regarding what she chooses to do with her fertility. Clearly this is not a method for everyone.

Thousands of women have, however, used wild carrot successfully as a contraceptive, currently and dating back at least 2,000 years, when Hippocrates called it an abortive. But it is not actually an abortive plant; it works preventatively. Used as suggested, wild carrot seeds and flowers prevent implantation of a fertilized egg from taking place. The oldest reported method of preparing and taking wild carrot for preventing implantation is to use the freshly crushed seeds in water, about eight hours after potentially fertilizing intercourse, as a "morning-after" herb.

Having experimented with tinctures and teas, and flowers and seeds, if I were still menstruating and ovulating today and concerned about conception, I would do that or, even more likely, roll the ground seeds (perhaps with flowers) into a sunflower seed or almond butter and honey ball (see recipe below). The fat in the seed and nut butters would help support the hormonal action of the plant, and keep it available in the body longer. I think this may turn out to be an important key. The honey is simply for pleasantness, and entirely optional. Powdered carrot flowers could be added, too. They are less astringent than the seeds, and add a gentle, soothing touch to carrot's overall medicine.

In the southern Appalachians, women's knowledge was passed down through the generations: Use fresh Queen Anne's lace flowers as tea for the morning-or-few-mornings-after. Appalachian herbalist Phyllis Light learned about it from her grandmother Rosie, and Phyllis has watched women successfully rely on this traditional use for quite a few decades now. I don't recommend using herbs as drugs, but RU-486 or "Plan B" (mifepristone) is supposed to prevent implantation, and wild carrot may act like an herbal drug when you need it. But she's not a drug—she is far more complex and deserving of your respect and gratitude.

The longest history of known use of the plant as a contraceptive is based on the use of the seeds rather than flowers or tinctures. Wild carrot was originally used in seed form in China and India over 2,000 years ago.

WILD CARROT RECIPE FOR NATURAL, CONSCIOUS CONTRACEPTION

If you wish to use wild carrot seeds, purchase them from a reliable source, or harvest the seeds in the fall when they are fully formed, whether green or turning brown, and store them in a paper bag. There are poisonous look-alikes in this plant family so be 100% certain that you have correctly identified *Daucus carota*.

Approximately 8 hours after intercourse, either chew one teaspoon of seeds (note that many women find this to be the least pleasant way of taking wild carrot) OR grind up one teaspoon of seeds in a coffee grinder dedicated for herbs, and do one of the following:

- · Stir the ground seed into water and drink it.
- · Roll the ground seed (and flowers if used) into a honey ball and eat it.
- · Roll the ground seed (and flowers if used) into a ball with nut butter (peanut, almond, etc) and eat it. It is possible that the fat content in the nut butter can aid the hormonal activity of carrot.
- · Take 15–30 drops of flower tincture and/or seed tincture in water. (This form has the shortest history of use, and is thus the least understood regarding its effectiveness.)

Grind no more than a week's supply of wild carrot seed at a time, to ensure freshness and potency. Powdered seeds should be stored in a jar or tin or other airtight container.

If you are having intercourse during your fertile phase, be clear in your intention and repeat the dosage of wild carrot several times approximately 8 hours apart, regardless of what form you use. Pay attention to sensations in your body and intuition regarding how many subsequent doses of wild carrot to take.

Finally, mugwort/cronewort *(Artemisia vulgaris)* or American and/or European pennyroyal *(Hedeoma pulegioides* and/or *Mentha pulegium)* can be safely taken as teas or tinctures, but *not* as essential oils, along with the wild carrot from time to time, as they may enhance carrot's effectiveness.

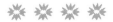

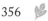

Wild carrot affects our estrogen and progesterone balance through its stimulating effects on the pituitary gland. Some women notice positive changes in their menstrual cycle and urinary system when using wild carrot.

I encourage any woman using wild carrot for contraception to first become intimate with her body's cycles and then to take wild carrot seeds and/or flowers just before, during, and after her fertile days, rather than daily.

To be intimate with your body, it's important and empowering to get to know the physical and emotional changes that accompany your ovulation, and to pay attention to when you are getting close to ovulation, since sperm can remain viable in a woman's body for three to five days. Also, ovulation can sometimes occur at unusual times in any given month—so when you know your body's signs and signals, you can use the wild carrot again at that time.

If you are new to wild carrot, I suggest proceeding with careful attention. If you feel uncertain, consider using a condom, diaphragm, or cervical cap while you are getting to know how wild carrot and your body fit together. That is how I started.

Fertility is magnified during lovemaking, and we can choose how to direct it, and what we want it to feed and generate. The natural tendency of a fertile woman's body is to create a new human being. If that is *not* what you want, it is vital to choose what you *do* want. You can work with your consciousness to create crystal-clear intention about what you wish to do with your fertility.

When making love, if you don't want to conceive, it helps to create an intention regarding how you are directing your fertility energy. Perhaps you want to invoke your own creative growth with your lovemaking, or send the life-force to the land somewhere, or to the water, or to another person for healing. Or imagine it nourishing your relationship with your beloved and yourself.

Speaking of beloved partners, if you are in a committed relationship, check in with each other about creating a conscious intention together. Remember that it is impossible to picture NOT getting pregnant, so make your intention affirmative. You might decide on a mutual image to visualize. And it's important to practice this ahead of time, and not suddenly try to conjure it up for the first time in the high heat of the moments right before or during an orgasm! As with anything else, you get better with practice.

CONTRAINDICATIONS FOR USING WILD CARROT AS A CONTRACEPTIVE PLANT

There are some contraindications regarding this use of wild carrot that I take very seriously, and I ask you to do the same. The first is that, if you experience discomfort of any sort when using wild carrot, particularly breast tenderness, it won't be a reliable method for you.

The second contraindication is, if your cycle suddenly changes when you start to use wild carrot, stop using it. The third warning is that if you have been on hormonal medications such as the pill, or have very erratic cycles or any other hormonal imbalance, this won't be an effective method for you until your cycles and hormones have been stabilized for a year or more. Fourth, if you are extremely fertile and have gotten pregnant using other common contraceptive methods, I would *combine* wild carrot with another, non-hormonal method for best results. Lastly, I don't think that wild carrot for contraception is best used daily for years and years, though it has worked this way for some women, including women with proven fertility.

The good news is that if you are going to have discomfort, or cyclical or other changes, from taking wild carrot, they tend to show up almost immediately. If those occur, stop using it and those problems will self-resolve just as quickly.

WILD CARROT IS A SAFE PLANT

Nursing mothers who have resumed their monthly cycles *for at least six months* have reported that wild carrot is a safe, effective ally for contraception. Wait a few more cycles if you are in any doubt. Some women start using it again after three cycles, but that is riskier.

There are women who have had unwanted pregnancies using wild carrot. This will happen with any method other than abstention from intercourse. Women I've known of who chose to bring those pregnancies to term have all had healthy babies. We are talking about a carrot after all—a healthful vegetable, not an experimental designer drug.

In more good news, women have also conceived easily and had healthy babies when they chose to become pregnant after years of using wild carrot as a natural contraceptive. Herbalist Jim McDonald has written that, in his experience, a woman can become fertile immediately after stopping wild carrot. I suspect this is especially likely if someone has been using wild carrot regularly as opposed to using it on occasion. It also raises the possibility that it could be helpful for women who have experienced difficulty conceiving.

I haven't studied using wild carrot to support conception, so anything I say here is pure conjecture—but if you want to try it I suggest you set your intention, ask her for help in creating and holding a pregnancy, and then use wild carrot seeds in a different rhythm than for contraceptive use. For *conception*, take the wild carrot seeds daily, except when menstruating, and remove them from your diet during your most fertile days.

WILD CARROT—A POTENTIAL ALLY FOR MALE INFERTILITY?

I have long held a strong suspicion that men may be able to use wild carrot for healing male-infertility issues. I look forward to finding out how this plant may be of benefit to men in this way. I would start an experiment by crushing the seeds and infusing them into wine to be drunk daily, if you want to try it—and please report on your results!

WILD CARROT AND OTHER HERBS FOR THE URINARY SYSTEM

Wild carrot is astringent, tones tissue, and is high in volatile oils that help support the urinary system, promoting the easy flow of urine. Carrot is used to break up and move gravel out of the bladder and kidneys, alone or combined with other herbs or on their own. I have used ginger poultices (see page 490) over the kidneys, along with the wild carrot internally, to good result.

Here is a helpful tonic for the kidneys, bladder, prostate, and urethra:

PEE TEA

4 parts dried corn silk

2 parts dried goldenrod leaves, stalks, and flowers

1 part dried wild carrot seeds

Bruise the wild carrot seeds and mix them together with the other herbs. Use a total of about 2 tablespoons of herbs per cup. Pour boiling water over the herbs. Let them steep about 30 minutes. Strain and drink.

In general I like teas and infusions for the urinary system, and think this recipe is best used as a tea, but a blend of tinctures of these herbs, in these proportions, can be made too. Goldenrod is a specific anti-inflammatory for the kidneys, and is pain-relieving and antibacterial. Corn silk is my all-around favorite urinary-system demulcent. It is soothing, moistening, and antiseptic for every part of our urinary system, and supports a healthy prostate and kidneys.

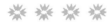

Other herbs that are classic helpers for the urinary system include the kidney strengtheners—nourishing nettles, mineral-rich horsetail, and tonifying sumach berries. Dandelion leaves, burdock roots and seeds, and parsley leaf and root tea are other favorites of mine that can be helpful for general urinary system health as well as specific problems such as inflammation, gravel, infections, or incontinence.

Herbalist Matthew Wood uses wild carrot to stimulate the pituitary gland, while Appalachian herbalist Phyllis Light mixes wild carrot flowers with black walnuts and chickweed for hypothyroid problems. I've used wild carrot with chickweed and oat straw for the same purpose. Phyllis also shares that wild carrot flower tea is used for weight loss in southern Appalachian medicine. She suggests one pint of the fresh flower tea, sipped slowly every day.

Wild carrot flowers are lovely to look at, and taste quite delicious in sandwiches and atop salads. They'll bring a light, uplifting energy into your house when you put them out in a vase alone or with other cut flowers. Inhale their delicate scent and invite them to delight you!

SEVERE MENSTRUAL CRAMPS

I was out of town when I received a disturbing letter from a dear young woman who was apprenticing with me. She was feeling desperately afraid of her monthly menstruation. She told me that almost every other month for the past two years she'd been having severe cramps that would eventually lead to a fast drop in her blood pressure. She would start to feel dizzy, then break out in a clammy sweat and become very pale. Her hands would begin to tingle, then cramp and spasm until they resembled claws, and she couldn't open them again until the cramping stopped. Sometimes the tingle would go down her legs, and more than once she hadn't been able to move at all. She was so fearful that this might happen again that the last few times she'd had her period she called her mother and asked her to come stay with her in her apartment.

She'd tried a variety of herbs, going from one to the other in desperation. She'd consulted with gynecologists who had recommended either painkillers or birth-control pills. From my window on the world, recommending the pill seems to be the standard response and prescription for virtually every menstrual problem! She admitted that she wanted the quick fix, but said, "My wiser woman knows there is a better way—I just haven't been able to find it."

Until this started to happen, she'd never had menstrual cramps. I wrote back and suggested she start with the herbal recipe that follows until we could arrange a session together. Every woman is different, and in the wise-woman approach you support a person uniquely as she heals herself with the help of herbs and other natural means, rather than focusing solely on what substances or interventions will "fix" her problems for her. So although any woman with menstrual cramps and related challenges could use and benefit from some of the herbs this client used, the specific choices made for her at each stage of her healing journey also grew out of her unique story.

REMEDIES FOR A PERSONAL JOURNEY
OF MENSTRUAL HEALING

2–4 cups red raspberry leaf infusion daily

2–4 cups hawthorn berry infusion daily

25–30 drops dandelion root tincture twice a day

I suggested that this woman drink 2–4 cups of hawthorn berry infusion daily for the first two weeks of her monthly cycle (from menstruation to ovulation), then alternate it with 2–4 cups a day of red raspberry leaf infusion for the next two weeks (from ovulation to menstruation). She was to take 25–30 drops (about one dropper) of dandelion root tincture in water or infusions, 2 times daily.

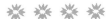

Red raspberry (*Rubus* species) helps to tone the uterus and is a womb-loving herb. Though it is most famous as a supportive herb for pregnancy, due to its womb-strengthening fragrine content, red raspberry and her little sister, strawberry, are also allies for menstruating women. Red raspberry reduces cramps by providing optimum nourishment for the womb, and helps regulate the timing of the menstrual cycle, especially when used rhythmically as described. If the uterus is contracting more smoothly, there will be less congestion and therefore less cramping.

Red raspberry leaf is also rich in mineral nutrients including calcium, iron, magnesium, manganese, phosphorus, and potassium, which feed the nervous system. Strengthening this woman's nerves was important. She was feeling frightened and helpless, and that's counterproductive when you want to initiate healing.

Hawthorn berries (*Crataegus* species) help the circulation and normalize high or low blood pressure. (Note that a small percentage of people with low blood pressure find that hawthorn exacerbates their problem. If that happens to you, discontinue it or lessen the amount you're using.)

Hawthorn berries are iron-rich and contain antioxidant bioflavonoids including vitamin C. The hawthorn tree was—not coincidentally—the medicine plant this woman had chosen as her herbal ally that year. It's wise to invite your allies on your healing journey!

I had observed that whenever we were working outside and she stood with a hawthorn tree, a great deal of emotion would well up in her, sometimes overflowing in quiet tears. There was clearly emotional healing work for her to do—perhaps old hurts to clear and release—and I knew hawthorn was up to the job. With her long, fierce thorns, hawthorn teaches us how to open the emotional and spiritual heart, and at the same time create healthy boundaries when necessary.

Dandelion root is often the herb I reach for when there is a need to nourish the liver and improve how well it is functioning, especially in relation to the female reproductive system. There are, fortunately, numerous helpful plants and foods for the liver, but dandelion is one of my favorites; whenever possible, I prefer to work with common, abundant plants that I know well.

The liver performs hundreds of functions in our bodies including the production of numerous hormones. When a woman has menstrual problems of almost any sort, it's reasonable to think that at least part of the problem is that the liver is overloaded to the point where it can't do its job as well as it should. If you are living on Earth in the twenty-first century, your liver needs extra nourishment even if you eat a great diet and don't smoke or drink. It is simply a fact that we have to deal with more chemicals and pollutants than our brilliant bodies were designed to metabolize, so we have to take good care of our filter systems.

Wise herbalists don't seek to use herbs to take over for the body's filtration systems, because that weakens those systems. That would also be bringing a conventional medicine-model mindset to traditional medicine. What we would much rather do is work *with* the body by nourishing and strengthening the body systems and filtration systems such as the liver, lymph, kidneys, lungs, and skin. These systems are designed to help deliver nutrients to and clear wastes from the cells, so whether the health challenge is one of excess (having too much of something) or deficiency (not having enough of something), these systems will help you remain healthy and/or heal when you are ill. If a system is too depleted or overloaded to respond to herbs or other natural therapies, then medical intervention, though not one's first choice, is sometimes the necessary and therefore wisest choice.

When I got together for a detailed consultation with this woman, I learned that she had a life-long struggle with weight, ate an excellent diet, exercised regularly, and was currently having trouble sleeping.

I asked for *her* perspective of what was going on with her health, especially regarding any emotional/spiritual connections she may have made regarding this sudden onslaught of such severe problems with her moon cycle. She shared her story freely, and a few key facts were revealed:

She had been in an unhealthy relationship for seven years.

She had been so relieved to get out of that relationship that when it ended she had never talked about it again.

Two years previously, she had started therapy and had begun talking about the relationship. She was actively trying to shift out of similar unhealthy patterns in her current relationships.

When she heard herself describe this, she made the connection on her own and said, "Oh, this could have a lot to do with what's been going on with my body for the past two years!" Bingo! Her body was expressing and releasing all the pain that had been stored inside it/her all this time. Once she saw this for herself, she was no longer fearful. She became curious and excited. *Releasing fear is one of the most healing things we can do for ourselves anywhere along the continuum of our healing journey.*

To my mind, she could have taken any number of herbs perfect for her situation such as relaxing motherwort, or anti-spasmodic cramp bark, and they may or may not have helped her. As she said, "I do hear my body screaming for my attention, especially during menstruation." We can take herbs to shut our bodies up, using them in a drug-like way, or we can take herbs in a way that helps us heed the messages of love that our body is always communicating to us whether we're listening or not. This doesn't preclude symptom-relief and healing—it encourages these in ways that tend to be more sustainable and longer-lasting.

Before the session she wrote, "I want to have a plan that I know will work for me. I want to know what my body needs, so that I can create a better partnership with it. Right now I feel helpless when I am feeling the pain, and I would like to empower myself with more knowledge and remedies so I can heal myself."

With her commitment and intention focused on healing rather than simply escaping from the pain, we devised a plan that included a lymph-, liver-, and nerve- nourishing daily infusion, an emotional heart-healing tincture, a lymph-moving breast-massage oil, and a pain-relieving womb-massage oil.

The oils for breast and womb massage were key here not only because of the herbal properties in the oils but because these self-healing, sensual massages offered her opportunities to touch herself with tender care and love. I find this hands-on aspect of self-healing to be important even though it can be challenging. It is almost always helpful to include it in some way when a woman is healing her reproductive/hormonal system and learning to love her body/herself.

I also suggested that she have as many orgasms as possible in the week before her period. Because she was currently on her own, this was an opportunity to heal herself through her own loving touch and, practically speaking, orgasms stimulate and then relax the womb, making for less cramps. Who says healing can't be fun and pleasurable?

LIVER-LYMPH-LOVE INFUSION

¾ cup dried red clover

½ cup dried dandelion root

¾ cup dried violet leaf

Combine the herbs in a half-gallon jar. Cover with boiling water, and steep overnight. Drink it warm.

She was to drink one quart of this tasty infusion daily.

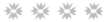

This woman also had breast swelling and tenderness before her period, which indicated a need to improve her lymph circulation too. All three herbs in her blend are great lymph-movers. Violet is also a tender, gentle healer; I turn to this herb when people are feeling vulnerable as they are entering into new places within themselves, or venturing into new territory outside. I also find violet to be one of the most helpful herbs for releasing grief.

Red clover provided a rich array of minerals for her, so important for nourishing and strengthening her nerves. She was bravely exploring what she had avoided up until then, and needed all the support she could get. Red clover also helps harmonize the female reproductive system generally.

Next we added the following tinctures. Here is a simple recipe if you want to make your own.

HAWTHORN BLOSSOM AND HAWTHORN BERRY TINCTURES

1 part fresh hawthorn blossoms

100-proof vodka, to fill the jar

———

1 part fresh hawthorn berries

100-proof vodka, to fill the jar

For the Blossom Tincture, pack the fresh flowers in your jar until the jar is full, and then cover with vodka. Label your jar. Shake it now and then. Top it up with more vodka as needed over the first week or two. Wait at least 6 weeks, and then decant the tincture.

For the Berry Tincture, cut up or mash the fresh berries and put them, seeds and all, into your jar. Fill it to the top with vodka, and follow the same directions as for blossoms. This woman used 25–40 drops of this tincture blend in four daily cups of herbal infusions.

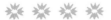

These tinctures are ideally made from fresh blossoms and fresh berries. These must be gathered and processed separately, because the flowers bloom in May and the berries aren't ripe enough to harvest until after a hard frost in the late autumn. If you don't want to make your own, or don't know where or how to get your own hawthorn blossoms and berries yet, the tinctures can be purchased and then combined together.

Hawthorn berries are sheer magic for healing heartache and heartbreak. She could have used berries alone for the physical and emotional healing that has been discussed so far.

The reason the hawthorn flowers were added into her mix was that they are helpful when a woman wants to healthily express her sexuality and illuminate her patterns of power dynamics in relationships. For another woman, roses or wild carrot might have been better choices.

VIOLET LEAF- AND DANDELION FLOWER-INFUSED BREAST-MASSAGE OILS

Fresh violet leaves and stalks–enough to fill a small jar

Olive oil—enough to fill the jar

Fresh dandelion blossoms—enough to at least half-fill a small jar

Olive oil—enough to fill the jar

To make either of these oils, gather enough fresh plant material to fill a fairly small jar. I guarantee it will hold more leaves or blossoms than you expect!

Spread out the leaves or blossoms and let them sit for several hours to a full day, out of direct sunlight, to dry a bit. Use the leaves and stalks of violet, and the entire blossom heads (inflorescence) of dandelion. Leave out most or all of the juicy flower stalk. (Don't throw out the stalks—eat them instead. They are bitter to taste, but help balance your blood sugar.)

For these and any infused oil, make sure your jar and lid are completely dry. The same goes for your hands, and the herbs too. Tear or cut up the violet leaves into small pieces, and fill the jar nearly full. For dandelion blossoms, pull the flower heads apart and fill the jar half-full. Cover with olive oil. Make sure the herbs are completely saturated, and then poke with a chopstick to release air bubbles. When you've done that for a while (you'll never get *all* of the bubbles) fill the oil to the tip-top rim of the jar and set the jar on a saucer to catch the overflow. Label the lid of the jar, and put it in a safe place.

For the first week or two, open the jar, poke the plant material down, add olive oil as needed, and wait about 6 weeks before decanting it for use. Don't leave your plant material in the oil for much longer than 2 months, as it is likelier to mold. That is definitely the voice of experience talking! (See Herbal Oils and Ointments, page 54, for trouble-shooting tips.)

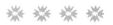

I love both violet and dandelion flower oils for breast massage, and suggested she alternate using them. I make my violet oil with the leaves and stalks, and the oil turns deep green, almost bordering on black. The dandelion blossom makes golden-yellow oil that smells and feels delicious. Both of these can be a little tricky to make, as they are moist plants and the water in them can cause mold. That's why I suggest letting the leaves and flowers dry out for a few hours to a day before infusing them.

Breast massage is a self-healing practice I encourage women to do as a regular part of their self-care. It helps any woman to know her breasts better, and is a pleasurable way to literally take your breast health into your own hands. Your breasts are filled with lymphatic vessels, and it's important to help the lymph fluid circulate freely and not get congested. Breast congestion can lead to swelling, tenderness, cysts, and tumors. There are women who teach breast massage (though any woman can feel her way, intuitively and literally), and these and other lovely herbal breast-massage oils are available for sale by herbalists. (See Resources, page 509.)

Womb Massage

Note: This is not related to the Arvigo Technique® of womb massage that Rosita Arvigo learned from her teacher Don Eligio Panti, in which she offers trainings. (See Notes, page 519.) Although I have learned that technique and recommend it, what I am referring to here is a simple, circular lower-belly massage that requires no special training, only love and gentleness.

I created an herbal oil I love to use for womb massage that I call "A-Z Oil." That name may sound as if it has a multitude of ingredients, but it is actually quite simple. It is made with *Artemisia vulgaris* (mugwort, aka cronewort) and *Zingiber officinale* (ginger).

A-Z (ARTEMISIA-ZINGIBER) WOMB-MASSAGE OIL

1½ cups dried *Artemisia vulgaris* leaves and stalks (If fresh, use 2½–3 cups. Make this oil with mature summer or autumn artemisia, ideally gathered when in flower, if possible.)

1 cup fresh ginger root

1 quart olive oil

Crumble up the mugwort/cronewort leaves and flowers, cut up the stalks, and grate the ginger. Put all the herbs directly into a pot made of stainless steel or some other non-reactive material (do not use aluminum unless it is the only option).

Cover the herbs with the olive oil. Heat it slowly and gently, while covered. If it threatens to bubble, turn it down or off. Take off the cover and stir it periodically with a wooden spoon throughout the process.

Then turn off the heat and let it sit covered for 1–3 hours; then repeat the warming process, being careful not to let it boil. Let it sit, covered, overnight.

Each day, repeat the gentle cooking, stirring, and steeping—ideally, for about 3 days. Then strain off the herbs, squeeze them, and bottle the oil.

If you are in a hurry you can make this oil in one day, but it gets better the longer and more gently it is prepared. Some women tell me they like to make it in a crock-pot that has a low temperature setting. I prefer not to infuse electricity into my medicine when I have a choice, but it is an option you may choose if you wish.

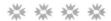

I originally created this recipe to use in a hands-on class I was giving at a women's spirituality conference. I have since used it for womb massages at women's herbal conferences and womb-wisdom classes around the United States. During these presentations, women of all ages give each other womb/belly massages in pairs, sometimes with great trepidation.

The youngest women I remember in one of these classes were thirteen-year-old friends who had come with one of their mothers. They *really* didn't want to do the massage, but I encouraged them, and they participated. Near the end of the class, one of them raised her hand and then said to the whole group, "I really hated having my period—hated everything about it; but after today, I love it. I can't believe how good that massage felt either. I want you to know I'll be doing that again."

Womb and belly massage is a tender thing to share with another woman. It is often approached very tentatively. And yet it is invariably healing to be gently touched with a sister's love and with the love of these plants. The combined heat (Artemisia is warming and Zingiber is heating) of these plants is soothing and helps release congestion. Both plants can (but don't necessarily) stimulate menstrual bleeding when used internally as foods, teas, tinctures, or vinegars. Externally, the oil will encourage healthy circulation and ease cramps.

It is a healing oil and a ritual oil that is warming, penetrating, and heating. Though it is a favorite for many women, and both of these plants definitely have a resonance with the womb, men can benefit from it too. It helps anyone with tired, sore muscles. I use it on stiff necks, calf muscles, or anywhere that it might be useful. A-Z Oil is pain relieving, anti-inflammatory, and enhances blood circulation. Not only that, but it is also delicious as a culinary oil on food! Try it on sautéed vegetables for a treat.

A-Z Oil helps with sprains, muscle-pulls, strains, and inflammation as well as with menstrual cramps and healing from sexual trauma. It can be massaged into one area or rubbed on the whole body. You can add it to a bath or put it on after a bath while your skin is still wet. It is fantastic for doing your own belly/womb massage. Massage your belly with the oil in a clockwise (sunwise) direction.

If your womb has been surgically removed, use this massage as an opportunity to reclaim the sacred space and energy of that area. The physical womb can be removed, but not your energy or womb-wisdom, which is innate and inviolate.

This practice of womb massage can help any woman reconnect with both her vulnerability and her power. It is helpful to note without judgment any feelings that arise. Write, draw, or do some other form of art about what arises for you. And please, after you make the oil, give those herbs back to Mother Earth. Ask her to help you in healing/reconnecting with your female core and the divine feminine energy (which contains the masculine within it) for yourself.

Please note that when a woman is pregnant I recommend a different oil to use over the womb or in a bath. A-Z Oil stirs up the blood in the pelvis, so it's best to err on the side of caution. Pregnant women in my workshops particularly loved infused rose oil and lady's mantle oil.

. . . .

Remember the client we were discussing? She did beautifully with her herbs and rituals; she did everything we set up for her to do. It has been almost two years since then, and she has never again had a painful period! After three months she wrote to me, "I didn't even know my period was coming. I can't tell you how relieved I feel!" Her flow was healthy. She had no cramping, no spasms, no blood-pressure drop, no feeling faint. She said she had had no more pain, extreme or otherwise.

Her understanding is that the pain she never expressed had gone into her body and stressed out her liver and lymphatic systems. She feels more and more confident in herself, her body, and her herbal remedies. I know she's on her way to healthier relationships, too. She tends to her "pale-ness" (a call for more iron) by eating more cooked carrots and beets the week before her period, and drinking nettles whenever she feels drawn to it—which, she tells me, occurs regularly.

Lady's Mantle (Alchemilla vulgaris)

I will at least consider the possibility of using lady's mantle for any illness of the womb, from fibroids, to pain, to infertility, and for nearly anything that needs tending to in a woman's cervix, uterus, ovaries, tubes, vagina, and breasts. It is a potent restorative herb.

The botanical name for lady's mantle translates to "common alche-mist," and I tend to turn to her most for times of transition when you need an alchemist's help! Lady's mantle is a lovely tonic that enhances fertility and strengthens the womb, supports a natural, healthy transition into and through menopause, and can help when there is a dire need, as with reproductive-system cancers.

Lady's mantle can be effective in quite a few forms, depending on your purpose. I most frequently use a tincture of the fresh leaves, stalks, and flowers in recipes or on its own, and also as a tea, poultice, sitz bath, or in anal or vaginal suppositories. Lady's mantle tincture (or dried leaves) combined with red clover infusion is a good hormonal tonic, and with red raspberry leaves added it increases its power as a fertility blend.

This strong, safe, gentle plant can also help a woman with uterine fibroids, especially those that cause heavy bleeding. I've had occasion to use lady's mantle to stop excessive uterine bleeding that even shepherd's purse couldn't stop. Shepherd's purse *(Capsella bursa-pastoris)* is a mustard-family plant once officially recognized in the U.S. pharmacopeia as a styptic herb—one that will slow down heavy uterine bleeding and even hemorrhaging—until it was removed some decades back, presumably for competing with more profitable pharmaceutical alternatives.

Lady's mantle has been called "Our Lady's herb." Could the lady be Gaia, the Earth Goddess herself, blessing us through the lady's mantle leaves, stalks, and star-like yellow-green flowers? I think so. When you look at, sit with, or take this herb, you may experience the feeling of being blessed. I experience lady's mantle as having a gentle, compassionate healing spirit, a kind of bodhisattva herb.

Down here on the Earth plane, lady's mantle helps heal both simple and inflamed hemorrhoids, and will help pain and tissue healing in an anal fissure. When more moistening is needed, I add chickweed internally and/or externally. In these instances I might use lady's mantle in combination with other vulnerary tissue healers such as plantain, yarrow, calendula, white oak bark, and/or witch hazel.

My great-grandmother was well-known in her day for a plant she used to help heal people's eyes. The details have been lost to time, but intuitively I suspect that it was lady's mantle, and imagine that she applied the softly furry, scalloped leaves as a healing poultice. They are soothing, anti-inflammatory, and antiseptic, helping anywhere there is infection with pus. The lady's mantle leaves on the plant are also well known for how they catch and hold the morning dew. The glistening drops of lady's mantle dew are sipped fresh from the leaves first thing in the morning to invoke healing and regeneration, physically and spiritually. It's one of my favorite magical things to do in my garden every morning. I also dip a finger into the dew and gently apply it over my closed eyes.

Lady's mantle is notable for being one of the rose-family plants that doesn't have any thorns. She excels at tissue repair, and clears heat and inflammation. Used internally, the tincture can help with insomnia, PMS, and swollen or lumpy breasts. I would use this plant for post-partum bleeding or heavy menopausal bleeding. It is definitely a plant to consider for healing from sexual trauma and from aftereffects of hysterectomy, abortion, miscarriage, and stillbirth.

A STORY OF HEALING AFTER A MISCARRIAGE

A mother of a one-year-old boy came to see me for help. She had unexpectedly gotten pregnant again one year after his birth, but she and her husband had been happy to learn she was twelve to thirteen weeks along. They were then deeply grieved when it turned out the little one had died inside her womb at around seven weeks. Labor was induced, and she had completed the miscarriage two months previously.

She came to see me because she had been on an emotional roller coaster since then. She was moody, often sad, angered easily, and would hold the anger inside. After the induced stillbirth, she had bled for a couple of weeks, stopped for a couple of weeks, and then had one period. At that point she had been bleeding lightly for five weeks and felt, in her words, "hopelessly miserable." The doctor had told her everything was fine. She had a history of depression, and had been on various medications over the past four years in order to be more functional; now she found herself afraid of her own grieving.

My heart went out to her. We reviewed her diet, lack of regular exercise, sleep patterns, etc., and I made a variety of suggestions. But as we were speaking about these important physical things, what really stood out to me was that she needed to mark the loss as genuine and allow herself to fully grieve it in order to have a sense of completion and be able to move on. She and her husband hadn't told anyone about her pregnancy or their subsequent loss. I suggested that she create a simple ritual with her husband.

Her grieving seemed utterly normal to me, especially given that her hormones were out of whack and in need of some soothing and nourishing. They had been in pregnancy mode, and she was abruptly no longer pregnant. Instead of getting ready to celebrate a birth, she and her husband were mourning a death, secretly. Not only that, but she had been holding death inside her for nearly six weeks while taking care of her baby boy. What woman wouldn't feel like an emotional yo-yo from all this? I wanted to help her trust her feelings and her body. What herb would help?

I suggested lady's mantle—*Alchemilla vulgaris*, the alchemical one. This plant is often put into gardens as an ornamental because it is so beautiful. The abundance of tiny green-yellow flowers are like little stars, and the leaves are furry, soft, and scalloped.

LADY'S MANTLE WOMB-TONIC TINCTURE

Fresh lady's mantle leaves, stalks, and flowers—enough to fill a jar

100-proof vodka

Use flowering lady's mantle. Cut the leaves and stalks up very small, and fill the jar with the leaves, the starry yellow blossoms, and the stalks. Pour the vodka over it and wait at least 6 weeks before decanting.

Lady's mantle is a great astringent and, like many plants in the rose family, very helpful to stop bleeding. But it is also a hormonal womb tonic, to bring strength and health back to this woman's womb. She was to use 25–30 drops of homemade tincture, 3 times daily.

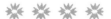

As I continued to listen to her with my ears and my heart, I had a sudden intuitive feeling that she couldn't stop grieving because she literally hadn't finished the miscarriage. It was unlikely that this was true because, upon questioning, she had absolutely no signs of infection such as fever, nausea, pain, or unusual fatigue. This was very fortunate. Still, I shared my feeling with her and told her that if that were the case, lady's mantle wouldn't stop the bleeding prematurely. Instead, it would help her body do what it needed to do, including clearing out any remaining tissue.

She would also add in a daily infusion of oat straw, nettles, and red raspberry. The profusion of vitamins and minerals in these three herbs rebuilds and strengthens blood, bones, and womb, to help this woman as they've helped so many women before. They optimally nourish the nervous system, enabling a person to become more adaptable and responsive to stressful situations with ease and grace. The oats bring physical and emotional peace and fluidity, and the nettles rebuild the overworked adrenals.

Together, they support emotional and physical stamina and vitality. When she felt stronger physically, I reasoned, it would be easier for her to feel stronger emotionally.

Finally, the red raspberry, a classic herb for childbirth, also in the rose family, would help heal and tone her womb. It could also help it to contract in the unlikely possibility that more tissue needed to be released.

WOMB AND WOMAN-STRENGTH INFUSION

¾ cup red raspberry

¾ cup nettles

½ cup oats

Put the dried herbs into a half-gallon jar and cover them with boiling water. Cap tightly. Steep the brew overnight. In the morning (or after at least 8 hours) decant the infusion by pouring off the liquid through a strainer or cheesecloth and squeezing out the herbs into the infusion, then using the spent plant material for compost.

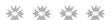

I didn't hear from the woman after giving her this recipe.

I finally called her two months later to ask how she was doing. She told me that she was feeling much better and was no longer, in her words, "grieving obsessively." She was still drinking her infusion daily and had no plans to stop, and was down to taking her lady's mantle twice a week. She had really liked the lady's mantle and taken it three times a day as suggested, and then stopped after a week or so. She hadn't been sure why, but felt that she should stop. She thought about what I had said about trusting her body and intuition, and decided to listen to her inner prompting.

Three days later she had begun to bleed more than before, and the bleeding increased until she finally passed some tissue that had not been expelled with the miscarriage. She felt better almost immediately after she'd released it.

She and her husband had done a simple, personally meaningful ritual. They planted a tree in honor of their daughter who had gone back to Spirit, and named her. They were now ready, she said, to tell their families. Then they would receive even more support.

As I write this, she is actively involved in sharing her gifts through positive community work, and she now has *two* beautiful, healthy children. Talk about green blessings!

The following story is an example of a situation where two common herbs, nettles and shepherd's purse (more readily recognized as nourishing herbs used to help build healthy blood through rich supplies of vitamins and minerals, to replenish a woman who has lost a lot of blood through her normal menstrual bleeding, or to help slow down and stop unusually heavy menstrual bleeding), were used as emergency remedies for an acute crisis.

HEALING FROM A BOTCHED LEGAL ABORTION

A woman I know had an abortion and began to hemorrhage at work the next day. She called me and asked for help. I advised her to go back to the clinic immediately. She informed me that she had called them, and was told she was not hemorrhaging—sounds unbelievable, but it's true. She said that at her age, thirty-two, she knew the difference between menstrual bleeding and hemorrhaging. She had bled through several menstrual pads, her clothes, and the cushion on her chair, right down to the carpet, and really needed help. They told her to come in the next day!

Her experience up to that point at this clean, respectable public health clinic had been good. She was astounded at their response, as was I. But she refused to go straight to a hospital emergency room, and asked me if I would be willing to help her. So we got to work.

Here's what she did:

She got home as quickly as possible and squirted a dropper of fresh shepherd's purse tincture into her mouth, directly under her tongue. In an emergency, this is a helpful way to take the herb, as it will get into the bloodstream more quickly, bypassing the digestive system. (That is the same reason I normally don't recommend taking tinctures that way in non-emergency situations. I suggest adding tinctures into water or infusion because you don't want them to by-pass your stomach and digestive tract and move through and out of your body fast.)

She repeated this every 10–15 minutes for an hour. She was "under orders" (mine) to go to the hospital emergency room without delay if her bleeding didn't slow significantly in this time; but it did slow down after the third dosage, and kept decreasing slowly but surely.

After this I suggested she boil a couple of big handfuls of dried nettles in a pot for about 10–15 minutes, and then let it steep for a while. She began to drink it freely, and felt her strength beginning to return. Meanwhile, she made a nettle infusion for later. When we spoke an hour later, she assured me that she was getting better.

I asked her if the bleeding had slowed down enough for her to be able to get into a bathtub. She responded that it would have been unthinkable before, when the bleeding was so heavy, but she could do that now. So she poured the nettle tea through a strainer into her full bathtub and soaked in a tepid/cool nettle bath, decreasing the bleeding even more as her skin directly absorbed the healing medicine of the nettles. (Rose-blossom infusion could have worked, too. Herbalist Rosita Arvigo tells the story of her first herbal experience—a woman had just given birth in a remote village and was bleeding to death. Rosita, guided by the village midwife, gathered roses and then watched as the cool rose bath saved the woman's life.)

By this point this woman was drinking the shepherd's purse tincture in water in much smaller doses every few hours, until she was finally putting about 5–10 drops of shepherd's purse tincture (which, by the way, she'd made the year before from weeds growing in her Manhattan neighborhood) into every other cup of nettles infusion that she drank the next day. Both the nettles and the shepherd's purse provided her body with astringency and a good supply of vitamin K to help stop the heavy bleeding. (See page 70 for more on stinging nettles.)

She was ultimately fine, and rebuilt her strength with herbs, cooked leafy greens, liver, beets, and other iron-rich, blood-building foods.

It's important to bring healing to your womb and hormonal system (and psyche) after intentionally or unintentionally releasing a pregnancy because it is not an easy thing for your body to go through. Some of the herbs I like to use for this have been discussed throughout this section, in particular the rose-family plants such as red raspberry, strawberry, lady's mantle, and rose, as primary womb-healing astringent tonics. Yarrow and nettles can be very helpful, too.

REGULATING THE MENSTRUAL CYCLE
WITH ALTERNATING INFUSIONS—ONE VARIATION

Infusion I: 1½–2 cups dried nettle leaf and stalk

Infusion II: 1½–2 cups dried red raspberry leaf

For each infusion, pour boiling water over the herbs in a half-gallon jar. Steep overnight and decant the herbal infusion in the morning.

The menstrual cycle is considered to begin each month at menstruation. Drink 2–4 cups daily of Infusion I for the first two weeks of your cycle, and then drink Infusion II for the next two weeks, taking a break during your menses if you like, and/or drinking whatever infusions feel right to you at that time. If your cycle is extremely rare or you don't cycle at all, use the new moon to mark the beginning of each cycle.

This variation is one example of alternating infusions, perhaps for a woman who wants her menstruation to flow each month as is natural. It could be appropriate for a woman who bleeds heavily during her menses and would benefit from taking blood-building nettles right afterward. For a woman looking to regulate her ovulation and menstruation in order to become pregnant in the future, I might reverse the order of the infusions, suggesting red raspberry for the first 2 weeks to begin tonifying her womb during the follicular phase in preparation for her eventual pregnancy.

Herbs I most commonly alternate in this cyclical way include: mugwort/cronewort, red clover blossoms, rose blossoms, wild carrot, red raspberry, strawberry, violet, lady's mantle, and nettles. For encouraging pregnancy, red clover blossoms, red raspberry and lady's mantle would tend to be my top choices, but again, individuals vary, and so do our needs.

Generally speaking, using two plants cyclically, for approximately two weeks each, follows the rhythm of the waxing and waning phases of the moon, and the follicular and luteal phases of a woman's cycle. It is a simple and effective way to re-regulate your menstrual cycle, whether it has never been regular, or has been thrown off by a hormonal experience such as a miscarriage or abortion, or if you recently stopped using hormonal birth control.

This healing can be helped by also learning to engage and work consciously with the cycles of the moon. (For more about moon magic and women's wisdom, read my book *Healing Magic: A Green Witch Guidebook to Conscious Living*.)

Simple Ritual Before Releasing Spirit Life from the Womb (or after, no matter how much time has gone by)

In a safe space, indoors or out, light a red candle to honor the sacred red thread of life, and the one who is (or was) held within your womb.

Meditate on the gift of life, and reflect on how humans spiral into and out of form, as all life does eventually. If it feels true for you, give thanks for this sacred gift that you may be unable to accept at this time.

Envision this being within you going home. This tiny spark of life is still primarily connected to All-That-Is and not yet fully attached to life in form.

Let the candle burn all the way down. Commune. Communicate. Express whatever is in your heart. Listen. Let go unconditionally. Imagine the briefly embodied spark of potential life reentering the womb of the Goddess, the Great Mystery, becoming one with the Universe, with God-Goddess-All-That-Is, or whatever you call the Divine Spirit.

You can imagine releasing this beloved Spirit back to the primal elements, Earth, Air, Fire, Water, and into the Void of All Becoming, the Center.

> If appropriate, you might choose to invite this Spirit to come
> back to you later, at a time when you are ready to have a child.
> (If inappropriate for you, don't include that.)
>
> When the candle is done, bury the remnants in the earth, either
> right away or later; or burn them in a fire pit or fireplace; or give
> them away to a flowing body of water. It is done in Beauty.

A woman may feel that acknowledging the life essence in her womb contradicts her right to release that life. It doesn't. It is still a woman's right to make her own choice, not least because it is *her* body that would be directly responsible for continuously nourishing the spark of potential human life that we call an embryo.

If you are feeling any guilt because of teachings you've received or stories you were told, do whatever you can to release that "emotion." Guilt is more of a mindset than a real feeling. It's a pattern of thinking that keeps you in the past, blinded by the fear that you are bad or wrong in some fundamental way. You are not.

Meditation, movement, and simple ritual can help you learn how to allow your feelings a space in which to be. Let them flow, including any honest remorse, anger, grief, and/or relief and freedom you may feel. Breathe in and out, and be present to what is.

A woman may fear that it will be too emotionally painful to connect with the spirit inside her womb. Many of us attempt to go through the process of aborting (by whatever means) with detachment, in an attempt to protect ourselves. But it is impossible to truly detach from what is happening, given the intimacy of the experience. Conversely, going through it with awareness can actually become an empowering experience and a rite of passage.

Here is what one woman, who works with young women at risk and is the mother of a toddler, had to say on the subject:

"Consciously choosing to abort with herbs was a difficult decision but, surprisingly, one of the deepest and most powerfully *positive* experiences of my life. I know it sounds almost like heresy, but it's true. I emerged through that process feeling deeply connected to my body, my partner, my ancestors, *and* my unborn child. Through meditation, visualization, prayers, and soul-baring communication, I was able to process my fear and regret, thank the life that had chosen us, *and* ask it to leave; to feel spiritually and emotionally connected to my foremothers (three generations of whom experienced abortions or miscarriages), and forge a deeper bond with my partner.

"The entire process took a few weeks, and while it was a very difficult time in my life, it also allowed me the time to truly process my emotions and to go deeper and deeper in my own herbal, spiritual, and healing journeys. We rarely hear real women's abortion stories, and particularly stories such as mine, where women leave stronger, more resilient, and more *whole*. I am blessed to have had the experience, and equally importantly the *guide*, to experience abortion as an empowering rite of passage rather than as a shameful trauma, and hope that more women consider *and* have access to this option for themselves."

Attempts to keep women from having full freedom of choice take many different forms, including legislative efforts aimed at making it increasingly difficult to obtain contraception, let alone abortions.

And then there are the women who want the freedom to have their babies but choose not to do so because financial limitations make it seem as if they don't really have that option. They are fearful that if they don't have enough money they won't be able to support a child, or another child, and there is no adequate safety net, nor community support, for these women and their families.

Our culture, including those factions that call themselves "pro-life," meagerly support women and children once they're born—least of all, women and children of color. But we are a culture in transition, a culture on the edge of eve-olution. As we each increase our sense of interconnectedness with one another through the help of herbs and simple rituals, and continue to empower ourselves in natural ways, waking up our hearts, we will gather the energy and confidence we need to guide the transformation of our culture with our visions, our voices, and our actions.

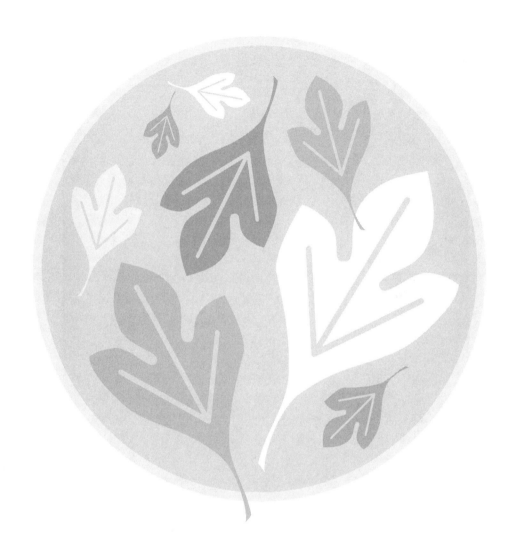

PART III

Everything Is Medicine

14

Kitchen Medicines—Common Foods, Herbal Honeys, Herbal Vinegars, and Herbal Medicine in Your Spice Rack

One of the most common ways of healing self, family and friends is with homemade herbal medicines called "meals." As Hippocrates said, "Let your food be your medicine, and your medicine be your food."

There is medicine all around us. Our kitchens, including our spice racks, can be an abundant source of effective medicine for us, and safer than what we find in the pharmacy. Open your mind and your senses to the broader possibilities for creating healing feasts in your own kitchen.

Common herbs, foods, and condiments such as basil, garlic, salt, onions, carrots, dark leafy greens, honey, vinegar, and so much more provide remedies for a vast variety of conditions. Mint plants, so rich in antioxidants and helpful for digestion, can help keep us well and in tip-top shape, which is to say, in mint condition! Many healing spice plants are in the mint family, such as basil, sage, rosemary, and lavender.

Some Common Healing Foods

Apples—for digestive health.

Basil—for good fortune, good spirits; helps the system heal in the presence of parasites, fungi, viruses, and/or bacteria.

Cinnamon—styptic, antiseptic; helps circulation, balances blood sugar.

Garlic—for respiratory, immune, cardiovascular, and digestive health.

Ginger—euphoric, stimulant, ant-spasmodic, and anti-inflammatory.

Honey—for wounds; rehydrating, anti-allergenic, provides amino acids.

Hot cocoa/dark chocolate—healthy comfort food; antioxidant, endorphin-stimulating.

Lavender—soothing, antiseptic; heals burns.

Lentils—phytoestrogen-rich, nourishing, and protective to female reproductive system.

Marjoram—antibacterial, warming, soothing to joints.

Mushrooms—immune-modulating, cancer-protective, anti-tumor.

Mustard—pungent, breaks up congestion in the respiratory system, brings heat to release pain (though too much mustard can cause pain).

Onions—drawing, anti-infective, anti-inflammatory, cough-relieving.

Rosemary—enhances cardiovascular circulation and brain functioning; memory tonic, liver tonic; helps ease headaches including migraines.

Sage—mineral-rich brain and nervous-system tonic for illnesses that cause paralysis; good in foot baths; throat-healing, strong antiseptic.

Salt—for wounds, anemia; protective against bacterial infections.

Seaweeds—rich in antioxidants, carotenes, calcium, and selenium; remove heavy metals and radioactive isotopes from the body.

Slippery elm—demulcent for throat and intestines; nourishing mucilage; helpful for constipation and/or diarrhea.

Thyme—warming, calming; bronchial antispasmodic, antibacterial.

Turmeric—for circulation; warming liver and digestive tonic; anti-inflammatory, immune-supportive.

Vinegar—helpful to acid/alkaline balance in body, restoring proper pH; digestive aid; helps joints remain flexible; menstruum for minerals.

If you're eating well and feeling gratitude for your food, you're already taking good medicine. Medicine is anything that heals, including and perhaps especially positive energy that comes from genuine kindness extended to oneself and others.

When our food is prepared with love and care, these foods and spices are among the best medicines in the world. Along with a sense of connection to nature and a community of people, they truly form the foundation of good health.

When you buy local food, it is fresher and more full of vitality than even organic food from a supermarket or big-box store. When plants or animals are raised as if they are "things" being manufactured in a factory, the generous essence of life-feeding-life is lost. The relationship chain is broken. There is something deeply satisfying about knowing where your food comes from, who grew the vegetables or raised the chickens, and how they take care of their land. It brings you into a more direct relationship with Earth, which feeds you. That is a healing revelation, especially to urban and suburban people who have access to twenty-four-hour markets and don't necessarily think about all the miles that the food they are buying has traveled to reach them, not to mention all the hands, trucks, and warehouses it has passed through.

At one point when I lived in New York City, I was lucky enough to live a couple of blocks from one of the most vibrant farmer's markets in Manhattan. I learned so much when I began buying my food there. For example, I would ask for a particular vegetable and would be told that it was not in season yet, or that its season had passed. And even though that seems obvious to me now, it wasn't then. It gave me new insight and information that became important to my health.

It also brings communities together when it is your neighbor who is growing food for you to buy in a local farmers' market. You know they care about what they are providing for you, because they will also see you in the post office or the bank, and if the food isn't good they will hear about it! And they are feeding you the same things they feed themselves and their families.

You also develop a deeper understanding about the risks they take to bring you tasty, nourishing food, and more appreciation for the uncontrollable effects of weather and climate change, for example. If you have your own garden, you know how much work it is to build the soil and keep it healthy for the plants, so you eat your food with more gratitude. You come to care more personally about the health of the ecosystem you live in because you understand more personally that its health and your health are inextricably linked.

On a more basic level, when simply looking at locally grown food you can see that the colors are more vibrant. And tasting it, there is no question that a simple food like a fresh tomato can range from bland to divine. Years ago, a friend who had only eaten conventional and processed foods from the supermarket came to visit me in New York. I remember him taking his first bite of freshly baked whole-grain bread. The look on his face was one of pure astonishment. He finished chewing and announced seriously, "I'm learning right now that bread is actually a food, not just something to put around the insides of my sandwich!"

Food is the basic medicine we take every day.

My student Barry told me the following story. Barry comes from a close Italian family. His sister, the mom of a young child, had been run-down and constantly sick or relapsing for almost two months. He had been taking herbal-medicine classes with me for quite a while by then, and knew how to help, but she would have none of it—herbal medicine was not for her.

Barry felt like he was at his wit's end. But he's a clever and determined guy, and came up with another plan. He remembered what I said about making food our medicine, and he made her a very large pot of healing soup.

It contained an assortment of fresh vegetables including parsley and carrots, celery and tomatoes, squash and cauliflower, and whatever other vegetables looked good to him. He remembered to put in as many colors of foods as possible. He sautéed lots of garlic, onions, shiitakes, and other healing mushrooms in olive oil, and added some oregano, basil, ginger, and other healing spices. He put in some astragalus roots, and added nettle infusion and herbal vinegar to the soup. I think he may have snuck some seaweed in there, too. He said it was delicious, and she never suspected a thing.

He reported that by the time she got to the bottom of the soup pot in about a week, she was well. She never made any connection between her soup and her sudden wellness. He smirked a little, happy with himself at having gotten his stubborn sister to take her medicine. "We're Italian," he said by way of explanation. "Did you think she was going to turn down my home-cooked food?"

A HEALING STORY

One day I began to cough strongly, and didn't at all like the sound of it, or the way it felt. The coughing hurt my throat and felt as if it came from smack in the center of my chest. It even felt like the inside of my heart hurt.

Then I got scared. I had visited a dear friend in her late eighties that day, who was very weak with both pneumonia and an underlying lung infection (acquired years before in the hospital when she'd had a hip replacement) and she, of course, had been coughing.

What if I had been exposed to some bacteria or virus that "got" me? I started to feel panicky, but then I reminded myself:

Love is stronger than fear. Love strengthens, and love is what heals.

Fear and anxiety, self-doubt and worry all provoke illness. They bog down the body's vital energy, feed the conditions that give illness a place to take hold. I reminded myself that I did the right thing, visiting and loving my friend, hugging her, touching her … yet I knew I needed to take care of myself too, emotionally and physically.

I was hurting emotionally myself, having a strong response to my beloved friend's deteriorated condition, to seeing her attached to an oxygen tank, growing weaker day by day. But the symptoms I was experiencing were also physical.

It was time for some self-care. I boiled water, and put a small spoonful of dried lavender flowers into a mug to make a soothing, anti-microbial tea. Now lavender may be the herb least commonly found in the kitchen among the herbs discussed in this chapter, but to me dried lavender belongs in the kitchen. Lavender is extraordinary. It is lovely to cook and bake with, and is any plant better for putting the mind at ease and calming the heart than sweet-smelling lavender? I find it to be an unfailing ally. After ten minutes, I poured off my tea through a little mesh strainer, and also stirred some homemade lavender honey into my cup. Lavender honey is so delightful, and so simple to make! All you need is lavender, honey, and a jar.

LAVENDER HONEY

Fresh or dried lavender flowers

Enough honey to fill your jar

Fill a wide-mouthed glass jar loosely full with fresh lavender flowers. Fill it half-full if using dried flowers. Cover the flowers with the best-quality honey you can afford, local and raw if possible. Pour the honey over the flowers slowly while poking them with a chopstick to make sure the honey completely saturates all the lavender. Stir it in as needed.

Close the jar and wait as long as you can. Then enjoy it, in tea, on toast, or simply by the spoonful. I try to wait about a month before using it, but that's not always "possible."

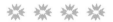

This antiseptic honey is also a wound-healer, and could be applied externally to a burn, scrape, or open wound to prevent and/or heal infection. Lavender soothes and comforts, brings ease, and cools things down physically and emotionally in her uniquely sweet way.

My cup of tea was healing and delectable! This simple homemade medicine soothed and softened my dry bronchia. It cooled down the irritated tissues, and deepened and relaxed my breathing. In a few more minutes I felt quite a bit more comfortable, physically and emotionally. I sighed a sigh of relief. As I relaxed, I realized I'd actually been "taking medicine" all night in my mostly organic, local food.

My meal that evening had been delicious, and almost everything in it had supportive medicinal properties for my respiratory, nervous, and immune systems. It contained immune-strengthening antioxidants, nerve-nourishing minerals, anti-infective vitamins and phytochemicals, and healthy fats to strengthen my cardiovascular system.

Consider the ingredients that made up the pesto I'd enjoyed. Though it's most commonly made with Genovese basil, you can make pesto with any greens, such as nettles, wild mustard, mint, catnip, lamb's quarters, or many others. I had made that one with half purple basil and half parsley, both from our own garden.

BASIC PESTO RECIPE

2 cups basil (or other) leaves

½–⅔ cup olive oil, or as much as needed for your desired consistency

3 large cloves garlic, or to taste

¼ cup walnuts or pine nuts

Sea salt, to taste

½ cup of Romano or Pecorino cheese (This is optional; I make mine without cheese, finding it rich enough as is, and it received a rave review recently from an "old-school" Italian apprentice whose family owns two restaurants; he said he couldn't believe how good it was without cheese.)

Combine some of the basil, garlic and olive oil and blend it coarsely in a food processor, or do it the traditional way, in a mortar and pestle. Keep adding your basil, garlic and olive oil bit by bit, blending or pounding it to your desired consistency. Then add the nuts, salt, and any remaining olive oil, and adjust the seasonings to your taste. Remember that it's going to be added to food and won't be as "strong" as it tastes on its own. (If adding cheese, use a food processor, or grate it finely and add it in).

You can use this immediately, and refrigerate or freeze any extra. Use a spatula to put it into small glass jars. If freezing them, make sure to leave about half inch to an inch of space at the top of the jar since it will expand as it freezes. The larger the jar, the more space you should leave—and regardless of size, close the cap loosely until fully frozen.

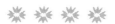

For a fabulous-tasting variation on the basic pesto recipe, add in some antioxidant-rich sun-dried tomatoes, and use raw pumpkin seeds instead of nuts. Pumpkin seeds are high in zinc, and superb for the prostate gland.

Basil and garlic both have antiviral, antibacterial and antifungal properties specifically helpful to the respiratory system, and therefore good for my cough. All species of basil that I've encountered lift your spirits as well. Basil is a truly magical plant.

Parsley has minerals galore, including a good supply of iron. It's high in folic acid, which helps relieve stress by strengthening the nervous system. Parsley is well-known for strengthening the functioning of the kidneys. (Kidneys are connected with fear and anxiety in Chinese medicine, as well as considered to hold our basic life essence.) The salt in the pesto is a great antibacterial. (That's one reason why we gargle with warm salt water for a sore throat; it's also soothing.) And olive oil is one of the healthiest, most nourishing fats available for daily use, providing essential fatty acids and benefiting almost every system in the body, beginning with the cardiovascular system. Olive oil is rich in monounsaturated fat and antioxidants including chlorophyll, carotenoids, and vitamin E.

Later that evening, I had a simple, delectable dessert.

BERRY-RICH DESSERT

1 cup plain, organic, whole-milk yogurt with live cultures

½ cup fresh or frozen blueberries

¼–½ cup fresh or frozen cherries

⅛ cup shredded coconut

Cinnamon powder, to taste

Vanilla extract, to taste

Cook the berries and cherries over a very low flame, if frozen—just enough to thaw them. Keep a watchful eye to ensure they don't get scorched.

Put the berries in a bowl when they're ready, and then stir in the yogurt and coconut flakes. Add the cinnamon powder and vanilla extract.

If you want to have this dish as a meal, you can add more fruit such as an apple or pear, and make it more substantial and protein-rich by adding your choice of walnuts, cashews, almonds, or pumpkin and/or sunflower seeds.

❄ ❄ ❄ ❄

Again, this is immune-enhancing food that tastes *amazing*. Freezing and cooking the berries actually makes their nutrients more bio-available. Blueberries are not only scrumptious, they are rich in anthocyanins (the antioxidant flavonoids that make the berries blue). And the plentiful live bacteria in the yogurt nourishes digestive- and immune-system functioning. I felt so much better later that evening, and went to sleep knowing I would most likely be well, come morning. And, come morning, I was!

Blueberry (*Vaccinium* species)

Blueberry is a well-loved, familiar fruit. It is tannin-rich, antioxidant, and provides potent medicine. Blueberry is strengthening to veins and capillaries, and especially healing to eyes. Blueberry is a food medicine, vibrating energy directly into our blood and our cells.

Eaten, tinctured, made into elixir or syrup, or even as an ingredient in dark-chocolate bars, blueberry is good medicine. Blueberry brandy tincture is helpful for digestive troubles from vomiting to diarrhea, and can help soothe an inflamed liver. The leaves can be used as a tea, dried, powdered and added to food, or taken in tincture form. They have been shown to help lower and regulate high blood sugar, making blueberry a plant medicine to consider for hypoglycemia and diabetes.

Alma Hutchens writes about the "blueberry-like bilberry" in her 1973 book, *Indian Herbalogy* [sic] *of North America*. Bilberry is a close cousin of our native American blueberries, so I'll quote her: "It may be of interest to know that in Russia, bilberry has a well-established reputation as being similar to insulin for sugar diabetes." More recent scientific research has confirmed this.

Spiritually, blueberries offer us the medicine of sweetness. They seek to remind us of the sweetness of life on Earth—the sweetness of flowers, of fruits, of friendship. Here on Earth we are part of the same living community as blueberries. I live at the edge of an oak and pine forest full of high- and low-bush blueberries. Their spring flowers are small, waxy, white-pink bells.

Once, when I was meditating with blueberry, she told me that she isn't from this planet but that she came here to help us and has now been here for a very long time. She said if I were to pick a berry and gaze into the star pattern at the bottom of it, I'd be taken to the star spaces inside myself. I tried it, wondering if I might be able to see where she was from. I sat quietly, letting my thoughts go. I felt pulled by a vortex of energy through a deep, dark spaciousness, and then floated far out into the cosmos. I don't know where I was, but I felt expansive and free.

Recently I found the following information in a Native American ethnobotany database from the University of Michigan: "The blossom end of each berry, the calyx, forms the shape of a perfect five-pointed star; the elders of the tribe would tell of how the Great Spirit sent 'star berries' to relieve the children's hunger during a famine."

Blueberries can be enjoyed fresh, or they can be dried or frozen whole for later use. Native peoples have often used dried blueberries in pemmican, a nutrient-dense, dried-food preparation that typically contains meat, fat, fruit, and spices. Pemmican is still useful to sustain a person on a long journey, or to sustain a community through lean times.

Science tells us that blueberry fruits contain anthocyanidins and proanthocyanidins, flavonoid molecules that give the fruits their deep-blue color and offer us a diverse spectrum of health benefits as discussed above, and more, including reducing inflammation and inhibiting the development of cancer cells.

Of course people have been benefiting from blueberries long before science took the plant apart in a laboratory to examine and determine its constituents. We learned about plants through our senses, and our sense of oneness with them. We can still do this. The plants remember why they are here, and when we approach them with love and respect they are our willing teachers and healers.

Singing has always been an important part of Earth-based healing traditions. Any plants or trees I've met so far love to be sung to, even off-key. I am told each plant has its own song, and I believe it, but I haven't yet developed the ability to hear them. Perhaps one day I will have that pleasure.

The following song is a call-and-response chant that my apprentice June taught to our circle when we were in the woods harvesting blueberries. I love singing with groups. Sincerity of heart matters more than perfect pitch, or even the ability to carry a tune! The author gave his blessings for this lovely song to be included here.

Sweetness Song by Jason Cohen

Sweetness is knocking on my heart's door.
Sweetness is knocking on my heart's door.
Sweetness is knocking on my heart's door.

(Call) I am home,
(Response) I am home,
(Call) I am home,
(Response) I am home.

(Call) Come on in,
(Response) Come on in,
(Call) Come on in,
(Response) Come on in.

(Call) We are home,
(Response) We are home,
(Call) We are home,
(Response) We are home.

(Call) Let it in,
(Response) Let it in,
(Call) Let it in,
(Response) Let it in.

Honey

There is evidence that people have been collecting honey at least since the Stone Age. Honey is an everyday, sacred miracle, as the bees that create it are themselves miracles. There is first the astonishing scientific "fact" that it is aerodynamically impossible for a bee to fly. Perhaps this is what Einstein meant when he said, "Reality can be tyrannical, but we can bypass it." Then there is the fact that bees communicate through dance to reveal the locations of water and pollen to other bees. And as if those weren't miraculous enough, bees give us honey, pollen, propolis, and beeswax.

Raw honey, which often contains bits of pollen in it, is antimicrobial, antioxidant, and a good antiseptic for a sore throat and for external wound-healing. One of honey's chemical constituents is inhibin, which reacts with the glucose in your body to form hydrogen peroxide, well-known as a common disinfectant. Interestingly, straight hydrogen peroxide can be destructive to skin tissue, whereas my educated guess is that the hydrogen peroxide that our bodies make in conjunction with honey doesn't have that destructive property.

Honey is a complex healing food, and a healthful sweetener. It is rich in minerals including calcium, iron, magnesium, phosphorus, potassium, and zinc. Earth poet/herbalist, Stephen Buhner writes that honey contains over sixty-seven different active constituents. This includes a range of B vitamins (no pun intended). Honey is also rich in amino acids, the enzymes that aid digestion and metabolism. It is well-established that the regular consumption of raw, local honey decreases the symptoms of pollen-induced allergies for many people. For that use, I'd suggest a half-teaspoon two or three times a day.

Honey is hygroscopic, meaning it draws moisture to it, and as such is a soothing moisturizer. This is part of what makes it an exceptional first-aid treatment for burns. Honey can also be used as a restorative facial mask for any type of skin: Simply apply plain honey (or infused herbal honey) to dry skin, wait ten minutes, and rinse off with warm water. Your skin will feel marvelous! Honey also reduces inflammation and redness.

Honey has been used for burns and wounds for millennia. On the National Institute of Health (NIH)'s website, there are numerous studies on the use of honey for healing burns and wounds. Here's an excerpt from one of them detailing clinical observations of the wound-healing properties of honey:

Fifty-nine patients with wounds and ulcers, most of which (80 per cent) had failed to heal with conventional treatment, were treated with unprocessed honey. Fifty-eight cases showed remarkable improvement following topical application of honey. One case, later diagnosed as Buruli ulcer *[a tropical bacterial infection]*, failed to respond. Wounds that were sterile at the outset remained sterile until healed, while infected wounds and ulcers became sterile within 1 week of topical application of honey. Honey debrided wounds rapidly, replacing sloughs with granulation tissue. It also promoted rapid epithelialization, and absorption of oedema from around the ulcer margins.

Translated into plain English, the honey caused the dead or infected tissue to be sloughed off without need for painful surgical intervention, promoted the growth of healthy new skin cells, and absorbed excess fluids held in the margins of the wound or ulcer. It did all this while helping to maintain (or create) a sterile environment for healing.

Honey is also soothing, and will relieve a cough. A December 2007 study from Penn State College of Medicine found that:

(A) small dose of buckwheat honey given before bedtime provided better relief of nighttime cough and sleep difficulty in children than no treatment or dextromethorphan (DM), a cough suppressant found in many over-the-counter cold medications. Honey did a better job reducing the severity, frequency and bothersome nature of nighttime cough from upper respiratory infection than DM or no treatment. Honey also showed a positive effect on the sleep quality of both the coughing child and the child's parents. *[I love that last detail!]* DM was not significantly better at alleviating symptoms than no treatment. These findings are especially notable since an FDA advisory board recommended that over-the-counter (OTC) cough and cold medicines not be given to children less than 6 years old because of their lack of effectiveness and potential for side effects.

Dark buckwheat honey was used in this study. The darker the honey, the higher the antioxidants it contains. Antioxidants are basically compounds that keep us from oxidizing, or "rusting," as we continue to age.

Golden honey is also excellent. It's simply that the richer in color a food is, the more nutritious and medicinally beneficial it usually is.

I love to infuse herbs into honey. Not only is it a pleasant way to take herbal medicine, but honey is also a fine preservative for the herbs. In fact, honey is so potent a preservative that for many centuries it was used for embalming.

Orange peel honey is an easy-to-make antioxidant treat. Herbalist Susun Weed calls citrus peel a potent longevity tonic. When you peel oranges to dry them for medicine, keep as much of the white inner peel intact as possible, since the most potent bioflavonoids in oranges are found there. You know they are fully dry when you bend them and they crack.

ORANGE PEEL HONEY

½–1 part dried organic orange peels

1 part raw honey

Break up the dried peels and place them in a clean, dry jar. Pour in the honey, slowly covering all the peels and filling the jar. Cap the jar and wait.

When you open the lid to check on your preparation, or to add a bit more honey if it has been absorbed by the peels, wait until the sweet orange-honey smell bowls you over in the best possible way, usually in 4–6 weeks.

Use your orange peel honey freely, alone, in tea, over yogurt and fruit, over ice cream, pancakes, or whatever you dream up. You can also use tangerine or blood-orange peels, but use organic fruit only, please.

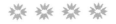

Orange blossom honey is commonly available for purchase. If you have access to fresh or dried blossoms, you could also infuse orange blossoms in honey in the same way as the peels for a nerve-soothing, libido-enhancing, delightful and sensual treat.

I got the following sweet recipe from Honey Gardens of Vermont:

CARROT HONEY SPREAD

4–5 carrots

¼ cup raw honey

¼ cup chunky peanut butter (I use almond butter instead)

⅛ teaspoon curry powder

Salt, to taste

Peel and finely grate the carrots. Stir in the remaining ingredients. Season with salt as needed. Enjoy!

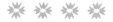

Salt

What is more basic than the salt of the Earth, the salt of our oceans? Salt, or sodium chloride, is a mineral-rich rock crystal that your body's systems depend upon. Salt is necessary to life.

Sodium is one of the primary electrolytes in the body, along with chloride, potassium, magnesium, and calcium. Sea salt adds these and other vital minerals and nutrients to your diet. Salt is sometimes the single most important missing nutrient for resolving anemia. When you perceive a salty taste in an herb, such as nettles, chickweed or dandelion greens, for example, that taste is telling you that it is a plant rich in mineral nutrients.

Sea salt is a general term that refers to unrefined salt derived directly from a living ocean or sea. It is harvested through channeling ocean water into large clay trays and allowing the sun and wind to evaporate it naturally. Traditionally, such salt is harvested by hand using wooden rakes, and some commercial salt is still harvested this way.

Table salt, the most common kind of salt found in the average kitchen, usually comes from salt mines. Once mined, it is refined, and most minerals are removed until it is pure sodium chloride. This makes it bitter and less nourishing than sea salt. Most table salt is also available in iodized form, where the salt is artificially spray-coated with iodine. I strongly suggest going with "real" salt—unrefined salt from the sea that is not pure white because its trace and other minerals are intact. It actually contains less sodium than table salt. Table salt may also be adulterated with sugar and other additives. The problem with excessive salt intake has mainly to do with the refined, adulterated salt that is added indiscriminately into processed and packaged foods of all kinds, where it does take a toll on our health.

Sea salt is an excellent antibacterial for wounds, and one of the first things I reach for when there is an open injury with a potential to get infected. (See Wound and Bruise Healing, page 471.) Salt can be dissolved in hot water and used to bathe a wound to prevent or help cure infection. Salty water can also be taken into the nose via a neti pot or by cupping some saltwater in your palm, bringing your nose to it, and inhaling it up into each nostril, one at a time. Either method of "snuffing" salt water is used to help clear the sinuses when allergies, infections, and/or acute or chronic inflammation cause the sinuses to get clogged. Additionally, this can be used to protect you from the potential harm of inhaled pathogens. Herbalist Susun Weed has written that salt water snuffed up the nose is a simple protective against anthrax poisoning.

On a more routine note, taking a bath in salt water is one of the surest ways to rewire your energy circuits and put your endocrine and nervous systems back into sync if you've gotten overwhelmed by anything or anyone, and especially if you've been navigating through hospitals, schools, jails, or any other institutional setting.

SEA-SALT BATH

2–3 cups sea salt

Bathtub full of warm-to-hot water

1–1½ cups baking soda (optional)

Stir at least 2 cups of good-quality sea salt into your bathwater *after* your tub has filled with hot water. Spend at least 20 minutes in the bathtub for best effects. Baking soda increases the energy-clearing and anti-radiation benefits of the bath. You could also choose to add it to your salt bath simply because it smoothes and softens skin.

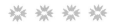

This bath is so helpful to both relax and re-energize yourself. A salt-water bath evokes the oceanic waters that are our ancient place of origin. We, like all life on Earth, evolved out of the oceans.

I read a lovely blog post written by herbalist Rachel Fee-Prince:

> Alchemists thought salt would "fix the volatile spirit," binding soul to matter. I share their belief that salt is akin to soul. As salt preserves food, so does soul preserve body, and life itself. Salt brings out flavors otherwise dull, while soul enhances the life experience, allowing us to savor all the morsels of goodness the universe has to offer.... Salt evokes the ocean, abundant primal mother of all.

Coarse salt can be heated up, wrapped in a muslin bag or old pillow-case, and applied as a poultice to a painful area. Salt can also be used as an invigorating scrub to encourage exfoliation, and increase circulation and a general sense of vitality.

Dehydration can have serious consequences. If someone becomes dehydrated, whether through diarrhea, too much sun, excessive sweating, or any other cause, it is important to restore the fluid and electrolytes that have been depleted. Electrolytes are responsible for the balance of fluids in our bodies. They are essential for the electrical signals to fire properly and stimulate the nerves that send communications to the muscles and just about everything else.

The first signs of dehydration are usually thirst, dry mouth, and very little urination, but dehydration can progress quickly to stomach or muscle cramps, disorientation, nausea, and dizziness. Here is a quick, easy recipe for immediate use:

SIMPLE ELECTROLYTE-RESTORATION REMEDY

⅛–¼ teaspoon sea salt

1 teaspoon honey

Dissolve salt and honey into a glass of water, and drink for immediate relief.

This, or any similar salt-and-sugar mix, offers a more natural alternative to Gatorade and the like. It is common belief that if you are dehydrated you only need to drink water; but your body needs the water *and* the combination of sugar, salt and minerals to maintain the fluids surrounding every cell, and to keep all those synapses successfully firing.

Apple (*Malus* species)

The sweet or sour crunchy fruits of the apple tree may be the ultimate digestive healing aid. Hildegard of Bingen is reputed to have used apples for everything. She prescribed raw apples as a tonic for healthy people, and turned to cooked apples as the first treatment for any sickness. That is saying a lot!

Rich in vitamins and abundant in minerals, apples improve your circulation, and the functioning of your nerves and brain. Hundreds of species (there are thousands) are used as both food and medicine. Apples are high in soluble fiber; they relieve constipation and/or diarrhea, benefit the liver, and are a fine source of quick, healthy energy, since their fruit sugar breaks down slowly to keep blood sugar stable.

Apples are rich in malic and tartaric acids, which help neutralize excess acid in the body. They help clear tartar from the teeth. Regular consumption of apples aids digestion, and can help with arthritis and gout. In France, the dried peels are used for gout both internally as infusions and externally as poultices. Herbalist and writer Dian Dincin Buchman writes that sweet apples help with an acidic stomach, while sour apples are the most helpful to increase stomach acid. She also recommends raw, peeled, grated apple pulp as a poultice for muscle strains or sore eyes.

Maud Grieve, author of *A Modern Herbal*, shares, "Ripe, juicy apples eaten at bedtime every night will cure some of the worst forms of constipation. Sour apples are the best for this purpose." Southern folk herbalist Tommie Bass used fresh apples for constipation, and dried apples for diarrhea.

In Ayurvedic medicine, green apples are favored for treating diarrhea. In Chinese medicine, apple bark tea is used for diabetes. The bark and

At this point I was pretty weak, having lost a lot of weight very quickly. It turns out barley is a perfect food for convalescents, deservedly famous as a supremely nourishing food, especially when the digestion is weak. Barley water is gentle enough for infants and elders, and I have used it for both.

The evening I cooked the barley, I stood in my kitchen and felt the presence of my great-grandmother guiding me, clear to me in a way I've never felt before or since. She occasionally corrected me as we went along. So I made it exactly how my great-grandmother Esther "told" me to. Here's her recipe, complete with her rather idiosyncratic directions in italics:

GREAT-GRANDMA ESTHER'S BARLEY RECIPE

1 part pearled barley

2 parts water

1 medium onion

1 tablespoon butter

Salt and black pepper, to taste

Put the barley and the water into the pot. Cut the whole onion into quarters, *but not all the way through*, and place it on top. Put the butter on top of the barley too; *do not stir it* in. Add salt and pepper.

Cook until the barley is soft; the onion will be soft by then too. Only at this point, and not before, stir everything together, and then adjust seasoning as desired.

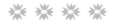

This barley went down nice and easy. I use pearled barley here because although it is less nutrient-dense than hulled barley, it is easier to digest. The first times I tried to eat the hulled barley I had stashed in my cabinet, it was impossible for me to digest. Maybe there had been some wisdom in my "never getting around to it" after all. If your digestive system is not yet strong, use the least-polished pearled barley you can find, as it will still have plenty of nutrients. There is also a middle cut called pot barley that is more easily digestible than hulled barley and less polished than pearled barley. They're all good, so you can see what works best for you.

Dian Dincin Buchman recommends barley broth for a tasty, restorative drink following surgery. Her recipe follows:

BARLEY BROTH

1 cup barley

6 cups water

Simmer the barley in the water. Bring it to a boil and cook for 2 minutes, then let it stand 15 minutes. Strain out the barley and set it aside for later use.

Drink this broth for strength. The barley can be eaten if desired; blending it with honey gives it a pudding taste. Or you can reheat it and add a little butter, salt, and tamari. If you like, stir some yogurt into it.

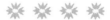

Barley seeds have been found in Anatolian tombs (in modern-day Turkey in Asia Minor, where barley is thought to have originated), and the seeds are believed to date from 3500 BCE. When people bury seeds with their beloved dead, it is a sure sign that those foods were highly esteemed and considered to offer sacred sustenance.

Herbalist Juliette de Bairacli Levy says,

Barley is a highly medicinal cereal, cooling to the blood, and heating to the internal organs, and especially beneficial to the kidneys. Because of this, barley is a favored cereal of Arabs, for themselves and their purebred horses.

Barley is rich in minerals, especially iron. It is reputed to benefit people with arthritis since its natural sodium content keeps calcium in solution, where it will not deposit into bones and joints. The minerals and B vitamins in barley make it a good nerve tonic. It is a calming and nutritive food for the functioning of the overall nervous system.

If barley itself is difficult to digest, barley water is a fine remedy for an infant, invalid, or convalescent. Barley water can also help bring down fevers. It is soothing when the chest or intestinal lining is inflamed. There are various recipes for it; some call for the addition of honey, lemon, figs, and other ingredients. Here is a simple recipe that can be used as is or embellished:

BARLEY WATER

2 ounces barley

5 pints water

Lemon peel (optional)

Honey (optional, but do not use for infants)

Wash the barley, and discard the water. Boil the barley in 1 pint of water for just a few minutes. Discard the water. Add 4 pints of boiling water to the barley. Simmer over a low flame, or boil it carefully until half the liquid is gone. Strain and use as is or add 2 ounces of honey.

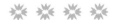

I use barley water (without honey) as a reliable remedy for infants with ongoing diarrhea from stomach or intestinal irritations, or when it is from eating foods that are too complex or rich for their newly developing digestive systems. It invariably soothes the digestion and helps it normalize again. For that purpose, yogurt can also be given. It will help restore healthy intestinal flora, cool and soothe inflammation, and make the digestive system stronger and healthier.

Some of the additional foods and herbs (along with sunflower seed butter and barley cereal) that I credit with helping me slowly but surely regain my weight, health, and full vitality after I moved from the Indian Point nuclear power plant area are: *Artemisia vulgaris,* turmeric, yarrow, garlic, red clover, nettles, horsetail, oat straw, lots of nourishing wild greens and roots, and immune-strengthening foods such as mushrooms, wild salmon, sardines, grass-fed beef, yogurt, squash, onions, yams, seaweeds, kale, collards, and aged barley miso.

Seaweeds

My beautiful, lustrous-coated cat Pandora, whose name means "giver of all gifts," was almost dead when we moved away from there. When she had come to live with me six months earlier, she was a powerful young cat who could run like the wind, chasing a red fox through the woods. She would walk with me anywhere I went in the forest, no matter how far. Living in that exquisitely beautiful yet toxic environment, she had utterly transformed in a matter of months into a weak, old-looking cat who was losing her teeth and hair, and barely moving out of the cabin.

One day I watched her carefully, and she never moved all day. She was lying in the exact spot where my first cat, healthy when I moved out of New York City nearly three years earlier, had lain down and died after wasting away very quickly and mysteriously. I knew in my bones that if we stayed there she would die soon too, and if she was dying, I realized I would be, too. Fortunately, we were able to move.

Pandora too regained her health with the help of herbs over the next year and a half or so. Seaweed (kelp) was her main healing plant. She ate tiny amounts on its own or in her wet food, and drank seaweed water frequently. I broke up about a tablespoon of dried kelp into water, and kept a bowl of that next to her fresh water. I'd top up the seaweed water as needed and change it every couple of days. She also ate yogurt and slippery elm, and bits of bright-colored foods like squash and corn, along with the best-quality cat food I could afford. When she got strong enough, she began to hunt again.

I never tricked her into taking medicine. I followed her lead, trusting her instincts as much or more than my own. That is always my approach now when working with children and animals. We adults usually need to work on letting go and listening before we trust our instincts as fully as children and animals do. That natural ability has been trained out of us—but with attention it comes back!

When we first moved to our new home, Pandora couldn't even climb up the ladder to my loft bed. She'd stand with one paw on the bottom rung and cry. It was heartbreaking. But by the time we moved again three years later, her coat was beautiful, she'd stopped losing teeth, and she could bound up the ladder, and anywhere else she wanted, at top speed. Maybe you can understand why I bless the herbs over and over again. They have helped me so many times, and likely saved my life. I know they saved my beloved cat's life and, more than that, they helped us become healthy again. Pandora's since passed, but that was years later.

· · · · ● ● ● · · ·

There are many varieties of seaweed to get to know. The two I use most are both green, though they are from the "brown algae" family. They are kelp *(Alaria esculenta)* and kombu *(Laminaria japonica,* or *Saccharina japonica),* another form of kelp. I also eat some red seaweed, such as dulse *(Palmaria palmata),* and enjoy mild-tasting hijiki *(Hizikia fusiformis),* the first seaweed I ever tried. Hijiki's milder flavor makes it a good seaweed to start with if you've never tried any before. Put a handful of it in some miso or vegetable soup, or try some cooked with burdock and ginger for a yummy, immune-strengthening meal.

Seaweeds are a nourishing everyday food, a healing plant *par excellence,* as well as an emergency remedy and a survival food. Everyone would do well to find ways to consistently incorporate some seaweed into their regular diets. All seaweeds are rich in minerals, including trace minerals that nourish the nervous system. They are high in essential vitamins such as vitamins A and C, and contain good amounts of protein and iodine. Seaweeds nourish and protect the endocrine system, the thyroid gland in particular.

Kelp contains a generous amount of fucoidan and alginic acid, which will be discussed below. These are part of seaweed's famed protective abilities, and contribute to its ability to strengthen our glandular and immune systems. Seaweeds also provide nourishment for our cardiovascular, reproductive, digestive, and musculoskeletal systems. They improve circulation, enhance fertility, support healthy assimilation and elimination, increase flexibility, and decrease aches and pains.

An American expert on seaweed is herbalist Ryan Drum, and I suggest that you read his writings online and/or take his classes to learn about hundreds of ways to use seaweed for healing. He teaches about many different kinds of seaweed, and I've bought his fantastic, hand-harvested kelp and other seaweeds for over twenty years.

I turn to kelp because it is gifted with a superior ability to remove damaging chemicals, heavy metals, and excess radiation from our bodies. It is reputed to provide protection from cancers that could result from radiation exposure. To quote Susun Weed from her informative chapter on seaweed in *Healing Wise:*

> Research at McGill University finds that alginic acid, one of the main components of seaweed, binds with radioactive strontium to form strontium alginate, an insoluble compound, which is rapidly eliminated from the gastrointestinal tract, reducing the absorption of strontium-90 by 50-90 percent. Strontium-90 is one of the radioactive isotopes released from an up and running nuclear power plant, and much more is released when there is a nuclear "accident" (disaster).

This information about seaweed is backed up by current research that confirms the immune-strengthening properties of kelp, as well as its ability to help the thyroid dump radioactive iodine as it uptakes the natural iodine in kelp. Shortly after the nuclear disaster at Fukushima, Japan, herbalist and naturopathic doctor Linda Page wrote, "Seaweed-based products do not contain as high of levels of iodine as pharmaceutical grade potassium iodide (K1), but they do help shore up deficiencies, and are a good choice to keep your thyroid gland nourished with organic iodine."

Susun Weed puts it succinctly: "Seaweed is a bodyguard." I like that. We could also call it a "lifeguard," since seaweed is a wild plant, a weed of the sea, growing prolifically in oceans all around Earth, guarding and protecting life. When you ingest seaweed, it brings the flowing energy of the ocean into your body.

Because seaweed is so talented at removing heavy metals and radiation from our bodies, we also need to be careful about what it may be absorbing from the waters it grows in. I buy seaweed from places that gather ethically and test their seaweed regularly, such as Ryan Drum's Island Herbs, and Maine Coast Sea Vegetables (see Resources, page 510). I also want to do everything in my power, physically and spiritually/magically, personally, and as a member of the collective of humanity, to protect our precious oceans along with all the waters of Earth. Please get involved in protecting our water—it is a sacred and essential resource that should belong to no one, be available to all, and be taken care of by everyone.

Seaweed is beneficial to our hearts. This may seem confusing, because seaweed is salty and we've been told over and over again that salt aggravates high blood pressure. Table salt certainly does. But the synergy of plant medicine is different than that of a manufactured substance. We evolved along with the plants; they are our elders, and our bodies know how to make use of plants far more wisely and safely than processed substances.

Some good-quality seaweed in the diet will help prevent brittleness and rigidity in the cardiovascular system and in the bones and joints. Seaweed, like nettles, helps tone blood vessels, and its moistening qualities help keep us from growing brittle as we age. Seaweed helps prevent the buildup of plaque in the arteries, and keeps capillaries softer and more flexible so that your blood can flow freely and your heart doesn't have to work harder than it already does to pump blood through your veins and arteries. Think again of the ocean—how the tide moves in and out, ebbing and flowing ceaselessly like the beating of a living heart, sending blood around the body again and again. This is the graceful, fluid dance of seaweed, both in the saltwater and in our bodies.

I hear a lot of people say that they don't like seaweed. They are convinced that it's too fishy and too salty. My mom said she really hated seaweed and wouldn't eat it in anything. Little did she know I snuck it into her food many times when I cooked her meals.

I wouldn't have done that under normal circumstances, but she was calling upon me to be her healthcare provider when she had metastatic lung cancer, and I had to use whatever tricks I could find to get healing substances into her. She lived far longer than her doctors said would be possible. My main point is that if you don't like the taste of seaweed, keep experimenting. It melds nicely into soups, stews, sauces and sautés. I often bake it in the pan with a roast chicken, or in with squash; and its taste blends smoothly with roasted vegetables in a pan or clay cooker.

You can add dried, crumbled kelp to garlic bread or toast. Put some into the delicious Japanese condiment *gomashio*. Gomashio is generally made with toasted and ground sesame seeds and sea salt. It is a tasty, calcium-rich seasoning blend that can be sprinkled onto any savory dish. You can buy gomashio in most health-food stores and some supermarkets. It's easy to make, too. Here's a recipe with a few extra touches:

FANCY GOMASHIO RECIPE

> 8 (or up to 10) parts sesame seeds
>
> 1 part sea salt
>
> 1 part nettles
>
> 1 part kelp
>
> Thyme, sage, and/or rosemary, to taste

Use whole, unroasted sesame seeds and pink or gray sea salt if available. Toast the sesame seeds in a cast-iron pan, stirring continuously with a wooden spoon or spatula until the seeds smell toasty and start to pop.

Separately toast and stir the sea salt for a few minutes.

Combine the toasted sesame seeds and sea salt in a mortar and pestle, or in a *suribachi,* a specially ridged bowl with a pestle, designed for grinding. Use the pestle to lightly grind the mixture in a circular motion. Then mix and grind the other dry ingredients, either in the suribachi or in an electric seed-grinder if you want them more finely ground. Stir everything together. Put the finished gomashio into glass jars with shaker lids.

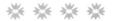

Gomashio, already nourishing to nerve and bone with its calcium and protein-building amino acids, becomes even more beneficial with the addition of the kelp and nettles. This recipe was inspired by Isla Burgess' suggestion to add nettles to sesame seeds in her beautiful book, *Weeds Heal.* In our home we keep a jar out in the kitchen for easy access and daily use along with the salt and pepper, olive oil, herbal vinegars. and other staples.

Shiitake *(Lentinula edodes)* and other favorite mushrooms

Shiitakes are rich, meaty mushrooms that can be incorporated into the diet in many ways, such as simply sautéing the sliced mushrooms in butter and serving them with sea salt.

You could also add a splash of white wine and tamari, mix in some chopped fresh sage, and suddenly you have a dish that's not only savory but a delicacy. A bit of seaweed could be added to make this an even more immune-fortifying dish.

SAVORY SHIITAKE DISH

Organic butter

Fresh shiitake mushrooms

Fresh sage leaves (dry can be used if necessary)

Tamari

White wine

Sea salt (optional)

Kelp flakes (optional)

Herbs de Provence (optional)

Marjoram (optional)

Twist the caps off the stalks ("stipes" in mushroom speak) and put the stalks aside for later use. (See Shiitake Vinegar Recipe, page 136.) Heat butter slowly in a cast-iron or stainless-steel frying pan. Slice the caps thinly, and put them in the pan when the butter has melted. Add freshly chopped green sage leaves, to taste. (Use about 1 tablespoon or less of fresh sage to every cup of shiitakes, and half that amount if using dried sage.)

Add a splash or two of white wine and tamari and a dash of Herbs de Provence, along with a teaspoon or so of marjoram and 1–2 tablespoons of kelp, and cook for 5–10 minutes, turning the mushrooms slices with a wooden spatula. Remove from heat. Add sea salt if desired, and enjoy your savory shiitakes.

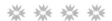

Shiitakes nourish us through an abundance of protein, an assortment of minerals including copper, selenium, and manganese, and a range of B vitamins. Shiitakes are also rich in vitamin D. If you place the mushrooms gills-up in the sun, from several hours to a couple of days, it increases their vitamin D, and you benefit from that when you eat them.

Shiitakes, like other fungi including delectable *maitake (Grifola frondosa)*, medicinally esteemed *reishi* or *lingzhi (Ganoderma* species), immune-supportive turkey tails *(Trametes versicolor* and other species), and an adaptogenic conk mushroom called *chaga (Inonotus obliquus)* that grows on birch trees, are cancer-preventative, helping the body reduce and eliminate existing tumors.

One of the best things to do with dried mushrooms (and the traditional method of preparation for many thousands of years) is to decoct them in water and use them as teas and infusions. These can be drunk and/or added to foods or used as soup stocks. Different dried mushrooms can be cooked anywhere from an hour to several days.

Seventh-generation herbalist and mushroom maven Christopher Hobbs suggests using dried, powdered mushrooms in tea (about 1 teaspoon of powder added to a cup of ginger tea, for example) or cooked into foods. He also recommends cooking dried mushrooms for about an hour to make mushroom tea. Spices can be mixed in to offset the bitter taste of some mushrooms. He suggests adding a small piece of ginger root and about half that amount of licorice root. Or you could take ½–1 teaspoon of homemade tincture. (See general guidelines on making tinctures, but note that Chris recommends blending vodka and dried mushrooms in a blender or food processor, and shaking the tincture every day.) In all cases, he suggests you use the preparation for at least three months to gain greatest benefit from it as an immune-strengthening tonic.

Kate Gilday, herbalist and cocreator of Woodland Essence, recommends preparing chaga mushrooms in a French press as a healthful alternative to coffee. I make mine that way, and use a touch of powdered ginger and cinnamon to enhance its taste and digestive healing properties, then top it off with organic cream or half and half.

Many mushrooms, including maitakes, honeys, puffballs, chantrelles, and oyster mushrooms are delicious and healthful cooked fresh, too. Oyster mushrooms are powerful land healers (as seaweed is to water), so be mindful of where you gather them. Generally speaking, do not gather these or any other mushrooms (or plants for that matter) from an industrial area where they may have absorbed runoff or pollutants. Leave them to do their land-healing work.

One of my favorite ways to ingest edible mushrooms is in the form of infused vinegar, especially when I've gathered them from the wild.

"The wild" takes many forms these days. One evening after I'd parked my car in New York City, I was walking through Riverside Park, heading to the Upper West Side apartment where I held my apprenticeship program. As I was passing an old oak tree I stumbled on something. Looking down, I was so excited to see that it was a beautiful maitake mushroom! My apprentices were amazed too, and after careful identification I cooked it; it was unanimously declared delicious.

As I mentioned earlier, shiitake vinegars (page 136) are particularly yummy and versatile. They can enhance many types of sauces, soups, stews, salad dressings and other dishes. The same is true for maitake vinegar. If you have the opportunity, do try it!

A note on preparing herbal and mushroom vinegars:

When you infuse your plant material in raw, unpasteurized apple cider vinegar, you may find that you've grown a life form akin to a *kombucha* "mushroom" in there. It will appear to be a somewhat slimy, pancake-shaped, gelatinous mass covering the top (or middle or bottom) of your jar! The first time I saw one, I assumed that my vinegar had spoiled, and threw it out. But it does not ruin your vinegar in the least. In fact, back when I learned about them, these "mushrooms" were being touted as a panacea for health and selling for $50 apiece on the Internet!

These mushrooms are actually vinegar "mothers" or starters, and you can compost them, make kombucha tea with them, or give them to someone else who wants one. If you are interested in learning how to brew kombucha tea, there are many good sources of information online. The kombucha "mushroom" is sometimes called a SCOBY, which stands for a Symbiotic Colony of Bacteria and Yeasts.

I also like to make infused oils with shiitakes and maitakes. The flavors, infused into good-quality olive oil, are deep and delicious.

MAITAKE MUSHROOM-INFUSED OIL

Fresh maitake mushrooms

Good-quality olive oil

Make sure your mushrooms (and jar and lid) are completely dry. Don't wash them; if they need cleaning, just use a soft rag, paper towel, or vegetable brush.

Simply chop or tear up the fresh mushrooms, fill a wide-mouthed glass jar with them, and then slowly fill the jar with olive oil. Set the jar on a saucer. Before you cap it, gently poke in and around the mushrooms with a chopstick to release any gas bubbles, and then be careful to top up the oil to keep the mushrooms covered, for the first week or so.

Wait about six weeks. After that, use the oil freely in food. You don't need to decant this preparation; you can use the mushrooms along with the oil. Try not to let the mushrooms stick up out of the oil, though. Keep them submerged as you use up your preparation, to prevent mold and keep the oil fresh.

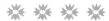

Shitakes (and other mushrooms such as reishi and maitake, and some seaweeds) contain polysaccharides called beta-glucans that help rally a person's immune system into action. This helps protect the body from invasive viruses, bacteria, parasites or fungal infections. In hospitals in Japan, where mushrooms have been recognized as potent medicine for thousands of years, shiitake's most-studied chemical component, lentinan, is administered as an IV treatment for some types of cancers.

Regular use of shiitakes in any cooked form (including "cooking" them by infusing them in vinegar, or making tea from dried shiitakes) will help prevent and offset the side effects of chemotherapy and radiation. Some countries, such as Australia and Korea, have begun to incorporate shiitake medicine into treatment plans for people with various cancers. Shiitakes help you adapt to long-term stress, too.

Shiitakes are a great antioxidant and, like all mushrooms, should be eaten cooked because our bodies are not equipped to break down the chitins and lignans that make up the mushroom's cell walls. (The cell walls of plants, by contrast, are made of strong but digestion-friendly cellulose.) Cooking also does wonderful things for the flavors and textures of mushrooms!

Interestingly, it turns out that we have more DNA sequences in common with fungi than with any plant, so in that sense we are actually more closely related to mushrooms than to plants. Like mushrooms, we inhale oxygen and exhale carbon dioxide and, also like mushrooms, we convert sunlight and ultraviolet radiation into vitamin D but not into food. Like mushrooms, we are also unable to make our own food (other than mother's milk, certainly a notable exception).

When we think of a mushroom, we typically think of the fruit of the fungus. The largest part of the organism, the mycelium, has hidden depths. Mushroom maven Paul Stamets wrote in his seminal book, *Mycelium Running: How Mushrooms Can Help Save the World,* "I see the mycelium as the Earth's natural Internet, a consciousness with which we might be able to communicate."

According to David J. McLaughlin, professor of plant biology at the University of Minnesota's College of Biological Sciences, human cells are surprising similar to fungal cells. And in 1998 it was discovered that fungi split from animals nine million years *after* plants did—another indicator that they are actually more closely related to humans than plants are. It has been speculated that this bond may be why so many mushrooms species have such profound medicinal benefits to us. Whether that is true or not, numerous clinical trials on humans have proven mushrooms' anti-cancer benefits, and medicinal mushrooms are widely used to support health; they have been documented as valuable for over 150 conditions.

Like mushrooms, people are fertile and creative, with great hidden depths of connectedness. In fact, who we really are is what we are here to find out and become, and every one of us possesses creativity and capacity to heal beyond our wildest dreams.

Mushrooms such as reishi, turkey tails, and chaga mushrooms are too hard and woody to eat. These can be mixed with any of the dried, edible mushrooms and prepared in a soup pot as a mushroom stock. This mushroom stock can also be made on its own, or with vegetables and spices. The key is long steeping on very low heat. I steep my mushroom or mushroom-and-vegetable stock for about 24 hours, either on the lowest possible heat on the gas stove, or on a trivet on top of the wood stove. It is then strained and squeezed out, and can be eaten on its own, seasoned however you like, or used to cook any other dishes that normally require cooking water.

You can also incorporate it into Bone Soup, a healing recipe I consistently use and recommend for both preventative and curative medicine. I consider Bone Soup to be a life-sustaining, immune-strengthening tonic, and one of the best food medicines available to us.

BONE SOUP WITH MUSHROOMS

4 cups of saved bones from any animal, preferably free-range or pasture-raised and organically fed (I accumulate bones in one large ziplock bag or jar in my freezer until I have enough to make soup. I don't clean them of scraps or gristle, as the soup will get strained; I also don't worry about who has gnawed them, as the long steeping time will take care of any contamination.)

1 large bone with meat on it, roasted

1½ cups dried astragalus slices

¼ cup mushroom vinegar (Apple cider or infused herbal vinegar may be substituted.)

1 or more cups seaweed

Optional ingredients:

1 cup or more mushroom stock

1 cup of dried mushrooms

Handful dried nettles

Vegetables such as carrots, celery, onions, leafy greens, etc.

Herbs and spices to taste such as marjoram, garlic, ginger, salt, etc.

4–6 Fu Zhang ice cubes (This is an immune-strengthening
blend of Chinese herbs and mushrooms, cooked for
three days and then frozen into cubes to be added to soups.
I buy mine from Woodland Essence—see Resources,
page 510.)

Put the large bone in the soup pot and roast it in the oven at around 350 degrees for 1–1½ hours. Don't use a pot with plastic handles! I sometimes do this step after I've started the soup because I'm pulling that raw bone out of the freezer. If that's the case, put it in a separate roasting pan and add it into the soup after it's roasted.

Put about 4 cups of saved bones and the large roasted bone into a large soup pot, and cover them with cold water, or a combination of cold water and mushroom or vegetable stock, so that your pot is close to ¾ full. Next, add the mushroom or herbal infused vinegar to help bring out the minerals in the bones. Turn the heat on high, and when it gets close to boiling, turn it way down to simmer.

After the soup has cooked for a few hours, add in the astragalus slices and the seaweed (any kind you like).

These are the essential ingredients. Everything else is additional.

If you stop here, simmer the soup on low heat from 12 to 48 hours. I always do the longer steeping when I have time to wait. The long, slow steeping (on your stovetop or atop a trivet on a wood stove, as for the mushroom stock, above) brings out all the gelatin and protein in the bones.

When you've waited as long as you can and you feel the soup is done, strain out the astragalus and the bones, making sure the marrow has come out into the soup. This broth can be seasoned and enjoyed as is, or used to cook rice or other dishes.

You can go on to sautee onions or leeks and garlic, perhaps along with mushrooms, carrots, and dark leafy greens, and add them to your soup during the last 8–12 hours to make it even more immune-nourishing and tasty. Warming winter spices such as ginger, turmeric, cinnamon, etc. are great too. I love to add marjoram, finding that its sweetness helps balance the flavors. I also add Fu Zhang cubes when I have them. If I put the veggies into the soup on the last day, I leave them in, but if I put them in at the beginning I strain them out because they are pretty lifeless by then.

Adjust the seasonings to your taste and, if you like, put the soup into a blender, or use an immersion (hand-held) blender. I like to do that, but it's entirely optional. Refrigerate some for use, and freeze the rest in labeled glass quart jars, being sure to leave an inch or more of head-space atop the soup, and to cap the jars loosely until the contents are thoroughly frozen.

Any version of this soup will warm and heal you deep inside your bone marrow. Take it as a strengthening tonic throughout the fall and winter, or take one or two bowls daily when healing from serious conditions.

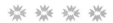

The Benefits of Vinegar

Remember to try the simple things, for they often work well. Folk medicine holds a rich repository of gentle and effective herbal wisdom, and apple cider vinegar is as much a part of folk medicine as any plant. In my kitchen, vinegar is a daily food and an indispensable menstruum for fresh herbs. I rely on these infused vinegars as much as on herbal infusions for daily medicinal food. Vinegar is a wholesome and strengthening food that excels at bringing out the minerals in plants infused into it.

Here's another true story about my dad's healing. He has given me lots of opportunities to learn by doing!

I was sitting at dinner next to my dad, and took his hand for a moment. I saw him wince with pain, and I was stunned to feel red-hot heat under my fingertips. I asked him what was going on, and he told me that his joints had started to swell all of a sudden. His hands had been hurting more and more over the past few weeks. I investigated with my fingertips and sure enough, on top of and underneath the joints in each of his fingers were hard, hot nodules.

I suggested he use the classic folk remedy that follows:

ARTHRITIS RELIEF RECIPE

> 1 tablespoon apple cider vinegar (store-bought, or see recipe below)
> 1 tablespoon honey
> 6–8 ounces water

Stir a tablespoon each of raw, unpasteurized apple cider vinegar and raw honey into a glass of water, and drink daily.

I asked my dad fairly regularly how he was doing, and he said he thought it might be working but wasn't sure. The next time I saw him, about two weeks later, I checked his hands, and the nodules were down by about half. He still wasn't sure it was working!

I see that this is a common reaction among people in the midst of their healing process. For some reason it is hard to notice, or acknowledge, gradual progress; we often need other people to reflect what they see. (This is true of both physical and emotional healing.) I showed him that they were half the size, and he noted that with some interest.

Two weeks after that, his hands didn't hurt anymore, and the swellings were gone! He said he likes the mix now, and will continue it anyway. That's great, because this old home remedy (a favorite of Doctor D.C. Jarvis, whose 1958 book *Folk Medicine: A Vermont Doctor's Guide to Good Health* sold over one million copies) is also great for digestion and the re-mineralization of bones. It is also immune-strengthening and nourishing, and helps with energy. With regular use over time, it will continue to increase flexibility in the joints. It is a simple medicine, filled with green blessings.

I haven't yet made my own apple cider vinegar, since good-quality vinegar is so readily available; however, I've just started my first one and will share the recipe I'm using in case you want to try it. I can't vouch for it yet, but it sounds good and is certainly easy enough. The author says it takes about two months to make this, as opposed to seven months to make vinegar from whole apples. This recipe (with slight adjustments) is from a website called TheHealthyEatingSite.com.

HOMEMADE APPLE CIDER VINEGAR FROM SCRAPS

Apple scraps—the cores and peels from organic apples

A wide-mouth jar

A piece of cheesecloth for covering the jar

Leave the scraps to air. They'll turn brown, which is exactly what you want. Add the apple scraps to the jar, and top it up with water. You can continue to add scraps for a few more days.

Cover with the cheesecloth and put it in a warm, dark place.

You'll notice the contents of the jar start to thicken after a few days, and a grayish scum will form on top. When this happens, stop adding scraps and leave the jar for a month or so to ferment.

After about a month you can start taste-testing it. When it's strong enough for you, strain out the apple scraps and bottle the vinegar.

It's OK if your vinegar is cloudy; there will be some sediment from the apples and what's known as "the mother." If you don't like the cloudiness, strain it through a paper coffee filter to remove most of the sediment.

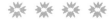

Vinegar can be jazzed up too, if you like:

CONCORD GRAPE VINEGAR WITH MOLASSES

Fresh Concord grapes to fill a quart jar

Apple cider vinegar

¼ cup blackstrap molasses

¼ cup buckwheat honey

Mash up the grapes a bit. Put them into the jar and cover with vinegar, leaving enough space at the top to stir in the honey and molasses, preferably with a wooden spoon. After stirring those in, top up any remaining space with one of the three ingredients—your choice.

Wait 6 weeks–6 months before enjoying.

Grapes are nature's vital circulation-enhancer, and the vinegar brings out the abundance of minerals in these blood-nourishing fruits. The molasses adds even more iron, and the whole combination will give you great energy. This vinegar can work in many different dishes, is delicious cooked with meats, or can simply be added by the spoonful to a glass of water. It is knock-your-socks-off good!

A Few *Real* Happy Meals

MARVELOUS MORNING OATMEAL
(makes 2 servings)

1 cup pin oats (you may use steel-cut oats, but first soak them overnight in cold water in the saucepan)

3 cups water (with more in reserve)

¾ cup frozen blueberries

½ cup frozen cherries

1 banana (or ½ apple or pear), sliced or chopped

2–3 tablespoons ground sunflower seeds

2 tablespoons chopped walnuts

1 tablespoon ground flax seeds

1 tablespoon ground milk thistle seeds

1–2 tablespoons shredded coconut

3 tablespoons slippery elm powder

1–2 tablespoons aged barley miso

½ teaspoon cinnamon powder

Splash of vanilla extract

1 cup plain yogurt (or more, to taste)

Put the oats in a stainless-steel or enameled saucepan, and cover with cold water. Cook, covered, for about 10 minutes, then stir in the blueberries, cherries and shredded coconut, ideally using a wooden spoon. Add water if needed, and put the lid back on. After another 5–10 minutes, stir in the fresh fruit, walnuts, seeds, and spices. When it's cooked to your satisfaction, turn off the heat, add the miso and vanilla extract, and let it sit, covered for about 5 minutes. Serve with organic cow, goat, or sheep milk yogurt. Yum!

Variety is the spice of life, so here are some options to rotate in or include as desired: 5-spice powder, allspice, cumin, almond butter (about 2 tablespoons), raisins, currants, cranberries, dried mission figs, brazil nuts, and/or almonds.

What a way to start a day! Along with one of your favorite infusion blends, this mixture of sweet and savory, fruit-sugar energy, seed and nut protein, anti-inflammatory EFAs, and digestion-strengthening yogurt will get your day off to a smiling start.

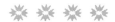

LUXURIOUS LENTIL SOUP

2 cups orange lentils

3 quarts or more water or stock (optional variation: Use bee balm or holy basil tea in the cooking stock.)

Cinnamon, curry, turmeric, cumin seed, cardamom, coriander

1–2 stalks lemongrass

Tamari, to taste (I use wheat-free.)

1 large yellow onion

Coconut oil

Garlic, to taste

Ginger, to taste (Use powdered ginger if you don't have fresh ginger root.)

5 medium carrots

3–4 stalks celery

1 cup kohlrabi (optional)

2 cups collards (optional)

Sea salt

Shiitake or other herb-infused vinegar (optional)

1 can whole, organic coconut milk

Put orange lentils in a soup pot with about 1½ quarts of water to start.

Apply a liberal amount of powdered cinnamon, curry, turmeric, cumin seed, cardamom, coriander, and sea salt. Cut up the stalks of lemongrass and stir them in. (These are fibrous and will need to be removed before serving, or as you're eating.) Bring the lentils just up to a boil, then turn down the flame and continue cooking on low, adding liquid as needed. Add a splash or more of tamari.

In a pan, sauté sliced onion in coconut oil. Add garlic and ginger to taste.

Add thinly sliced carrots and celery into the soup pot. Add (optional) collards and kohlrabi, and additional water and (optional) vinegar. Adjust seasonings as desired, and cook for 15 minutes or more.

Stir in the sautéed ingredients. Add sea salt and adjust seasonings again. Cook till all vegetables are soft and flavors are melded. Stir in coconut milk.

You may choose to make a simpler lentil soup, but if you make this recipe I trust you will find it delicious that same night and even better the next day. Lentils cook quickly, and they are high in soluble fiber and low in calories. They are also a great source of phytoestrogens. These plant chemicals can help keep our bodies from taking in more harmful, exogenous (external) estrogens that come to us through plastics and other damaging conveniences of modern life. Phytoestrogens keep the estrogen receptors in our cells busy. Imagine the harmful forms of estrogen calling us, but getting a busy signal that tells them we're unavailable. Lentils are also a good source of protein and B vitamins.

The healing power of these mostly Indian spices is legendary. Turmeric nourishes the liver and is a restorative anti-inflammatory, as is ginger. Both these herbs benefit the blood vessels by dissolving fibrin (fibrous protein tissue) that can otherwise build up inside blood vessels, impeding blood circulation. Garlic is antibacterial, antiviral, antifungal, and beneficial to the respiratory and digestive tracts. Cumin and coriander both aid digestion and warming, and delicious cardamom improves appetite, sweetens breath and prevents gas. Coconut oil and milk taste great, and provide us with healthy fats and antiviral compounds.

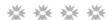

And here's a treat for a cold day. After stacking some wood, or taking a winter walk, there's nothing better than a cup of hot cocoa. Not that you need an excuse.

BEST HOT COCOA

1 cup organic whole milk

¾ tablespoon organic cocoa powder

¼–½ teaspoon cinnamon powder

⅛ teaspoon ginger powder (or to taste)

⅛ teaspoon turmeric powder (or to taste)

Dash grated nutmeg

Splash vanilla extract

Cinnamon stick (optional)

Vanilla bean (optional)

Gently warm the milk. Add all the other ingredients, heat slowly and gently, and enjoy this extra-healthful, warming and stimulating hot cocoa, beloved by seven- to ninety-seven-year-olds! (And if they're not adventurous eaters, don't feel you have to tell them what's in it, if they don't ask! I didn't, and my company loved it.)

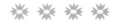

MY TOP RECOMMENDED FOODS FOR VIBRANT HEALTH

Understanding that everyone is different, here are my recommendations:

- Bone broths, wild and cultivated mushrooms, astragalus root, garlic, onions, dark, leafy, well-cooked greens, bitters such as arugula and watercress, assorted vegetables including cabbage family plants, carrots, and seaweeds, olive oil, coconut oil, fresh eggs, fermented foods including yogurt, tamari, and miso, sunflower seeds, sesame seeds, raw honey (with and without herbs infused into it), aromatic herbs like basil, rosemary, sage and thyme, pungent spices such as turmeric and ginger; herb-infused vinegars, brightly colored berries; lots of fruits, lentils, and beans.
- Variety is key. Eat some of all the different-colored foods and, if possible, eat some of all different kinds of foods—seeds, nuts, animals, milk, cheese, fruit, fish, raw and cooked vegetables, whole grains, and, most especially—
- Wild foods including meat, mushrooms, dandelions and other wild edible roots, leaves, flowers and seeds.

RANDOM FOOD-MEDICINE TIPS

- Cook your leafy greens such as kale, collards, and mustard greens in water for a good, long time (at least thirty minutes; more is fine), and season with vinegar to get more minerals out of them. (If you are not fond of vinegar, cook tomatoes with your greens, or season them with lemon juice.) Drink the cooking water, or use it for soup stock, cooking grains or in other recipes.

- A good all-purpose greens seasoning is a mixture of coconut oil or cold-pressed olive oil with tamari and herb-infused vinegar.
- Add turmeric powder into eggs.
- Add slippery elm powder into any of the following: oatmeal, eggs, yogurt, applesauce, and anything else you can think of!
- Add shatavari, ashwaganda, or maca powders into anything that you're cooking (even eggs) to keep your nervous system strong and your love life spicy. Shatavari, a member of the asparagus family, is "she who possesses a hundred husbands," and is cooling, lubricating, and restorative to the sexual-reproductive system, especially for women. Ashwaganda, or "the smell of a horse" is a renowned nightshade-family herb that tonifies the male nervous system and improves sexual vitality. I like the taste of maca best of all. It is a mustard-family plant grown at very high altitudes in South and Central America, and is touted for its libido-nourishing gifts to men and women. (I've never met a plant that is only a "men's" herb or a "women's" herb anyway.)
- Add seaweed into almost anything you're cooking.
- Add fresh or powdered ginger and turmeric freely to vegetables.
- Eat some garlic and onions cooked, and some uncooked. (Think pesto!)
- Add herbal vinegar to all your stir-fries, soup, sandwiches, sauces, and stews.

Herbal Medicines in Your Spice Rack

Many spice herbs are aromatic, antioxidant, soothing and nourishing to the nerves, and good digestive aids. They often contain volatile oils that make them antiseptic as well. Classic aromatic spice herbs are often also anti-spasmodic and uplifting.

Black Pepper *(Piper nigrum)*

In some times and places, black pepper was used as currency, and considered a measure of a person's wealth. It has also been used as a sacred offering in rituals.

Native to India, true pepper comes from a climbing vine with tiny white flowers that are followed by the peppercorns (the seeds). These are harvested at different times to give us black, pink, or white peppercorns, much like sweet bell peppers, which can be harvested when green (unripe), red, purple, or brown, or like tea, harvested at different times (and processed differently) to be green, black, or white.

Black pepper is a heating stimulant rich in several nutrients including manganese, vitamin K, and iron. It is reputed to aid digestion, acting as a carminative and a stimulant for the production of hydrochloric acid in the stomach.

Black pepper is often used in Ayurvedic medicinal preparations and cooking, usually in small amounts. Medicinally it is considered, along with cayenne, to be an activator, helpful for getting nutrients and other herbal constituents zipping through the circulatory system to where they're most needed.

For some people, any amount of black pepper acts as an irritant. If you are one of these people, don't worry, because fortunately there are other spice plants that can provide stimulation without irritation. If you like it and find it beneficial, use it; but if black pepper doesn't agree with you, leave it out of your spice-medicine shelf and explore the alternatives.

Red Pepper (*Capsicum annuum* and other species)

All peppers act as stimulants to circulation, including red peppers. Did you know that the red pepper isn't really a true pepper at all? It's a member of the nightshade family that includes tomatoes and potatoes, and it comes from a tropical American plant that has been cultivated for millennia to give us both sweet and hot red peppers. This plant grows wild in some parts of Africa and South America, and is grown in gardens everywhere.

The hot red peppers, or chili peppers, give us the familiar kitchen spice cayenne. According to the George Mateljan Foundation newsletter, bell peppers contain a recessive gene that omits capsaicin, the component that gives cayenne its infamous heat, measured in Scoville Heat Units (SHUs). The hottest red pepper is African bird pepper, which typically measures from 200,000–300,000 SHUs. Still, it is said that the burn of cayenne is only healthful inside our bodies, and never harmful.

Sprinkling cayenne powder into food stirs the blood, and has a tonic effect on the heart and cardiovascular system. It is a good source of vitamins C and E. Cayenne has the reputation of being an emergency stimulant remedy after a heart attack when someone can't get to, or is not yet at, a hospital emergency room. I can't personally attest to that, but I have read that it can be administered repeatedly on the tongue as powder in such an emergency.

Cayenne is used in heavily diluted gargles for sore throats, and in small amounts in tea recipes for colds, fevers, and flu. It is also famous as a styptic, staunching the flow of blood in emergency first-aid situations. It will sting like crazy when applied to an open cut, but it will stop the bleeding.

One of my students came into class and told us the following story: Her knife slipped as she was chopping vegetables, and she cut herself badly, causing profuse bleeding. She reached for something to help her and the next thing she knew she'd knocked down her spice shelf, breaking some bottles. One of them was cayenne, and the powder got in the cut. It made her yelp aloud with its profound sting, but it also completely stopped the bleeding in less than sixty seconds. I'd only use it that way for emergency first aid—and I prefer other herbs for stopping bleeding—but it's always good to know our options!

Cayenne is a disinfectant, often used as a condiment in hot climates to overcome the dangers of eating spoiled food, especially meat. Juliette de Bairacli Levy writes of learning from the Romany people (commonly called gypsies) how to use cayenne as an intense but safe fumigant herb to get rid of harmful insects and rodents. She says to "sprinkle several tablespoons of the powdered pepper on a flat tin lid, place it over a low flame, seal the room and allow the pepper to fume until it is all used up.

Repeat as necessary." (I need to add: Leave the room at once when the pepper is lit!) She says that the room will be habitable again in a very short time. Similarly, cayenne-infused water is often used as a form of natural pest control in the garden. Be careful not to inhale any of it!

Dian Dincin Buchman lists cayenne as one of her favorite herbs, and the most important food herb in her pantry. She suggests adding a few grains of cayenne to hot chamomile, linden, or peppermint tea to instantly correct sluggish digestion and flatulence, to reduce a mild fever, and as a whole-body restorative. She also uses it along with apple cider vinegar and salt, in tiny doses, as a preventative gargle during epidemics.

My personal favorite use for cayenne is external rather than internal. Cayenne can keep your feet warm in winter. Sprinkle cayenne powder liberally, alone or mixed with white dusting powder, into your socks (or shoes, if your feet are very sensitive). It will stain, but it will keep your feet toasty-warm while you shovel snow, ice-skate, and cross-country ski, or simply take a walk on a lovely winter day.

Regardless of how you're using cayenne, treat it with a healthy dose of respect. Remember that less is more, and be careful not to touch your eyes after you've been handling red (or any other) pepper, fresh or dry.

Cinnamon (*Cinnamomum* species)

When I met a cinnamon tree in the tropics for the first time, I was so excited that I kissed it and gave it a big bear hug, much to the amusement of our guide. Cinnamon is a delicious, warming spice, and one of my all-time favorites. The powder can be ground from the bark of any species of cinnamon tree and added to many foods. It blends well with everything from vanilla to curries. It is also potent medicine, both antimicrobial and a clinically proven moderator of blood sugar.

When I was a little girl, one of my favorite comfort foods was "cinnamon toast"—toasted white raisin bread with margarine melted on it, with a blend of refined white sugar and cinnamon powder sprinkled on top. Though I remember it fondly, that is definitely not the best way to take your cinnamon as medicine! Here's a healthier, more delicious variation:

CINNAMON-RAISIN TOAST

1–2 slices whole-wheat cinnamon raisin bread

Butter or coconut oil (organic if possible) to taste

¼ teaspoon cinnamon

¼ teaspoon raw sugar

Rose or orange blossom honey (optional)

Toast the whole-wheat raisin bread, and spread butter or coconut oil on it while it's still warm. Sprinkle the cinnamon and raw sugar on it freely, to taste, or pre-mix them in a mortar and pestle or small dish and sprinkle a thin layer over the toast. If you want to add another layer of delight, add a touch of the infused honey, too.

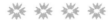

STOMACH-SOOTHING CINNAMON INFUSION

6 cinnamon sticks

1 quart water

Put cinnamon sticks into a mortar and pestle and break them into pieces. Put the pieces of broken-up cinnamon bark into a quart jar. Cover them with boiled water. Cap and let sit for about an hour. Strain and drink warm or hot. This can be refrigerated and gently reheated if desired.

Cinnamon-stick tea is often the quickest help I know for nausea and vomiting during and after the flu. It will allay fierce nausea. This fragrant, spicy tea is warming and great for a simple upset stomach or an acute case of diarrhea too.

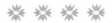

Cinnamon can also be tinctured as a simple:

SPICY CINNAMON TINCTURE

10–15 cinnamon sticks

1 quart vodka

Break up the cinnamon sticks in a mortar and pestle. Put them into a wide-mouth quart jar. Cover them with 100-proof vodka, and fill the jar to the top. Wait about 6 weeks. It isn't necessary to strain the cinnamon out as it will settle on the bottom of the jar, but you can if you like. Otherwise, simply pour the cinnamon tincture through a strainer when you want to use it. This tincture can be added to tea or coffee, diluted into water, or served neat in shot glasses.

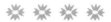

Cinnamon tincture, straight or diluted, is strong, tasty and warming, a winter-party favorite. It lifts the spirits, balances blood sugar, and stimulates digestion. Cinnamon is also a good antiseptic herb. I had reason to be grateful for this on a trip to the tropics. A large tropical centipede bit my partner when we were visiting the Caribbean island nation of Dominica. Centipedes are the only poisonous creatures there, but one managed to find him, crawl up under his shirt, and bite him under the arm. This compounded the challenge, because it invited the poison to circulate directly into his lymph system! I was quite alarmed, and gave him whatever antibacterial tinctures I had in my travel kit—some echinacea and some yarrow, first directly under the tongue and then in water.

I ran to our next-door neighbors to find out how poisonous the centipede venom was. I needed to find out whether or not I had to get him to an emergency room. He was pale, and felt anxious and a little woozy. Everyone there was familiar with centipede bites, and I was informed that the site would inevitably swell up and turn red. He might have some systemic symptoms, such as headaches. He'd certainly be in pain, or at the very best feel quite uncomfortable for four or five days, but then he'd be fine. I was told I shouldn't worry.

Well, that was easy for them to say. I was relieved he wasn't in danger, but I didn't want to give up four or five days of the holiday that we'd worked so hard to afford ourselves—at least not without doing whatever I could to help him heal faster!

I wanted to supplement the internal herbs with a topical drawing medicine, a fresh leaf applied directly to the site of the bite. But I was unfamiliar with the local plants, so what leaf to use? I wracked my brain for something I could use, and then remembered that I'd gathered some cinnamon leaves that afternoon. Now, everyone I know uses the bark and not the leaves, but I'd smelled them and they seemed strong to me, so I had gathered some. I pounded up one of the leathery leaves and poured boiling water over it to soften it and open up the cell walls to release its antiseptic compounds. He held it over the site while I bandaged it so it would stay put.

Well, the story ends quite happily, as he had no more pain, no swelling, no infection, and was completely fine by the next morning! Our local friends later told us that they had never seen a bite from a large centipede not swell and hurt for days. They were very impressed. My poor guy had to show off his armpit to everyone, and the next thing I knew folks were asking me for consultations! Of course I said yes—and there went the holiday! (Later, on the other side of the country, we met local, indigenous folks who work with healing plants. I didn't get a chance to ask, but I'm sure they have their own favorite effective remedies for centipede bites.)

Here's a blended cinnamon tea for you to try:

BELLY BLISS TEA

½ cup dried hawthorn berries

1–1½ dried cups marshmallow leaves and flowers

6 cinnamon sticks

Break the cinnamon sticks into pieces with a mortar and pestle. Mix the herbs into a half-gallon jar, cover them with boiled water, and let the brew sit out on a counter overnight.

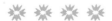

This overall sweet, yet complex mixture offers a combination of good effects in the body. It is soothing, stimulating and nourishing. Hawthorn adds a healthy supply of Vitamin C, digestive enzymes, and iron. Marshmallow is nutritive, and its moistening mucilage soothes the stomach and inflamed mucous membranes in the digestive or urinary tracts. Cinnamon's stimulating oils help warm and stoke the digestive fire, and increase blood circulation. Drink this blend to soothe and nourish your digestive system and bring more warmth into your belly. It can also be enjoyed as a yummy infusion that supports your general wellness.

Thyme *(Thymus vulgaris)*

The body system most strongly affected by the herb thyme is the respiratory system. I generally use "regular" culinary thyme for medicine, but you can use any of the variations, such as lemon thyme, as long as the species you use has the strongly aromatic, camphorous smell characteristic of thyme. The tiny, leathery leaves are used before or during flowering, and provide specific medicine for the bronchia. Thyme is an anti-spasmodic, antiseptic, and expectorant herb that is drying and warming. It can be used to effectively ease both dry and wet coughs.

I've had the most success using thyme for people with dry, lingering coughs that are deep in the chest and also tickling the throat. Thyme leaves make a great steam for bronchitis. Thyme contains, and therefore is sometimes confused with, thymol, a powerful phenol obtained from thyme. This volatile oil is safe as part of the whole herb because it's buffered by other constituents of the plant, but less safe by itself when it's concentrated in the essential oil of thyme that's popular for steams. Dried or fresh thyme leaves and stalks are not only safer, they're more effective than the essential oil (the same goes for eucalyptus) because the concentrated oil is irritating and dries out mucus membranes too much. Try it and see.

The fresh or freshly dried herb is easier on you; not coincidentally, it's easier on the planet, too, because it takes a huge amount of an herb or flower, plus energy expended, to make a minuscule amount of essential oil. You could use a tiny amount of the essential oil for steaming if it's your only option, but that's unlikely as long as you have a spice cabinet! I've seen that in a pinch even older, less-alive medicine can sometimes work wonders. Of course, as always, use the best-quality herbs available.

THYME STEAM

½ cup dried thyme leaves (or one cup fresh thyme)

1½ quarts water

Soup pot

One or two large towels

Put the thyme leaves and stalks into a 3–4 quart pot. Add cold water.

Cover the pot and bring the water just up to a boil. As soon as it begins to boil, turn heat down to the lowest level and simmer, covered, for 5–10 minutes.

Turn off the flame and let steep for another 5–10 minutes with the cover still on. You could pour off a cup to drink before sitting down to the steam.

Arrange things so you can set the hot pot down safely where it won't slide, or burn the surface it's on. A kitchen or dining table with a mat or one of the thick towels on it will work well. You want to be able to sit down in a comfortable place that's a good height for you to be able to relax as you lean over the steaming pot.

Set the pot down and remove the cover. In a couple of minutes or so, when the thyme preparation is still steaming hot but not hot enough to burn you, sit down in front of it and drape the other big towel over your shoulders. Pull the towel up over your head, pull the corners around your neck from behind and hold it closed snugly in front, letting the rest of the towel drape over the outside of the open pot to catch the steam. Lean forward and wrap your arms around the towel-enclosed pot to make a snug tent for yourself.

The more airtight you make the towel tent, the hotter it will be, and the more helpful. However, if it's uncomfortably hot at first, leave some air space between the towel and your neck, or loosen your arms from around the pot. As soon as you are good and comfortable, relax and breathe deeply in and out for 10 minutes or more, or until the liquid cools. You can reheat it and repeat this process 2–3 times in a row for maximum benefit.

The thyme steam feels so good; besides being lovely for your skin and circulation, this steam will quiet your coughing, open your bronchia, and ease chest pain. At the same time, you'll be breathing thyme's healing oils deep into your sinuses, and down into your windpipe, bronchial tubes, and lungs, facilitating symptom relief and more. This warming spice plant, used as an anti-infective steam and also as a simple tea, will help your respiratory healing, calm you, and gently lift your spirits too.

The following recipe provides a tasty way to benefit from thyme's anti-spasmodic, immune-strengthening gifts.

THYME-GINGER EUPHORIC ELIXIR

1 cup fresh thyme (or ½ cup dried)

2–3-inch piece of fresh ginger root

Unflavored brandy

Honey (raw, buckwheat if possible)

Cut up the fresh thyme, and grate the fresh ginger (if organic, include the peel). Put the herbs into a pint or slightly larger jar.

Pour brandy to cover the herbs. Top up the rest of the jar with honey. Stir it all in together well. Cap the jar and wait 6 weeks. If you can't wait, use it by the teaspoon or tablespoon, and then top up the jar again with brandy or honey.

When it's ready, pour off the liquid and squeeze out the herbs; or leave them in and use just the liquid.

Take 30–60 drops of the elixir in tea or hot water, or drink it straight by the teaspoon, tablespoon or shot glass.

This elixir can be used as a digestive calmative for stomach or intestinal cramps, or to help fight a respiratory or gut bug. It will open up the bronchia and lungs, and promote easier breathing. Each ingredient helps both your respiratory and immune systems. Thyme, ginger, and honey are all antibacterial and anti-inflammatory. Brandy is calming, and gently antispasmodic. The thyme and ginger together have a calming and euphoric effect at the same time!

This delicious respiratory tonic is beneficial for anyone, and especially for those with particularly vulnerable lungs. I've found it strengthens the respiratory tolerance of folks who are more susceptible to becoming ill when they're in cold, damp weather. It eases the symptoms of colds, coughs and painful constriction in the lungs and bronchia. You can make this medicine in advance to have it on hand when you need it. Or use it as preventative medicine—it will warm you up on a cold winter night. It's fortifying, and so yummy!

Thyme is also one of my favorite anti-hysterics, and not just because I like to say "anti-hysteric." It is effective taken as a simple tea. Perhaps you know someone you'd like to share it with—or perhaps someone you know would like to share some with you! I've read that thyme helps ward off nightmares, and though I haven't experienced using thyme that way, I can easily imagine thyme's aroma being strong enough to pull someone back to themselves, away from a nightmare—especially if it's mixed with some lavender to sweeten those dreams, and/or hops to invite deeper sleep.

Basil (*Ocimum* species)

If it were only for the smell and taste of the plant, basil would be worthy of note! But of course there is more. Basil is a broad-spectrum, antimicrobial plant that helps the body heal when it has been overloaded with harmful bacteria or infected by parasites, fungi, and/or viruses. And like many of our mint-family plants, it's a great tonic for the digestive system, helping to allay nausea and settle an upset stomach. Basil is also an ally to help transform a bad mood into a more cheerful one.

Basil leaf can be used externally as a poultice against the itch and inflammation of poisonous bites. The infusion is used, mixed with Castile soap, to repel insects from other plants, and basil leaf juices rubbed on the skin are used to repel flying insects. Basil plants can be placed near windows, or outside on a patio or porch, to help repel mosquitoes, flies, and gnats.

RINGWORM REMEDY

Fresh basil poultices, applied frequently along with basil tea or infusion, are effective for helping eliminate the common skin fungus known as ringworm. Listen to your body; but a general guideline is to leave a basil poultice on for about thirty minutes at a time. A clean rag, bandanna, or band-aid can hold it in place if you're moving around.

Make a strong tea with dried leaves; bathe the infected areas, and allow them to air-dry between fresh plant poultices. If the ringworm is extensive, you could take some basil baths and let your whole body air-dry. Finally, dust the affected areas with herbal antifungal powder (see page 158), which is soothing and keeps the ringworm patches dry, giving your skin time to fully heal. Other immune- and skin-supportive herbs, such as calendula flowers, can be used internally and externally with the basil, depending on the person and situation.

Basil tea is spirit-lifting and anti-depressant. Basil is prized in many cultures as a plant that brings not only happiness but good fortune and prosperity in business. Simple rituals such as strewing basil in a new shop, or placing basil plants in the front window, are said to draw good luck and financial success.

Basil is a boon to the immune system. I mostly use it before it flowers, though I understand some herbalists use it in flower. The leaves are sweeter before flowering. A cup of basil tea is often the first thing I suggest to someone who calls looking for help because they feel miserable from a head cold. Most people will have a jar of dried basil in their kitchen cupboard even if they aren't "into" herbs. Basil can be brewed as a simple 10–15 minute tea, but it's even more tasty and effective brewed for about one hour as a full-strength infusion.

BASIC BASIL INFUSION

½ cup dried basil leaves (or 1 cup fresh leaves, including small stalks)

1 quart water

Put basil leaves and stalks into a quart jar and cover with boiling water. Cap to be airtight, and let steep for one hour.

Strain; reheat gently and serve. Refrigerate the rest, or put it into a thermos hot, for drinking.

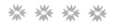

SIMPLY SUBLIME CULINARY OIL

2 parts fresh basil

1 part garlic

½ part sun-dried tomatoes

Olive oil

Fill a wide-mouth jar with chopped fresh basil leaves (any fragrant basil will do; I've mostly used Genovese), chopped or thinly sliced sun-dried tomatoes, and chopped or pressed fresh garlic cloves. Pour cold-pressed, extra virgin olive oil in to the top of the jar. Stir the ingredients gently with a dry wooden chopstick, and when the bubbles settle, fill the jar to the top again with a little more oil. Let this sit in a cool, dry place with a saucer underneath it, and wait at least a month before using. It will get better and better with age.

You can decant this oil, or simply let the herbs come out onto your dish as you use the oil; but always be sure to keep your plant matter down below the surface of the oil. I've been making and sharing this oil recipe for over twenty years, and never had it spoil.

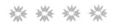

This medicinal, culinary oil can be used for dipping whole-grain bread, topping pasta, drizzling onto cheese and crackers, a salad, sandwich, or any cooked dish, especially one with cooked tomatoes and melted cheese. My partner likes to put in on sandwiches as a spread along with or in lieu of pesto. Sometimes I use it as the cooking oil to add a lovely flavor to whatever I'm making—even sunny-side-up eggs become a special treat cooked in Simply Sublime Culinary Oil.

. . . .

There are several species of basil that are called "holy" or "sacred" basil. These species are also collectively known in India as "tulsi, the incomparable one." This herb is grown in virtually every home garden in India. I had a lovely client from India who said, "I don't use any herbs."

I was incredulous. "Not even tulsi?"

"Oh, of course I drink tulsi," she said dismissively. This profound medicine that nourishes nearly every system in the body is such a part of daily life that it was impossible for her to conceive of it as an "herbal medicine." That's understandable, even though holy basil has been found to be adaptogenic and immune-supportive, and helpful with a range of health challenges from asthma to stress-induced hypertension. Most people don't think about pesto as medicine either. But—as discussed earlier in this chapter—it certainly is!

Personally, I think every species of basil should be called holy or sacred basil. I love all of the many kinds of basil that I've tried. I'm particularly fond of lemon basil, and lime basil—but then there's purple basil, and Thai basil, and—well, you get the idea!

Parsley *(Petroselinum crispum)*

Parsley roots, leaves, and seeds are most esteemed as a urinary-system medicine for the kidneys and bladder. They are a good tonic for the prostate gland, too. This lovely leafy green is used as a potassium-rich diuretic to help urine flow freely without depleting the body of potassium. Parsley is reputed to help dissolve bladder and kidney stones. One of its old nicknames is "breakstone." Parsley also helps the body as a carminative, easing flatulence and colicky pains. It is often recommended to freshen breath after eating garlic.

Parsley can be eaten, drunk as tea, or put into soup, and is quite delicious infused as medicinal vinegar. (See more on parsley in the chapter on cardiovascular health, page 63.) Parsley leaves can be bruised or pounded and then warmed, to use on the body as a poultice. A parsley poultice is helpful applied to swollen glands, and can be safely used by nursing mothers to relieve the pain of sore, engorged, or hard, knotted breasts. Or a cloth can be dipped into strong parsley tea and used on the body as a fomentation.

In general, applying the herbs themselves to the body yields the strongest, quickest results, but sometimes you need to use an herb the easiest way rather than the best way. It still works.

Parsley contains an oily chemical called apiol (or apiole) that is a stimulant to the kidneys and uterus. Because of this, it should not be eaten in large quantities or used medicinally during pregnancy, though normal culinary use is fine. Caution should be exercised during the first trimester, or if there is any history of miscarriage. Parsley can be used reliably as an emmenagogue, to stimulate the menstrual flow when a woman is not pregnant. It has also been used as an abortive herb, both internally as tea and topically, with fresh sprigs inserted into the vagina as a pessary (vaginal suppository). It is not a strong abortifacient, however, and is not considered reliable used on its own for that purpose.

Parsley is rich in bets-carotene and is an excellent source of both vitamin C and iron, especially if it's eaten as a bona-fide green vegetable rather than a garnish. When I lived in an apartment in New York City, it was often hard to get motivated to cook for myself after a long day at work. The temptation to call up a restaurant and order in food was compelling. But not only did it get expensive, I also never felt as well-nourished eating takeout as I did when I cooked for myself. I set out to find and create some simple, one-pot meals that could be prepared quickly, but that would also be nourishing and delicious. Here's one that features parsley:

PERFECTLY EASY PARSLEY PASTA

Whole-wheat, quinoa, rice, mugwort, or black bean pasta (your choice)

1–2 cups parsley, curly or flat

Olive oil, to taste

Tamari, to taste

Herb-infused vinegar, to taste

Garlic powder, to taste (optional)

Cook your pasta according to the package directions. While it's cooking, finely chop up your fresh parsley, including all but the largest stalks. Put the chopped parsley into a colander.

When the pasta is ready, pour the boiling water over the parsley and then let the pasta fall out of the pot on top of it, cooking it just a touch more—that is enough cooking for parsley. Stir in olive oil, and add these seasonings and/or any others you may desire. Stir it all together well. Serve and enjoy!

You can elaborate on this dish by adding more sautéed vegetables, such as onions and garlic, but this is how I make it when I want minimum time and effort to make a satisfying, nourishing meal—and have only one pot to wash when I'm done.

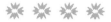

Garlic *(Allium sativum)*

Garlic's healing powers are legendary, and well-deserved. Garlic is a member of the lily family, which includes the sulphur-rich, smelly alliums such as shallots, onions, leeks, ramps (wild leeks), scallions, and chives. Garlic is a powerful, pungent herb, and studies have shown that it offers particular protection against stomach and colon cancers. Garlic generally supports the immune system, and the life-force or innate vitality that animates the body. It also has particular affinity for bringing healing to the cardiovascular, respiratory, and digestive systems.

Through strengthening these vital systems, garlic helps the body to fight off virtually any kind of microbe it encounters—bacterial, viral, fungal, or parasitic. Garlic is rich in antioxidants that help cardiovascular circulation and the lungs, and it contains a chemical called allicin that is anti-microbial, especially when garlic is used fresh in tea, soup, syrups, tinctures, or poultices. (Before applying garlic, protect skin with olive oil.)

Here are two of my favorite recipes. I keep these items on hand in case they're needed, in the same way people keep cough syrup and aspirin in the medicine chest.

SIMPLE GARLIC HONEY

Fresh, peeled, whole garlic cloves

Honey

Fill a clean, wide-mouthed jar about ¼–½ full of garlic cloves, depending on how strong you want it to be. If you want your garlic honey to be even stronger, chop the garlic cloves finely or use a garlic press. Cover the garlic with the best-quality honey you can afford, pouring it slowly until you've filled the jar to the top. Poke with a chopstick or sturdy twig to release as many gas bubbles as you can from this sulphur-rich preparation.

Place your garlic honey jar on a saucer. The mix will bubble out of your jar no matter how many gas bubbles you remove, and no matter how well-capped your jar is!

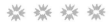

This homemade medicine is powerfully preventative of respiratory ailments. When you feel vulnerable to a cold or flu, take a teaspoon of the infused garlic honey 1–2 times daily as a preventative tonic. Something I've heard numerous times from grateful people I taught about garlic honey is, "Everyone in my office/home got this bug but me!" Another nice way to use it is as an ingredient in sauce for baking chicken or vegetables. It won't be quite as antimicrobial cooked, but it is still great preventative medicine.

You can also eat the cloves, whether you put them in the honey whole or minced. (If you leave them in there long enough—maybe a year or more—they will liquefy and the entire preparation becomes *really* pungent.)

If you are sick, garlic honey can be taken throughout the day. It can be taken straight, by the teaspoon, or mixed into hot water, tea, or anything you want. Whew—strong stuff! For babies, use smaller doses. For infants under one year, conventional Western wisdom warns us not to use honey at all.

I've observed that people who don't like this blend when they are feeling well will actually crave it when they are ill. This is true of many of the strongest, most "medicinal-tasting" herbal teas as well.

Please note that garlic-infused honey is not the appropriate garlic preparation to use for parasites such as worms, because parasites are generally nourished and energized by sugars.

DELUXE GARLIC HONEY

Fresh, peeled, whole garlic cloves
Grated ginger root
Honey

Make the same recipe as for simple infused garlic honey: Fill the jar ¼–½ full with garlic, and add grated ginger to fill it an additional ¼ full. Then add honey as above.

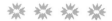

Thanks to my student Leslie for telling me that she liked adding ginger to the garlic honey. I like the taste of this blend even better than the original! And it adds the incomparable medicinal gifts of ginger to the blend.

Here's a traditional healing recipe with both garlic and ginger that is as hot as it sounds:

FIRE CIDER

¼ cup grated fresh horseradish

⅛ cup chopped fresh garlic

½ cup chopped fresh onion

¼ cup grated fresh ginger

Garlic mustard, mugwort/cronewort, epazote/Mexican tea (optional)

(You can add pungent garlic mustard *(Alliaria petiolata)* roots in place of, or in addition to, the horseradish. Add mugwort/cronewort *(Artemisia vulgaris)* leaves and stalks and epazote/Mexican tea *(Chenopodium ambrosioides)* leaves and stalks to turn your Fire Cider into a potent anti-parasitic. For the latter application, leave out the honey.)

Chop or grate all the herbs. Put them into a quart or smaller jar, depending on how strong you want your preparation to turn out, and cover them with apple cider vinegar to fill the jar. Let it sit for 4–6 weeks. Decant the herbs out of the vinegar. Add honey to your Fire Cider after decanting, if desired. If you want optimum flexibility for various uses, leave the honey out and only add it to individual servings or doses as desired.

A lot of people like to put cayenne in their Fire Cider. To me, that's overkill, but go with your own tastes!

This cider is very useful to have on hand if you find yourself outside for long periods of time on cold days or evenings, or during a chilly rain. It will fortify you, ease a sore throat, and keep you warmer than you'd be without it, for sure! You could also use this in winter soups, or as a respiratory stimulant if you are ill with a cough or flu. A spoonful in water can be used once a day to stimulate circulation.

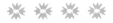

Ginger *(Zingiber officinale)*

This tropical beauty, native to Southeast Asia, is a classic. It is a food, a spice and an herbal medicine, all rolled up in one plant. The rhizome of ginger is most frequently used, whether in food, as an infusion, or in other medicinal preparations. I use ginger—fresh, dry, and powdered—and make it into baths, oils, honeys, glycerites (extracts using glycerin as a menstruum), and vinegars. I generally prefer infusions to tinctures, though ginger tincture is effective too.

Ginger tea or infusion is helpful for warming your body when you have a cold with chills, and for helping to relieve simple indigestion, gas, or digestive or menstrual cramps that come from congestion. It is helpful for the flu when you are nauseated as well as chilly.

Ginger has long been used to alleviate motion-sickness, and modern studies have found it more effective than popular over-the-counter medications such as Dramamine®. I turn ginger powder into honey balls for that purpose, as they travel well, whether by plane, car, or boat, and need no refrigeration. Candied ginger can work, too. Ginger tea is also used to effectively relieve morning sickness during pregnancy, though in pregnancy it is safest to take ginger infusion in small, frequent sips rather than by the cup.

I frequently use ginger to heal injuries such as muscle pulls, strains and sprains, especially externally as a poultice, compress, or fomentation. Ginger stars in one of my favorite pain-relieving baths, too, as it's especially helpful for stimulating circulation in the pelvis and lower back.

GINGER BATH

6-inch length of fresh ginger root
½ gallon boiling water

Make a ginger infusion in a half-gallon jar by cutting up the ginger root (you can leave the peel on), putting it in the jar, and filling the jar to the top with boiling water. If you want it stronger, grate the ginger. Let the infusion sit, covered and steeping, for 1–2 hours.

Pour the infusion through a strainer or cheesecloth, squeeze out the herbs, and add it into your full bathtub. Soak in the spicy luxury of ginger-infused bath water.

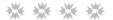

This bath is relaxing and pain-relieving for sore muscles, sore backs, and swollen joints. I suggest taking this bath just before you are ready to get into bed and pull up the covers, as you probably won't feel like doing much else. You will sleep well after soaking for at least twenty minutes in this soothing bath. It may seem odd, but it's true: Ginger is stimulating when ingested, but soothing used for a soak.

A ginger footbath is another great home remedy to try when you need it.

ANTI-NAUSEA GINGER FOOT BATH

6-inch length of fresh ginger root

1 gallon of water

Grate the ginger into a large soup pot. Add about one gallon of water. Bring the water to a boil; then turn it down and steep, covered, on the lowest heat for 1–2 hours. When it's ready, pour the infusion through a strainer into a container you can fit your feet into, such as a roasting pan, dishpan, or large soup pot. Add enough hot water to put your feet in up to your ankles. Also keep the top part of your body and legs covered and warm. This preparation can be reheated and used several times before a new one needs to be made.

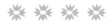

This simple remedy has helped many people who were vomiting, including intense projectile vomiting, whether from flu, food-poisoning, or any other reason. When you can't keep food or tea down to alleviate nausea, make the ginger into a foot bath and steep your feet in it. It nearly always resolves the nausea quickly. A foot bath also provides an alternative for someone who can't safely get in and out of a bathtub, or who doesn't have a tub. It will relieve muscle and joint pain and inflammation. You can make this preparation for yourself—but if you have the option of asking for help, please do that.

Ginger is high in anti-inflammatory compounds called gingerols. These antioxidant molecules are part of why ginger has been shown subjectively and objectively to help reduce the pain and swelling of osteoarthritis. In one double-blind, twelve-month study published in *Osteoarthritis and Cartilage*, people with swollen, arthritic knee joints found that their pain was reduced with the ingestion of even small amounts of ginger, and the circumference of their knee(s) was also reduced. The perception of pain is subjective, but the measurement of a swollen knee is objective. Furthermore, when the ginger was switched with placebos, these benefits diminished, indicating that the relief was objective and not imaginary; and when ginger was reintroduced, the benefits resumed. Consuming more ginger yielded even greater results.

The antioxidant molecules in ginger help neutralize the free radicals that aggravate various chronic illnesses that are associated with normal aging—but are not necessarily normal or inevitable. Rather, these chronic illnesses such as arthritis are far more prevalent when free radicals are left unchecked by antioxidants.

Antioxidants are abundant in nature and well-utilized by your body when you eat and drink them in a variety of foods and medicinal plants. Herbalist Mimi Hernandez offers this simple imagery to clarify the relationship between free radicals and antioxidants: Free radicals are needy because they lack an electron; they scavenge around in your body looking for that missing electron. Antioxidants are generous; they have extra electrons, and give them to the free radicals to satisfy that need, eliminating the need for the free radicals' to take vital nutrients out of your body. *Voilà!* A perfect if codependent relationship where needy-and-greedy meets giving-and-generous—yet in this case no one gets hurt, and the person in whom all this is going on benefits!

The following recipe for ginger and rosemary tinctured in brandy makes a good herbal medicine that I think you will enjoy:

GINGER-ROSEMARY BRANDY

2–3-inch length of fresh ginger root (or to taste)

1 cup fresh rosemary leaves (or ½ cup dried)

Any good aged-in-oak brandy

Chop or grate the ginger, and cut up the rosemary leaves. Put them into a one-pint jar. Amounts can be adjusted to your taste (and adjust accordingly if you use a larger jar). Fill the jar to the top with brandy. Wait 6 weeks or longer. Decant.

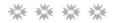

This is a great-tasting, warming blend that serves well as a digestive remedy and an anti-inflammatory cough remedy, especially when the body is aching from indigestion or coughing. Ginger and rosemary stimulate healthy cardiovascular circulation and promote liver health. This natural immune-boosting recipe is filled with antioxidants and antiseptic, antibacterial oils. I use it "neat" or diluted in hot water. I especially like to add it to cold or cough syrups, using the infused brandy as both a natural preservative and to bring additional healing qualities to the medicinal syrup.

Both herbs are warming and antispasmodic, as is the brandy. (That's part of the medicinal magic of an old-fashioned "hot toddy.") You can make this preparation as described, or make each tincture separately and then combine them afterward to give you the greatest flexibility in using them.

Ginger's anti-inflammatory properties make it useful for relieving pain, swelling, and congestion in the musculoskeletal system. Here is another blend I make with the same two common kitchen herbs. It can be used on food as a delicious cooking or seasoning oil, but is also useful for external application for pain relief.

GINGER-ROSEMARY INFUSED OIL

2–3 inches of dried ginger root or ¼ cup ginger powder

1 cup fresh rosemary leaves (and flowers, optional), cut up

Put the ginger and rosemary in a clean, dry pint jar. Cover them with olive oil, filling the jar to the top, and let sit for 6 weeks. Decant and use freely as needed to increase circulation and decrease muscle and joint pain.

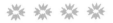

I find that ginger root is apt to spoil if infused fresh into oil, so I either use a powder that is still fresh enough to be pungent, or dried pieces of root. Dried ginger is also hotter than the fresh root. It you are using this oil to encourage circulation to the heart, massage this oil into your legs using upward strokes. It can also be massaged in circular motions over the abdominal area to encourage healthy digestion, through warmth that gently stimulates the abundance of blood vessels throughout the digestive system.

Finally, here's a satisfying lunch recipe featuring ginger:

GINGERED GREEN BEANS

2 cups green beans

Olive oil, to taste

1 tablespoon dandelion root, leaf, and/or flower vinegar

1 tablespoon tahini

½ inch or more length of ginger root

Tamari, to taste

½ teaspoon gomashio (see recipe, page 412)

2 tablespoons grated raw cheddar cheese

Serves one as a substantial main dish, two as a side dish. Cook green beans in just enough water to cover them for about 10 minutes, until fully cooked yet still a bit chewy. Stir in finely minced ginger. Splash with tamari, dandelion vinegar, and olive oil. Drizzle on the tahini, and sprinkle on the gomashio. Lastly, grate the cheese into the dish, and stir it all together. Adjust seasonings if needed.

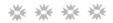

Rosemary *(Rosmarinus officinalis)*

I adore the taste of this aromatic beauty, and like to include rosemary in anything from an avocado sandwich or salad to an omelet, or atop a buffalo burger. Her botanical name, *Rosmarinus*, means "dew of the sea."

For cooking and/or tea, you can use fresh leaves, or the stronger dried leaves. If using the dried herb, crush and sniff a few leaves to check for the characteristic pungent rosemary fragrance. Replace old rosemary that's no longer fragrant, especially if it's to be used for medicine.

If you've never done it—or even if you have—rub a fresh leaf of rosemary and inhale deeply so you'll know what it's supposed to smell like. It's good for your brain too.

Famous as Shakespeare's herb "for remembrance," it's true that rosemary helps increase memory and improve concentration. This common culinary spice is a vascular stimulant, and rich in antioxidants that strengthen the brain and liver. Rosemary will help with depression related to poor digestion. This is more common than is generally realized, but is prevalent now because of poor diets and ongoing stress, which impair digestion as well as contributing to illnesses such as irritable bowel syndrome (IBS).

Rosemary is warming and stimulating, and benefits circulation in the liver, aiding digestion. Rosemary tea or tincture excels in treating liver stress and overload, which cause indigestion that includes "digestive headaches." These are headaches you get from eating too much, or eating something that isn't good for you or doesn't agree with you—or simply because your digestive system needs help to work optimally.

SIMPLE ROSEMARY TEA

1 teaspoon dried rosemary leaves (one tablespoon if using fresh leaves)

Put the rosemary in a cup or mug. Cover with boiling water and steep, covered, for 15–20 minutes. Reheat if desired.

Rosemary tincture can also be made into tea, using about one dropper of fresh rosemary tincture (25–30 drops) per cup of boiled water.

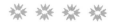

In one memorable case, a woman came to me who had been to see "everyone" and wasn't able to get any relief from her irritable bowel syndrome. She'd tried elimination/allergen diets for months, homeopathy, conventional medicine, herbal products, psychotherapy and more. But she achieved tremendous improvement with two cups of rosemary tea daily, and within a month she was able to resume her life without always needing to know where the nearest bathroom was. Bless that rosemary! It also cleared her mind, improved her memory and helped her with a long history of depression. (Her familiar problems and some new ones came back several years later, however, after she stopped doing lots of good things she'd been doing for herself, including drinking her rosemary tea.) I love simples—they are often far more effective than you might think.

I like to dry lots of rosemary so I'll have it around all year to enjoy in food and as tea. I also use fresh rosemary to make infused vinegar and tincture. Last but definitely not least, fresh rosemary infused oil comes out very yummy, and can be added to pasta or cheese dishes, salads, and more. It also helps hair health and growth, and is reputed to be especially beneficial for dark hair. The oil is massaged into the scalp and, ideally, left on overnight about once a week as a tonic. Apply it after a nettle rinse for optimum results. As often happens to me, the first time I was making rosemary oil for my hair, I ended up tasting it and found it so delicious that I left it in the pantry and had to make another bottle for my hair.

ROSEMARY HAIR OIL

Fresh rosemary leaves and stalks (flowers optional)

Olive oil (first cold-pressing)

Pint jar

Chop the rosemary finely, and fill the pint jar to about a half-inch below the rim. Next, slowly fill the jar with the olive oil, poking down into and around the herbs to insure that the oil gets thoroughly distributed and saturates all of the plant material. Fill the jar to the very top with the oil, continuing to poke with the chopstick to allow any air bubbles to rise to the top. When you've removed most of them, let the contents settle for a couple of minutes, then cap your jar and label it. Set it on a plate or saucer, because it will often ooze out as gas continues to be released from the infusing herbs.

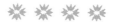

Here's a shampoo recipe I created that features rosemary as well as many of the herbs I've discussed:

DELUXE HAIR-RESTORATIVE HERBAL SHAMPOO

    ½ cup dried black walnut leaves

    ½ cup dried burdock root

    ½ cup dried horsetail (equisetum)

    ½ cup dried nettle leaves with stalks

    ½ cup dried St. J's wort leaves and flowers

    ¼ cup dried lavender flowers and/or leaves (the flowers are more fragrant)

    ¼ cup dried rosemary

    1 quart aloe vera gel

    1 small fresh lemon

    (Optional: A few drops each of lavender and rosemary essential oils. ¼ cup sage can also be added, especially for dark hair.)

Mix the herbs in a saucepan and pour three quarts of cold water over them. Bring just to a boil, and turn down immediately. Simmer for about one hour, and then let stand overnight.

The next day, strain out your herbs and stir in the aloe vera gel, either from a bottle of the purest gel you can purchase, without added ingredients or, if you have a lot of aloe plants, scraped from inside the leaves.

Squeeze and strain the juice of a small lemon, and add that in. Stir it all together well, and store most of the shampoo in a labeled glass jar in the refrigerator. You can leave a small usage bottle of about 4 ounces in your bathroom. You make a smaller quantity by adjusting the herb amounts so that you use approximately 1 cup of dried herbs for each quart of water (and about ⅓ of the other ingredients).

This recipe is helpful when hair is thinning, growing dull, and/or falling out due to stress, menopausal challenges, and/or dietary deficiencies. The blend is a mineral-rich bonanza that helps nourish and strengthen the shafts of your hair, and improves circulation through the blood vessels in your scalp, encouraging natural oil production so that your hair can grow in glossy, rich, and full.

Turmeric *(Curcuma longa)*

This celebrated member of the ginger family is indigenous to India, and has naturalized throughout much of Southeast Asia. The rhizomes are used extensively in Ayurvedic and Chinese medicine as well as in cooking and as a natural dye. Turmeric is widely available in North America today, and can be found in many forms—fresh or dried root, encapsulated powder, tinctures, extracts, and standardized extracts, which I'll talk about below.

Curcumin is the carotenoid that gives turmeric its characteristic orange color and its botanical name, and is the antioxidant reputed to be the main source of turmeric's healing abilities.

These well-known healing abilities include soothing inflammation in the muscles and joints, protecting the health of the liver, helping the body protect itself from infection, increasing peripheral circulation, and more. Turmeric is such a good anti-inflammatory that it would likely be used externally more often except that the skin turns bright yellow and orange for awhile after applying it—explaining, I'm pretty sure, its lack of popularity as a massage oil! I know that when I've tinctured fresh roots, my hands turn a lovely shade of orange until it wears off over time. How much time? That depends on how much tincture I've prepared!

The powder can be a handy first-aid remedy to stop bleeding. Turmeric is also classified as an "anti-angiogenesis" agent, meaning that it can help stop the blood supply to tumors, depriving them of the nourishment they need to grow and spread. This bitter, warming herb stimulates bile production, thus improving digestion. It also reduces cholesterol. I've found it to be helpful in the presence of parasites, supporting the liver as it works to clear the body. But is it just curcumin that does all this, or is it the whole herb, with all its component parts working together?

Standardized extracts are products that, through special manufacturing processes, concentrate the so called "active ingredients" in the plant, and standardize the amount of these "active ingredients" with an eye towards making the medicine stronger. This way of viewing plants is, in essence, a reductionist viewpoint that seeks to make plants more drug-like, equating these concentrated substances with increased effectiveness. But this conclusion is often simply not true. In fact, it often makes herbs more drug-like in the worst ways, rendering them less recognizable by your body and therefore less effective, and increasing the risks of side effects. It also has the added disadvantage (or advantage, depending on your point of view) of taking plant medicine out of the hands of people and putting it under the control of manufacturers. Science is also fickle, and changes what it considers to be the most active ingredient(s) depending on the latest research, whereas traditional knowledge and usage evolves much more slowly and naturally and, in my view, is generally more dependable.

Turmeric products are now sold that have had their curcuminoids concentrated and increased to a standard amount—but what that standard is based upon is entirely made-up, and other products exist where curcumin has been extracted and is sold alone, severed from the rest of the plant altogether. Science examines plants to find their so-called "active ingredients" because there is a fixation on reducing plant medicine to less complex forms that will be more predictable and less variable.

But plants work differently in your body than drugs do. They're variable because they are alive, like us. Plants are complex life forms. They are whole, multi-faceted beings, like us. The so-called "active ingredients" of plants are often alkaloids, its harshest chemical parts, and nature provides other constituents in the plant to buffer them and make them gentle enough to use safely.

It is not necessarily the best idea to have medicines made super-potent. Once herbs have been altered they are not the same, and are often not even really "herbs" anymore. They are more prone to cause unexpected side effects too. Herbalist and acupuncturist Karen Vaughan writes, "Standardized curcumin should not be given to people with gastritis or ulcers, while the herb itself protects the mucosa while addressing any infection."

Even when a standardized extract isn't necessarily harmful, I simply don't trust it as much as nature's own "product," produced by nature's own ever-evolving processes. I have seen unpleasant reactions to some standardized extracts, such as to standardized St. John's wort, for example, as contrasted with how favorably people generally respond to tea or tincture. St. J's wort *(Hypericum perforatum)* is one herb in which first one and then another chemical component was claimed by laboratory scientists to be "what makes it work."

This spicy plant turmeric is said to be able to help us with over 500 conditions—and personally, that's good enough for me!

LATE-NIGHT TURMERIC SNACK

1 cup whole milk yogurt

1½ teaspoons slippery elm powder, or to taste

1 teaspoon cinnamon powder, or to taste

¾ teaspoon turmeric powder, or to taste

½ teaspoon honey, or to taste (orange peel or rose blossom infused honeys are especially nice)

Splash of vanilla extract (optional)

This is a nice, creamy snack you can indulge in before bed (or anytime). Use all ingredients to taste to get the blend that you like. This tasty snack supports the immune system in your digestive tract, helps stabilize your blood sugar, and encourages a healthy bowel movement when you arise in the morning.

This recipe can be enhanced (or actually made palatable for people who are unused to such a strong flavor as turmeric) by the addition of a generous splash of vanilla extract. It can also be a substitute for the honey, especially helpful for people who can't eat honey or who find that sugar in any form, eaten at night, keeps them awake.

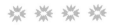

Fennel *(Foeniculum vulgare)*

Fennel is well-known as a digestive aid. Tea made from a teaspoon of seeds steeped for 10 minutes can help relieve cramps and indigestion. Mix fennel powder with ginger powder and honey, and roll up some honey balls in slippery elm powder. This is a good preventative remedy for sea sickness.

Fennel (or dill) seed tea eases insomnia brought about by indigestion. The seed tea can also increase the quantity of a woman's breast milk. Like dill, the aerial parts make a warming, aromatic, antispasmodic herb for the gastrointestinal system. Cooked fennel leaves and bulbs freeze beautifully, and can be a lovely touch added to soups, stir-fries, and stews, especially when it's early in the spring and you can't wait to begin eating out of the garden again.

Sage *(Salvia officinalis)*

This is the regular green garden sage that is commonly used in cooking, not "white sage" *(Salvia apiana)* that is more commonly used for burning. The name "Salvia" comes from the Latin "salvare" meaning "to save," and many species of sage provide antiseptic medicine due to the high content of volatile oils in the leaves and, to a lesser extent, in the flowers. I love to cook different wild and cultivated mushrooms with sage leaves. The flavors complement each other so well.

I use sage leaf tea for sore throats, with or without honey and lemon. It can also be gargled with salt (but skip the honey). Sage is helpful for mouth health in general; used as a rinse it can tighten loose gums, and a fresh leaf massaged over the teeth helps whiten them. Rubbing the leaf along the gum lines will not only help tighten gums but will help to prevent bacterial mouth infections too.

I make a tooth powder for daily use with sage (sometimes mixed with salt and/or rosemary), which does all of the above and is also particularly helpful if there are chronic periodontal problems.

SAGE TOOTH POWDER

1 cup dried sage leaves

(Optional: Mix this blend half and half with rosemary leaves. I often also mix the sage with high-quality ground sea salt such as Celtic salt, at a ratio of about 10:1 sage to sea salt.)

Grind sage leaves to a fluffy powder. Put in a jar in the bathroom, and use twice daily: Put about ¼ teaspoon on your toothbrush, with or without the natural toothpaste of your choice. I alternate between mixing in toothpaste and not. Moisten the powder on the brush with water, and brush teeth as usual, paying special attention to the gum lines and to being gentle.

Regular use of this tooth powder can help prevent and heal gum infections, tighten loose teeth, and generally promote good mouth hygiene and health.

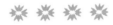

Sage is for sagacity, or wisdom. Its high mineral content nourishes the central nervous system, including the spine and brain. Herbalist Maria Treben recommends gathering sage leaves in full sunshine at midday for the highest concentration of volatile oils. She suggests frequent consumption of sage tea to prevent stroke. You may recall that I used it to good effect as an over-the-heart-area fomentation for my father when his blood pressure had risen alarmingly.

Sage can be helpful with restless leg syndrome, muscle cramps, and spinal-cord injuries. I use sage in combination with other nerve-regenerating herbs such as nettles, St. J's wort, and oat straw whenever there is any degree of paralysis, whether from accident or illness. I found it helpful for a friend with a severe spinal-cord injury and for a client with multiple sclerosis. It combines well with St. J's for both external and internal use. Externally, a tea or diluted tincture mix can be applied with a washcloth. For these uses I suggest blending sage tincture into St. J's infused oil, and rubbing the spine with it at least once daily. The tea can also be taken in to the body through means of a foot bath.

SAGE FOOT BATH

Dried sage leaves

1 gallon water

Tub, pot, or dishpan to fit your feet in

Put about 3 large handfuls of sage leaves into a pot on the stove. Add water and bring to a boil. After 1–2 minutes, turn off the heat and let the tea sit, covered, for about an hour. Reheat if necessary, and then strain the tea into a big pot or square washtub, or even a bathtub. (That will require more water, though, to get the sage infusion to cover the feet up to the ankles.)

Soak both feet in the warm tea for about 15–20 minutes. You can gently reheat and reuse the mixture once or twice more if needed.

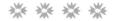

Sage also helps to keep your hair and scalp healthy. Hair needs lots of minerals to thrive and be glossy. In addition to drinking sage and cooking with it, fresh leaves can be infused into olive oil, or the tea can be applied to the hair as a final rinse; or you can use sage as part of an herbal shampoo recipe. (See recipe on page 452.)

Sage is well-known for helping dry excess perspiration. It generally dries fluids, including the night sweats that can be a part of menopause. Try a cup of cooled-down sage tea in the evening before going to bed.

Here is a less well-known use of sage: My mother lost her sense of smell, and with it most of her enjoyment of food. I investigated and was told to try giving her zinc supplements, as zinc deficiency can sometimes be the cause of this problem. I decided to recommend sage tea as her zinc supplement. She drank one cup of sage tea daily, made by infusing 1 teaspoon of dried sage in boiled water for about 10 minutes. She had been suffering with this loss of smell for over a year, and doctors had been unable to help her or determine the cause. After three weeks of sage tea her sense of smell returned, never to disappear again. Hooray!

Here is a caution about sage. It is rightfully famous for drying up breast milk, so it should not be used in medicinal quantities by nursing moms unless you are using it for that purpose, in which case it is effective.

One of my apprentices was leaving her two-year-old girl for the first time to go to the annual women's herbal conference in New England. She was quite concerned about her breasts leaking, and the possibility of being in pain all weekend. She started drinking sage tea a few days before she began traveling, and I brought some homemade sage leaf tincture for her to use during the conference.

A few experienced herbalists told me my plan wouldn't work, that the sage wouldn't be enough. Well, my student's happy smile at the end of the conference refuted that—she said it had worked like a charm. And when she went home and stopped using her sage, she resumed nursing her baby girl with no problem.

In challenging healing situations both large and small, I often find that working simply really works.

Here is one of my favorite recipes:

SAGE-LAVENDER HONEY

1 part sage leaves, with or without flowers (I prefer fresh, but it will come out beautifully with dried sage as well.)

1–2 parts fresh lavender flowers (and leaves, optional)

Honey (best quality you can afford)

If using fresh herbs, fill your jar 100% full, first with the herbs and then with honey. If you use dried herbs, crumble or grind them and fill your jar about halfway full and then drizzle the honey over the herbs until the jar is completely full. Whether they're dry or fresh, poke around and through the herbs with a chopstick to make sure you get the herbs completely saturated; then cap the jar and label it. Let the herbs infuse for at least a month. It doesn't need to be decanted, though you can if you prefer.

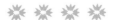

This joyful sage-lavender honey is delightful medicine, antiseptic and delicious. It can be used by itself, on a wound, or taken in hot water or tea for a cold, sore throat, or cough.

There are a variety of ways you can enjoy your infused herbal honeys. Sometimes I enjoy having pieces of herbs in my honey, especially when they're soft and lovely to look at, and spread well on crackers or toast, like fresh sage, lavender, or roses. But you can grind the herbs finely if you prefer that. I strain some batches—pine needle infused honey, for example—and others I make as honey "pastes" or spreads of varying thickness by stirring in dried, powdered herbs such as turmeric or ginger.

Marjoram *(Origanum majorana)*

Sweet marjoram is also called "joy of the mountain," and I love her very much. She is a close relative of the better-known oregano *(Origanum vulgare);* they are like sister and brother. His (oregano's) taste is sharper and a bit more pungent; hers is sweeter and gentler. But the medicine they provide is similar—both are nutritive, antiseptic, anti-inflammatory, healing tonics for the digestive organs, and soothing to the heart.

I generally prefer marjoram's taste, and frequently cook with it or sprinkle it on cooked food as a condiment. It is a great boon to the digestive system. Juliette de Bairacli Levy recommends marjoram for "sour stomach, fermentation, and bad breath." I have read that it can also aid in upset stomach, colic, and abdominal cramps. Gail Faith Edwards sings the praises of infusing marjoram in both vinegar and honey. She also informs us that the infusion can help lower blood pressure, and that the tea is an emmenagogue (to start or increase menstrual flow) and helps menstrual cramps.

I also find marjoram a boon to the musculoskeletal system. Marjoram gently stimulates circulation; it is warming and diffusive, relaxing the muscles and the mind at the same time. Rub infused oil or liniment into sore, aching muscles or joints. Apply it externally as a compress for swellings and joint pains, cramps, and spasms. The tea can be added to baths.

MARJORAM LINIMENT

Fresh marjoram leaves with stalks

Apple cider vinegar (or rubbing alcohol)

Cut up marjoram. Fill a jar with them nearly to the top. Fill the jar again with whichever menstruum you are using. Cap it. If you use vinegar with a metal lid, protect the lid with a piece of unbleached parchment paper between the jar and lid—or use a glass jar with a plastic lid or cork. Shake it well. Wait 6 weeks, shaking it periodically while it's steeping. Decant the liniment. Label it with a notation "for external use only" if you used rubbing alcohol.

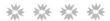

I sprinkle a good amount of dried marjoram onto salads and into soups and vegetable dishes. I add it, along with garlic powder, to whole-wheat vegetable pizzas that we buy at our local farmer's market. I cook marjoram into eggs and casseroles, and sometimes mix it with turmeric or curry in bean and lentil stews.

Another of my favorite ways to take my marjoram medicine is as an infused oil made with the fresh herb. I remember the first time I made a small bottle of this oil "for joint pain." I opened it and found the smell so intoxicating that I tasted it before rubbing it on; that bottle went right into the kitchen and stayed there until it was empty, and never got rubbed on anywhere! It's delicious on garlic bread. If you don't eat bread, put it on veggies, or rice and beans. Or—oh yes, you can rub it on inflamed joints, and it can be quite pain-relieving.

MARJORAM OIL

Fresh marjoram leaves
Cold-pressed olive oil

Put the marjoram, well cut-up, into a jar nearly to the top, and cover the herbs with olive oil. Label your jar and let it sit infusing atop a small plate or saucer for about 6 weeks. At that point, I suggest you decant this oil in a timely manner for the best flavor.

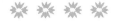

MARJORAM-GARLIC OIL BREAD

Marjoram oil, to taste (recipe above)
Fresh garlic cloves, to taste
Bread—your favorite kind

Brush the marjoram oil liberally onto bread, add slivered or pressed or fresh garlic, toast it, and *voilà*—you have an easily digestible, anti-inflammatory, antibacterial gustatory delicacy!

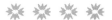

It seems that with marjoram, like rosemary, you need at least two bottles of everything—one bottle each of herbal oil and herbal vinegar in the kitchen, for the medicine you enjoy eating, and one set for the medicine chest, for the herbal medicine you put *on* your body when you're indulging in herbal beauty treatments, or hurting, or ill.

Mustard Family *(Brassicaceae)*

This plant family, important for both food and medicine, contains over 3,000 species, including numerous wild varieties in addition to well-known foods such as cabbage, turnips, and broccoli. Mustard, including the wild mustards, is used as food and medicine in various Native American cultures, and is a traditional medicine in various Latin American, Asian, and European countries.

The lines between food and medicine cross constantly in this family. For example, cabbage leaf, a staple food, is protective against colon and other cancers (as are all mustards), and cabbage is also a traditional and effective anti-inflammatory herb, used externally for swollen joints, skin ulcers, infections, and for relieving engorged, sore tissue in the breasts and elsewhere. Cabbage leaves can be heated in boiling water before applying, or a raw cabbage preparation can be prepared as follows:

CABBAGE POULTICE

Green outer cabbage leaves, ideally from organically grown plants
Rolling pin or bottle

Cut away the thick cabbage stalks, and use a roller pin or bottle to press flat and squeeze the cells and juice from the cabbage leaves.

Layer the inside of the leaves (the smooth side) directly on the skin, around the entire affected area, root-side down so the shape will more naturally conform to the body. You can cover it and snugly—not too tightly—wrap the poultice with cotton flannel or muslin, and pin that closed. If there is an infection, it will feel hot as it pulls the infection out of the cells.

Leave on for about an hour or longer.

Do not reuse.

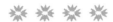

Before it was called *Brassica,* mustard's plant family name was *Cruciferae* ("cross-bearing"). You can easily recognize species in this family by the way the flower petals grow in fours, roughly in the shape of a cross. Additionally, the seedpods of mustard stand upright on the plant, and surround the stalk in whorls. According to wilderness expert Thomas Elpel, wild mustards are all edible (though not all are palatable!). Mustards get the blood moving while they nourish and fortify it. The leaves contain nutrients such as magnesium and calcium, vitamins A, E, and K, carotenes, flavonoids, and a great variety of other antioxidants. Current wisdom says that raw mustard-family plants may be inappropriate and harmful for people with hypothyroid illnesses, but cooked mustard greens are helpful. The seeds are an excellent natural source of omega-3 oils.

Mustard is stimulating, pungent, and warming, and mustard's seed oils are hot. It's just a question of hot to what degree? (Watercress, another well-known mustard-family member like arugula, has the botanical name of *Nasturtium* or "nose-twister," which refers to its peppery pungency.) In the kitchen, I enjoy the intense flavor of a variety of mustard greens and flowers, both in salads and well-cooked as potherbs, often mixing mustards with sweeter greens to cut the pungency a bit.

Mustard is a valuable medicine, unsurpassed for breaking up congestion in various parts of the body and most especially in the lungs. I turn to mustard seed powder as a plaster to break up entrenched congestion in lung or bronchial infections. The most common mustard seeds are black, brown and white (actually yellow). I use the yellow mustard for plasters as it is the least hot, and less likely to cause blistering of the skin.

I also make sure that the mustard doesn't touch the skin directly unless it is highly diluted as in a foot bath. Remember, mustard has also been used as a terrible chemical weapon. Mustard gas causes skin-blistering and respiratory damage. However, as long as you are not burning and inhaling it—which I strongly advise you never do—this is a great remedy as old as the hills, to be used with attention and a degree of caution, discussed in detail below.

MUSTARD PLASTER

2 parts yellow mustard seed powder

1 part flour (optional)

Warm water

Olive oil

Mix powdered yellow (or other) mustard with enough warm-to-hot water to make a paste. If you wish to make it less strong, add the flour to the paste. Coat skin on chest or back (over the lungs) with olive oil. (Pure mustard powder will burn the skin.) Wrap the paste in a thin cotton cloth, and carefully place it over the chest or back, taking care that every area it touches has been covered first with oil. Leave the plaster on for 5–20 minutes, checking regularly with the person to be sure it does not become too hot. When you are helping someone with a mustard plaster, stay close by!

Do not add heat to a mustard plaster by using a hot water bottle or heating pad. *Do* remove a mustard plaster immediately if someone complains of pain or burning. Start with a short duration and check in every few minutes, leaving it on for a maximum of 20 minutes. This poultice will break up painful congestion in the lungs and bronchia, and help ease breathing. It can also help to clear infection.

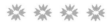

In one Russian study, 150 patients were treated with mustard plasters for painful and difficult breathing due to pneumonia, bronchitis, asthma, or other causes. The great majority had improved expectoration, decreased pain, and increased lung capacity.

The mustard chest plaster isn't a treatment to do on your own. If you want to use mustard powder to relieve your congestion, I'd suggest taking a mustard foot bath. A ginger footbath will work similarly.

MUSTARD POWDER FOOT BATH

2 or more tablespoons mustard seed powder

1 gallon hot water

Tub, dishpan, or pot large enough for your feet

Stir the mustard powder into the water and mix well. The amount to use will depend on the heat of the species of mustard you're using, and the sensitivity of your skin.

Soak your feet in this bath to relieve congestion. It warms and heats your body as it increases your circulation and draws the congestion in your chest down and out, helping to clear the lungs and bronchia. This foot bath should feel "good-hot," not "burning-hot." If you feel like you're burning, take your feet out immediately and dilute the footbath with more hot water.

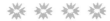

Vanilla *(Vanilla planifolia)*

Vanilla is a lush, climbing vine native to Mexico, though now widely cultivated, whose blossoms are white orchids that only bloom for one day. I saw these beautiful flowers growing on the Tahitian island of Taha'a, nicknamed the "Vanilla Island." There is no natural pollinator living there, so each flower must be hand-pollinated on the one day that it's open. Quite a nice job! Without this, we wouldn't have the vanilla bean, the elongated pod that is the fruit or seedpod of the orchid.

This herb, and the extract made from it, is uplifting and relaxing. It is often cited as being an aphrodisiac. Interestingly, the Latin root words for vanilla and vagina are the same! Both come from a word that means "sheath." The smell of vanilla is certainly appealing to the senses, and the tropical locales where it grows are lush and sensual—so perhaps your natural eroticism is evoked when you ingest vanilla in food or drink. Vanilla is used extensively in baking, and can also enhance dishes such as yogurt and fruit, hot or cold cereal, herbal elixirs, fruit drinks and smoothies, and many desserts, including ice cream.

Here is an example of its sensual delights:

ROSE VANILLA BEAN HONEY

Fresh rose blossom or buds of any fragrant species—unsprayed

1 dried vanilla bean, as fresh as possible

Wildflower, linden, or clover honey

Cut off the ends of the vanilla bean, open it up lengthwise, scrape out the insides, cut it up into small pieces, and place every part of the bean into a pint jar. Fill the rest of the jar with fresh rose blossoms or buds. (If you are using dried roses, use about 1 cup to fill the jar half full.) Cover the herbs with honey and stir gently, poking here and there with a chopstick to make sure the honey saturates the herbs completely, and continue filling the jar to the top.

Cap it and wait 6 weeks or more before decanting. You can leave the herbs in there as long as you like; when you're ready, decant them by gently heating the honey until it pours like water, through a strainer into a fresh bottle.

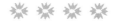

Rose Vanilla Bean Honey is an earthly taste of divine delight. Enjoy it in the Sophisticated Hawthorn Berry Elixir (recipe below) and any other ways that you like!

This elixir increases the natural aphrodisiac qualities of all its herbal ingredients. It makes an exciting wedding gift! But you don't need a special occasion to enjoy this elixir with your beloved. It will add an extra sparkle to a romantic encounter anytime.

And one more thing—please don't feel you have to be with someone else to enjoy this elixir. Both hawthorn and rose also increase your desire and openness to love your own sweet self. How they do that is a mystery to me, but that is among their most profound gifts, so please don't wait for anyone. Enjoy it on your own, and with your friends, too!

SOPHISTICATED HAWTHORN BERRY ELIXIR

Fresh hawthorn berries, cut-up

¼ cup rose and vanilla bean honey

3 tablespoons hawthorn blossom glycerite

2 tablespoons rose blossom glycerite

Brandy (any reasonably priced nice brandy that's been aged in oak barrels)

Fill a 24–32 ounce jar about ¾ full with hawthorn berries. Cover them about halfway up with brandy. Then add the infused honey (see recipe above) and glycerites.

The infused honey and glycerites will have to have been prepared in advance, (or the glycerites can be purchased) since they need to be made separately—in the spring and summer when the hawthorns and roses are in bloom, and then in the fall when hawthorn berries are harvested.

If necessary, add additional brandy, Rose Vanilla Bean Honey, and/or rose or hawthorn glycerites (your choice) to bring the elixir up to the top of your jar.

Wait a minimum of 6 weeks before decanting—longer if you can. This brew will benefit from long steeping.

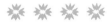

Even after you've decanted it, this preparation will continue to improve with age. It is one of the most delicious medicines I've ever tasted, and certainly will encourage someone to take their hawthorn medicine, if that is your aim! But since it's a bit complex to make, I use it more as a special, uplifting treat that just happens to also be medicinal.

For everyday medicinal purposes of heart nourishment and increased health of veins and arteries, there is absolutely nothing wrong with pouring brandy and a bit of honey over fresh hawthorn berries to make a simple, medicinal hawthorn berry elixir. In fact, I would recommend that elixir to anyone.

This "sophisticated" elixir requires a few more ingredients and more preparation time, especially if you count the time you wait for the glycerites and honey to infuse, and the fact that you make it over three seasons. These extra steps are worth it, though, as the additional ingredients give it a more complex taste and aroma. Adding the soothing yet uplifting medicines of hawthorn's flowers, along with the roses and vanilla beans, takes it to another level altogether!

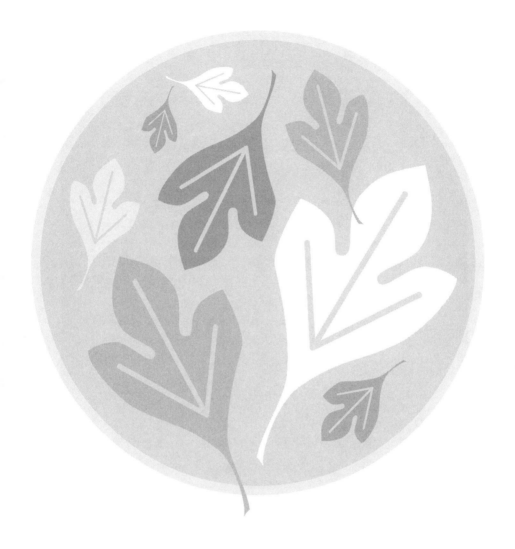

PART IV

Additional Remedies, Tips, and Thoughts on Healing

15

Wound and Bruise Healing

There are many situations that call for external treatments as part of a person's herbal healthcare, but nowhere are hands-on-healing treatments more primary than in first aid for injuries. Here is some general information to start with:

Fresh herbs for poultices can be mashed or cut up, or sometimes chewed (depending on the herb) and then applied directly to skin. Or the herb(s) can be steeped in boiled water for just a few minutes before applying to the skin. Generally speaking, depending on where a wound is located on the body, and how large an area is being covered, you can either leave it at that or, if that's impractical, wrap a piece of clean, comfortable material such as soft cotton flannel or a thin towel over the area, and secure it in place with a tie or safety pins.

You can also cover the herb(s) with gauze, and use surgical tape to hold them in place. I prefer the first method because sometimes the adhesive in surgical tape or band-aids can be a mild-to-severe skin irritant, which can complicate the healing process.

Dried herbs for poultices need to be steeped in boiled water to release their healing properties, unless they are powdered (see below). For a poultice, use just enough boiling water to cover the dried herb(s), and steep them for anywhere from 3–10 minutes. Any leftover liquid can be used to rinse the wounded area after removing the poultice or, if the herb(s) being used are suitable for internal use, you can simply drink it. If the dried herbs are applied as *powder*, they don't necessarily need boiling water. But they do need to be moistened before being applied to the skin, with water, aloe gel, an herbal oil, or saliva.

Tinctures can be applied topically for healing injuries and bruises. I tend to not use tinctures on open wounds because they hurt like crazy when applied, and the alcohol can increase bleeding. However, in an emergency situation, always use the best option available. A folk herbalist I met recently told me he applied yarrow tincture straight onto a fresh chainsaw wound. Though the poor man yelped with the stinging pain of alcohol in a gaping wound, the yarrow tincture actually stopped the bleeding, and they were able to bring the skin together; the man healed without infection.

I had a client in her forties whose mother had gone through chemotherapy when she was pregnant with her. As a result, she'd been dealing with a compromised immune system since she was born. Among many other manifestations, she had recurring bouts of shingles, the painful rash also known as herpes zoster. She found that St. J's tincture *(Hypericum perforatum)* worked remarkably well when applied topically to the lesions that erupted on her neck. I had suggested infused oil, but when she'd run out of oil and tried the tincture, she found it healed them much faster. I love when my students and clients open my eyes to new ways of using the plants. Flexibility and adaptability are vital keys to lifelong learning and healing.

Infused oils and ointments work well on bruises, and I use them frequently. I keep them handy in my first-aid and travel kits. Every situation is unique and can be evaluated on its own; however, generally speaking, the herbs themselves applied to the body as a poultice, bath/soak, or compress are my first choice. I often follow up poultices (or soaks and baths) by applying oils in-between.

I also find that adding tincture into oil can be an excellent way to enhance the healing properties of the oil. I do this in small batches, so that the oil won't spoil. I share examples of this in other chapters, such as adding arnica and/or lobelia tincture into the Ease Oil recipe (page 176), and I've mixed echinacea tincture into infused violet leaf oil to heal precancerous spots that were on the skin. I use infused oils and ointments on injured tissue that is closed or scraped, but don't recommend starting with oil on deep wounds, as there is a risk of infection. It's better to use the oil to aid healing after the risk of infection has passed.

IMMEDIACY OF TREATMENT

I've found the most helpful factor in healing wounds and bruises successfully is immediacy of treatment—sometimes even before it looks like there is any problem at all. The second most helpful is to continue all the way through to the completion of healing even when the obvious signs of trauma are no longer obvious.

I've noticed that quite often, if an adult or teen falls, they will say, "Oh, it's nothing; I don't need any help." Then their knee swells up later, and turns lovely shades of red, purple, and eventually yellow. Or someone may diligently take herbs to treat an injury such as a broken toe or a sprained ankle until it's about seventy, eighty, or even ninety percent better, and then get lazy or simply forget because the swelling is down and it doesn't hurt as much any more.

It's one thing to taper off the number of daily treatments as a wound or bruise gets better, but stopping altogether before it's fully healed, though understandably tempting, isn't a good idea. The first approach (denial at the start) is guaranteed to make healing take longer and generally be more difficult to achieve. The second approach (not completing the treatment) is more likely to invite problems later on that could have been avoided.

· · · · ● · · · ·

Some of my favorite herbal allies for healing wounds, bruises and injuries are: violet leaves, grape leaves, plantain leaves, yarrow leaves and flowers, witch hazel leaves, St. J's leaves and flowers, elder blossoms, motherwort leaves and flowers, goldenrod leaves and flowers, calendula blossoms, chickweed (aerial parts), lobelia (gathered in flower and seedpod stages), comfrey leaves, mullein leaves, chamomile flowers, agrimony leaves, coltsfoot leaves, mint leaves, lavender flowers, burdock leaves, prunella leaves and flowers, ginger roots, onions, maple-leaved cramp bark leaves, and hyssop leaves and flowers.

For additional information on internal herbs for pain-relief, skin-healing, and to prevent or heal infections, please reread the entries about these herbs and others, especially in the sections on the skin, immune, and musculoskeletal systems.

The following is a story of how well your body can heal when you tend an injury immediately and follow it all the way through.

HEALING A BURST BLOOD VESSEL IN THE EYE

I had some burst blood vessels (a subconjunctival hemorrhage) in the inner corner of my left eye. Even though I know these can happen spontaneously for no obvious cause, or just from a particularly strong sneeze or cough, it had never happened to me before, and I was a bit freaked out. It hurt a little, and was deep red and quite noticeable.

The next afternoon, when my apprentice Suzie came over to fulfill her work-exchange time with me, she recoiled when she saw it and exclaimed, "Holy cow!"

Later that day, an herbal friend of mine saw me and said, "That happened to me. It never went away."

I felt my fear engage and my energy sucked down and out. Then I thought to ask, "Did you treat it?"

"No," she said. "I didn't do anything—maybe just put some ice on it."

Another friend with us, also an herbalist, said, "That happened to me once, and I took care of it and it did go away." Immediately, I felt my trust restored, and my energy returned. We human beings are such suggestible creatures!

The first thing I did was to eat blood vessel-strengthening blueberries and hawthorn berries. Taking them in any form would have been fine, so I used what I had—frozen blueberries (thawed first) and a hawthorn berry-solid extract, a concentrate that can be stirred into food (Avena Botanicals, page 509). I picked out some of my favorite wound-healing plants, plantain (*Plantago* species), elder *(Sambucus nigra),* and witch hazel *(Hamamelis virginiana)* to use as eyewash. I drank an infusion of calendula and plantain, and added a tincture I'd made with my three primary allies—elder, rose, and plantain—to each cup of infusion, because they were appropriate for the situation and also to support me.

EYEWASH FOR BURST BLOOD VESSELS IN THE EYE

> Small handful dried plantain leaves
>
> Small handful dried elder flowers
>
> Small handful dried witch hazel leaves, twigs and flowers

Pour boiling water over the dried herbs in a quart jar, or put the herbs in a pot, cover with cold water and bring to a boil. Turn the flame down and simmer the herbs for half an hour or more. Strain well. When it's cooled down enough, use this eyewash frequently, tilting the head back to get the liquid all the way into the corner of the eye. The more frequently this is done, the better; 4–5 times daily is great.

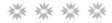

I put the witch hazel flowers into the blend even though I'm not sure that they are as tannin-rich and blood vessel-healing as the leaves or twigs. I did that because the petals (rays) of the spider-like blossoms resemble leaky spider veins and capillaries.

INFUSION FOR BURST BLOOD VESSELS IN THE EYE

> ½ cup plantain leaves
>
> ½ cup calendula blossoms

Put the herbs in a quart jar. Cover them with boiling water and let sit for about one hour. Drink about a quart a day until healing is complete, and then taper off as it feels right.

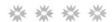

ROBIN ROSE'S PLANT-ALLY BLEND

> Elder blossom tincture
>
> Plantain leaf tincture
>
> Wild rose blossom tincture

Combine equal parts of these tinctures. I drank about a quart of the Burst Blood Vessel infusion above daily, with 2 droppers or so of my special tincture blend added to each serving.

The burst blood vessel happened on a Sunday night. On Monday it was very red and obvious, and it hurt. I started the herbs then, and by Monday night the color had lightened considerably. By Tuesday, it was barely noticeable and only hurt a bit after I began looking at the computer screen late at night after a long, busy day filled with driving many miles too. Over the next couple of days it healed fully, and I used the herbs for another couple of days after that, reducing the dosage intuitively as I went along.

Sometimes I wonder if we hurt ourselves in order to learn how to be nicer to ourselves. Bruises offer a metaphorical as well as an actual opportunity to tend to your hurt places, and have them tended to. As you learn to respond to your (body's) needs in the moment, it can help you to be more present in general, and remind you to tend to your inner hurts in the present, too, rather than unnecessarily dragging them along with you for years. This is another benefit of overcoming SCDD (Self-Care Deficit Disorder, in case you forgot)!

For the greatest results in terms of both the most immediate relief of symptoms and long-lasting healing, use your herbs internally as well as externally whenever possible.

Hyssop *(Hyssopus officinalis)*

This purple-flowering mint-family plant is one of my favorite herbs for healing bruises and wounds. I first wrote about hyssop in the sections on the respiratory and immune systems, but this additional aspect of my good friend hyssop's healing gifts is less well-known, and highly deserving of recognition.

The following story tells how I became acquainted with hyssop's wound-healing gifts. It also happens to have been my very first experience of guiding someone as they healed themselves with the help of herbs.

MY FIRST HERBAL-HEALING EXPERIENCE

My mom and one of her best friends (my adopted "aunt" Florie) were having a cup of coffee at our kitchen table as they talked about what had just happened to Florie at our local hospital. She and my mother had shooed me away as usual, but I was eavesdropping to hear why she was so distraught. Florie had slammed the tip of her index finger in a car door earlier that day. At the hospital she'd been told that her fingertip was so damaged they would likely have to amputate the bruised and blackened tip.

Hearing this, and being a brashly enthusiastic, budding herbalist even though I'd only read books so far, I burst in, blatantly revealing my eavesdropping and excitedly asking, "How many days do you have till the surgery? Can we get to your finger to soak it?"

She held up her bandaged finger and I saw it was merely wrapped, so still accessible. "I'm sure herbs can help! Give me five days!" This was the first time, but not destined to be the last, that I used this sort of healing battle cry to get someone to try herbs before surgery. I'm glad to report that herbal healing has been successful many times when surgery was deemed to be the "only" option. And as I wrote in the section on the musculoskeletal system, even when surgery proved unavoidable the herbs helped hasten the healing process, so it's a win-win situation.

Florie let me see her finger: The tip was crushed, black and purple, but there was no open wound. They must have given her strong pain pills! She agreed to give me five days, as she had no desire to give up part of her finger if she didn't have to. I ran to my herb books, and decided to use hyssop since Jethro Kloss described it as helpful for black and blue bruises. He wrote, in *Back to Eden,* "The leaves, applied to wounds and bruises, will remove the pain and discoloration." I decided to treat it as a terrible bruise.

I got her a bag of loose hyssop and a bamboo tea strainer, and gave her instructions to fill the strainer with hyssop and make tea (recipe below). She was to make the tea and simply stick her fingertip in the moistened, softened herbs as soon as they had cooled enough for her to do that. She was to keep her finger in the herbs for 10–15 minutes, as many times a day as she could but at least 5–6 times. At other times she could dip a cloth in the tea and wrap it around her finger. I suggested that she also drink the tea left over from making the poultices and compresses.

Well, Florie's finger healed beautifully, and she didn't need to have surgery. Maybe she wouldn't have had to have surgery anyway—there's no way to be sure—but that's the nature of preventative medicine. When you take medicine and it keeps you from getting sick, or from having to have surgery, the result is tangible but not necessarily visible. I'm grateful to hyssop because it showed me how well herbs could work, and drew me forward on my path as an herbalist. This beautiful plant will always have a home in my gardens, and a special place in my heart.

Following are several options for applying hyssop (or other dried herbs) externally.

HYSSOP POULTICE AND TEA

> 2–3 tablespoons dried hyssop leaves (or enough to generously cover the area)
>
> 1 cup boiling water

Pour boiled water over the dried herbs, and steep until it's cooled enough to apply the soaked herbs to the body part in need of healing. Strain and save the tea for drinking. If you don't want to have tea left over from the preparation, use just enough boiled water to cover the herbs, as in the recipe that follows.

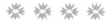

In the case above, I purposely had her make the tea in a bamboo strainer so she could put her fingertip right into the middle of the warm, softened herb, since the strainer was, conveniently enough, the perfect depth for that application. More typically, you would put the herbs on the affected body part and then wrap a cloth around them to hold them in place.

HYSSOP COMPRESS

> 2–3 tablespoons dried hyssop leaves (or enough to generously cover the area)

Pour enough boiling water to just cover the dried herbs. Let the herbs soak for 10 minutes. Wrap the soaked herbs in a piece of clean gauze or muslin. (You can dip that in the tea if there's any liquid left over.) Place the wrapped herbs over and around the area that needs healing for at least 15–30 minutes.

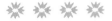

HYSSOP FOMENTATION

1 cup dried hyssop

1 quart water

Pour boiling water over the herbs in a glass wide-mouthed quart jar that you can close airtight. Let the herbs steep overnight.

Strain out the leaves and compost them, as they've had the majority of their healing properties drawn into the water due to the long infusion time. Dip a clean cloth into the strained infusion, and apply it over the bruise or injury. If it is an open wound, be careful not to let any bits of plant material get into it that might be irritating. It is less messy to place a wet cloth on the body than actual plant material, so sometimes people are more willing to do a fomentation than a poultice or compress. It is easier, so it can be a good option if you're on the road. It's not as strong as a compress or poultice, but can be helpful, just the same.

Make an herbal bath, such as a hand, foot, or full-body bath, if you want to put the affected part right into the infusion. Adjust the quantities according to what you need to cover. If you are healing a whole-body injury, make a half-gallon of infusion and add it to a bath.

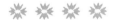

The severity of the injury should be the guide to how many times a day to treat it. Generally speaking, the more times a day you treat a wound or bruise, the faster the healing will occur. If it is not an open, infected cut, you can reuse your herbal poultice, compress, bath herbs, or herb-dipped cloth (fomentation). If there is an infection or an open wound, do NOT reuse any of these.

Many years later, I got a call for help from my then-new boyfriend, a cabinet-maker. A burly young man working for him had nearly severed the tip of his finger with a belt sander. My friend had taken him to the hospital emergency room, and then called me.

They stitched up the finger and were sending him home with pain medication and antibiotics. In that case, because the wound was open and severe, and could quite easily become infected (not to mention that by this point I actually had some knowledge and experience to draw on), I added a few more herbs into the recipe below, to make sure he'd have good use of his finger in the future. If he hadn't been taking antibiotics, I would have added internal herbs such as echinacea and yarrow to prevent an infection.

We again turned to hyssop for this severely injured fingertip. When the bandage came off, it was a finger of many wounded colors.

TRAUMATIC WOUND HEALING—TOPICAL TEA

1 teaspoon dried hyssop leaves and flowers

1 teaspoon dried yarrow leaves and flowers

1 teaspoon dried St. John's wort leaves and flowers

1 teaspoon dried calendula blossoms

(Later in the healing process: 1 teaspoon dried comfrey leaves and stalks)

Combine the herbs together and pour enough boiling water over them to cover the herbs. Steep this for about fifteen minutes. Soak the injured finger in the tea for 15–30 minutes at a time, as frequently as possible. At other times, it would be wise to keep a clean cloth dipped in the tea (a fomentation) wrapped around the finger.

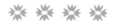

Yarrow, nicknamed "carpenter's weed" for good reason, is an extraordinary first-aid herb. It helps with closed bruises, but also with wounds that are or were bleeding. Yarrow helps normalize the circulation, relieving stagnation that can keep a wound from healing. Yarrow's beautiful, bitter, aromatic flowers bring astringent, anti-inflammatory, pain-relieving, and antibacterial properties to any herbal blend. I use dried yarrow for old or new bruises, swellings from poisonous bites and stings, and fresh wounds. I use fresh yarrow leaves or tincture of the flowering tops on poisonous stings when it's available.

Herbalist Matthew Wood writes of yarrow, "Through numerous devices—clotting, unclotting, neurovascular control, flavonoids, etc.—it regulates the flow of blood to and from the surface, in and out of the capillaries and venules, thickening and thinning. Through this it cures all manner of wounds, bruises, hemorrhaging, and clotting."

St. J's wort, as has been discussed previously, is superb at easing pain and inflammation, and is a specific for repairing nerve damage. St. J's helps with nerve damage that presents as pain, tingling sensations, or numbness, and helps the nerves to regenerate. The nerve endings of the specialized nerve cell retreat and retract back toward the cell body when trauma strikes. St. J's penetrates into these nerve endings, and helps them to relax and release again. As this happens, any muscles that have tightened in reaction to the pain can also let go and relax, thus increasing circulation to the area and helping it heal.

The antiseptic calendula (pot marigold) is a classic wound-healer, and can be added whenever there is damage to the skin surface, or when there is a need to prevent or help heal infection.

Finally, several days after this man had been soaking his finger in a tea made of the first four plants, I added comfrey leaf and stalk, since it is one of—if not *the*—foremost botanical healers of tissue. When a wound is deep and there is any chance of infection, I wait before adding comfrey. It is so good at closing up a wound that it could actually close it before the wound has become completely clean and clear. Once it's ready to close, comfrey—rich in gooey, soothing allantoin—can be safely used. It will not only relieve pain and repair damaged skin and connective tissue but will help repair tendons, ligaments, bone, or cartilage if they suffered any damage.

This young man healed beautifully, and continued to work at carpentry and cabinetry when he moved out of New York City.

Again, please remember that in many situations, simpling (the art of using one herb at a time) works very well too. Whether using one or more herbs, apply them with gratitude, and use them in the appropriate form to address the problem you're confronting. Use them both outside and inside the body whenever appropriate. Use the best options that you have available, and give thanks for the plants you use. Make sure to use your herbal medicine frequently enough to stimulate and work in conjunction with your body's innate healing energy. These are all vital keys to success when you use herbs to heal injuries. If you feel uncertain, get help.

More on Lacerations (Open Cuts)

I strongly suggest that you only take on the treatment of a wound if you feel competent to do so, unless you are somewhere so remote that you have no choice. Having said that, there are many things we can do for ourselves once we have knowledge of some commonly available plants and see for ourselves how well they work. The best way is to start with small everyday things like a skinned knee, a small cut, or a bumped toe. That's how you learn and build confidence.

· · · · ● · · · ·

Some of my favorite herbal allies for open cuts and lacerations:

Agrimony leaves *(Agrimonia* species)—a renowned wound healer; cool tea applied topically helps stop bleeding. Internally, it strengthens the liver to prevent or heal an infection. This plant is in the rose family, and like other rose family wound-healers and tissue tonics such as rose, avens (geum) and lady's mantle, agrimony is astringent, which helps stop bleeding.

Calendula flowers—a classic vulnerary (wound-healer); rich in tannins that create a protective layer over an open wound, allowing it to heal without infection.

Plantain leaves relieve pain and itching, reduce swelling, stop bleeding, cause new skin cells to begin growing; antiseptic.

Witch Hazel twigs, leaves, and flowers—tannin-rich vulnerary; stops bleeding, swelling, and bruising, and is antibacterial. **Oak** leaves and bark are also exceptionally tannin-rich and can be used similarly.

Yarrow leaves and flowers. In the open-wound healing realm, I think of yarrow as a stronger version of plantain; it is pain-reducing, anti-inflammatory, anti-microbial, and more effective than plantain for stopping bleeding. In relation to other systems of the body, they have many differences.

PLANTAIN, YARROW, AND SEA SALT FOR
A HAND LACERATION

I turn to these herbs consistently because I have found them to be reliable. I like plantain and yarrow best because they are commonly accessible weeds, growing abundantly just about everywhere.

I once had the experience of cutting myself with an old, dirty pocketknife. I was using it to cut a label off a candle right after I woke up in the morning and was still sleepy. (Note to self: No more handling of knives when not fully awake!) The knife slipped off the smooth surface of the candle and plunged deep into my left palm. Insides were hanging out, and blood was copious. Panic began to set in. But I gathered my wits to figure out what to do.

I went in my mind to the "Six Steps of Healing" as articulated by Susun Weed in her fine book, *Healing Wise:*

Step Zero: Do nothing. "Ok," I told myself. "Breathe. Now, move on." (That step lasted about one second.)

Step One: Gather information. "I see that I need to stop this bleeding, and I need to get help because I'm terrified and may be in deep trouble here." (That step took about three seconds.)

Step Two: Engage the energy. This was helpful. I took a deep breath and began to engage my imagination. I visualized my hand healing perfectly (three seconds).

Step Three: Nourish and tonify. Deep breaths would have to be my nourishment for the moment. It certainly wasn't time to sit down and brew a cup of tea—but knowing I had herbal allies to draw on was a form of nourishment. It nourished my confidence (three seconds).

Step Four: Stimulate and sedate. I held my hand high up above my heart, and kept placing it under a strong flow of ice-cold water. This was to slow down and ultimately stop the bleeding, and reduce or at least numb the pain. Ice and/or ice water can be effective sedation in many first-aid situations.

Step Five: Use supplements and/or concentrated substances. I didn't see any way to apply this at that moment.

Step Six: Break and enter/intervention. Ah! Though this step usually refers to approaches like surgery, I decided that in this case it meant, "Let help enter from the outside, and ask for help!"

I called herbalist 7Song at his home school in Ithaca. I knew he had a lot of experience with first aid, and loves to engage in trauma medicine. I realized that I was in danger of going into shock, and needed an outside perspective. Thankfully, he picked up the phone, and when he told me he was leaving town in about half an hour, I felt very blessed. I described the wound to him, and what I'd done so far.

He said I could take care of it, but would always have scar tissue. I asked him, "Would I do better to go to the hospital, then?" He told me that I'd have the same situation after stitches, so of course it was up to me, but he thought I could deal with it, based on what I was telling him. Then he reminded me of what I knew: Yarrow and plantain, along with sea salt, would save the day, and my hand!

When we hung up, I followed the instructions 7Song had just given me. I gently put all the tissue that was outside back into my hand, then immediately went outside and picked fresh plantain. (If you don't yet know how to recognize the common plants that grow where you live, I hope you'll be inspired to want to meet and get to know them by the time you've finished reading this book, if not this chapter!) Fresh leaves are my preference for this kind of first-aid medicine, but if only dried plantain leaves are available, pour boiling water over them, let them steep for 5–10 minutes, and then apply them to the cut.

7Song told me to boil the fresh plantain leaves so as not to risk infection. This was his only instruction that I didn't heed, because I checked in with myself and got the feeling that I'd do better if I chewed up the leaves as usual, since mixing them with an enzyme in the saliva increases plantain's anti-microbial potency. So I chewed up a bunch of leaves and put them on the wound.

I was still bleeding, and needed to slow that down and move the healing process along. I continued to hold the arm high above my head to help slow down the flow of blood. Then I made a soup pot full of yarrow tea and sea salt. 7Song wisely suggested that I make the brew very strong, so with my one working hand I put a few very large handfuls of dried yarrow in a soup pot along with about a cup of good Celtic sea salt. I covered these with water, brought it all to a boil, then turned it way down, put the lid on, and let it sit and steep.

After a few minutes, I poured a bowl of the brew through a strainer so that I could use it right away, while the rest of the medicine got stronger. I soaked my hand in the yarrow/saltwater mix, as by now the blood had slowed down enough for me to do that. The immediate pain relief from the plantain poultice and this hand soak were very welcome indeed.

Then I called my next-door neighbor who, upon hearing the story, was horrified that I was not in the emergency room. I told him that if I didn't think I could take care of it I'd be happy to go, but meanwhile, I was doing okay and just needed his help. He finally agreed to go to the drugstore and get me bandages called Steri-Strips™ that 7Song had recommended I use to pull the sides of the wound together for better healing. But he did this only after he had my promise that he could take me to the emergency room if I looked as if I were going into shock. (Later I found out that after we hung up the phone he'd immediately called his girlfriend, and said, "*You* make her go!" To his dismay, she replied, "I trust Robin and her herbs. She'll go if she needs to. Hurry and get her what she asked for!")

He got me the bandages and helped me pull the skin together and close the wound with those marvelous steri-strips. I continued to do the washes and poultices constantly for a week or so. I also took a tincture blend of anti-infective herbs internally, starting off with high dosages and then decreasing the dosages as I continued to heal without complication. These tinctures included echinacea, yarrow and calendula. (See "Some of my favorite immune-strengthening and anti-infective allies," page 108.)

The best part is that my hand healed 100%. There is no scar tissue, and no decrease in mobility or dexterity. I showed it to a friend who is a family-practice doctor a few months after it happened. There was still a scar (now gone), but no pain. She examined it, and said that if I'd gotten stitches there would surely have been scar tissue, and she was thrilled with the progression of the healing. What a wonderful affirmation!

Now, I'm not suggesting that you take on something like this if you're new to healing and working with herbs. I would not, for instance, apply this approach to a deep chainsaw wound. Some herbalists might be competent to do it, but that is beyond my skills and I wouldn't take it on unless I were the only available option. But I tell this story to illustrate how the simplest herbs can work even in a relatively serious situation—so you can use them confidently for everyday cuts and wounds.

MULLEIN MÉLANGE POULTICE FOR A NECK INJURY

One day Joanne, a woman in my apprentice program, came to our circle a few days after being in a car accident. She had been diagnosed with whiplash. The whole area around her neck was inflamed, and she couldn't turn her neck at all. She was in severe pain. She was moving so stiffly that she seemed robotic, and looked like she wanted to cry—but that would hurt too much, so she didn't dare.

We gathered fresh herbs and made her an herbal neck pillow out of the heated and moistened herbs to wrap around her neck for comfort and healing. It was a combination compress-poultice-fomentation.

You can use fresh or dried herbs, or both. There are great herbalists who say to use only one or the other. Maria Treban says only fresh leaves will work for medicinal teas and infusions. Susun Weed says to use only dried leaves. Others disagree with both of them and have their own perspectives. Not knowing whom to believe, I finally came to see that *the plants keep working in all sorts of surprising ways while people disagree, debate and argue about how best to use them. Fortunately for all of us, plants neither read books nor attend herbal lectures.*

FRESH HERBAL NECK PILLOW

Coltsfoot leaves

Comfrey leaves

Mullein leaves (set aside 4–5 whole leaves)

Motherwort leaves

Witch hazel leaves

Violet leaves

St. J's wort tincture

Yarrow tincture

Lobelia tincture

After cutting up the first six fresh herbs, pour enough boiling water over them to cover the plants, and leave them to steep with a lid on for about 10 minutes before taking off the lid.

As soon as they cool enough to handle but are still warm, pull out the leaves, wring out the excess moisture and gently knead a liberal dosage of about a tablespoon each of the tinctures of St. J's wort (for nerve repair), yarrow (for anti-inflammatory pain relief), and lobelia (a superb sedative and anti-spasmodic) into the leaves to make the medicine even stronger.

Pound 4–5 whole, large mullein leaves to make them more absorbent; let them steep, whole, in boiling water for about 3–5 minutes until thoroughly softened. Roll the rest of the herbs into a roughly 2-foot-long snake shape, and wrap them up inside the softened mullein leaves—true to their nickname "flannel dock," they will enfold the other herbs like soft pieces of flannel. Drape a towel over the shoulders to catch drips.

Protectively coat the neck skin with oil so that neither the fiberglassy hairs on the comfrey leaves nor the scratchy hair on the mullein leaves can irritate it. (We chose anti-inflammatory, pain-relieving mullein leaf and flower oil for this woman because mullein was her chosen herb—her ally—and therefore the star of this recipe. You could also use other pain-relieving oils such as yarrow oil, St. J's wort oil, or goldenrod oil, a good muscle relaxant.) Plain olive oil is perfectly fine if no appropriate infused herbal oil is handy.

Place the poultice around the neck and wind snugly. Dip a single piece of soft cotton flannel into the leftover liquid, squeeze it out, and place it over the entire mullein mélange poultice to help hold it all together, turning the poultice into a compress by tucking the thin cloth over and under the mullein leaves.

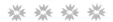

The coltsfoot leaves are helpful for bruises and pain relief. The comfrey provides multi-tissue healing. Mullein is anti-spasmodic, pain-relieving, and specific for spinal injuries. Motherwort is included as a calming nervine, smooth-muscle relaxant, and for her comforting spirit. Witch hazel is included for her superb anti-inflammatory powers, while violet's salicylic-acid content is pain relieving and anti-inflammatory, and this plant too is a super soother.

"Flannel dock" and "velvet dock" are two of my favorite common names for mullein. But the funniest nickname I heard was when I was in the mountains in southwestern Colorado. I was extolling mullein's virtues to a masseuse named Karen, and she exclaimed in surprise, "Wow, I had no idea the penis plant does all that!" In response to the look on my face, she added, "I've always called it that." We both laughed. To me, with mullein's wide, open-leaved, womanly rosette, and her second year's manly stalk rising out of her center, it's as if mullein is both *yoni* and *lingam*, and is making love with herself.

Speaking of love, Joanne sat in the center of our circle for a time, with her mullein mélange poultice around her neck, as we shared healing energies with her. She told us she felt her neck muscles being soothed and her spine relaxing as pain was released to the warmth of the poultice, and of course to the warmth of everyone's caring and tending to her. She looked like a different person by the time she took the poultice off about forty-five minutes later. She was still hurting, but it was as if a block of cement had been taken off her neck and shoulders.

She continued the poultices at home using far fewer herbs, focusing on mullein as the constant, and was very satisfied with the pace of her healing. When we met again, one month later, she felt completely recovered.

. . . . . ● ● . . . .

The following are a few more helpful herbs that are useful for external applications.

Chamomile. Add this dried herb to a bath to soothe spasmodic pain from almost any kind of injury. Chamomile flowers can be added to an oat or ginger-root bath for stronger pain-relief. Herbalist Doc Garcia swears by chamomile for kidney-stone pain; use it internally and externally. The chamomile will also act as an antibacterial in the bath. A woman came to me with a wound that had led to a potentially serious infection on her vulva. Using a blend of dried chamomile, hyssop, and calendula in a series of baths, along with internal anti-infective herbs, she healed completely and was in much less pain while the healing was underway.

Chickweed. This moist little herb, especially used fresh, is great for drawing out foreign objects and healing infections. Use on blisters, cold sores, or pimples, and to draw out any embedded object from under the skin. Tincture and oil can be used topically, too.

Fresh coltsfoot leaves *(Tussilago farfara)*. These super-smooth leaves feel like soft skin on one side and downy felt on the other. Put them into your shoes if you've bruised your feet by walking barefoot on rocky ground or in new shoes that aren't broken in yet. I recently used them when someone's eyelid mysteriously swelled up and turned red and dry for no known reason. It might have been from a bite, but we were unable to positively determine the cause. The coltsfoot leaves, rubbed and placed with their smooth side facing the skin and changed every 5–10 minutes, cooled off the eye, moistened the lid, and started to bring the swelling down immediately, taking about an hour to bring it down completely. Coltsfoot does infuse well into oil, though it's not my first choice to use oil on eyelids. The oil is helpful for aches and pains that follow strenuous physical activity.

Comfrey, horsetail, mullein, Solomon's seal, and St. J's wort. As discussed in the musculoskeletal section, use these dry or fresh herbs singly or in combination. Apply them as a poultice (you can include oils and/or tinctures blended into the herbs) on the spine to help heal spinal injuries that have led to slipped or herniated discs. Horsetail and comfrey heal the connective tissue, and plump up the discs. Comfrey and mullein leaves relieve pain and add moisture. Matthew Wood teaches that Solomon's seal literally helps seal the protective coating around the discs, and I originally learned from Susun Weed that St. J's acts like a chiropractor in a bottle—and it's true. When it penetrates into the nerve endings, the muscles that have tightened in response to the spinal pain can relax, and as the tension and inflammation in the muscles and nerves subsides, a slipped disc is encouraged to slide back into alignment. Remember, the body knows *how* to heal, and is oriented to heal itself. Provide the right support and you will be amazed again and again at what the body can do!

Ginger. Use fresh, grated ginger as a poultice for healing many types of injuries including muscle pulls, strains and sprains. It increases circulation to the area, and brings down inflammation. If using it on tender areas, put some oil over the area first. You can also use it as a compress or fomentation. I have used it to great effect on joints that are inflamed, whether from arthritis or infections such as those caused by tick bites. In one memorable instance, a woman whose knee had been twice its normal size from Lyme disease for a month or longer found that ginger poultices brought the swelling down almost to normal within a week, and reduced the pain substantially. She was amazed.

Perhaps this is a good time to remind you that the body speaks truths for us that we may be unaware of, or simply unable to express. This woman hated driving, and hadn't wanted to move out of an urban area to the country. But she and her family had moved, and with her knee swollen up she couldn't drive—and therefore didn't have to. She realized that this was one way she'd found to express her dissatisfaction to her husband. Having realized this, she shook her head in further amazement as she determined that she would have to be brave and find healthier ways to express her needs and feelings!

Grape leaf. Imagine the various colors of dark grapes; they range along a continuum from red to purple, blue, and black. Then think of how much like a bruise this is. When bruises turn many shades of black, blue, purple, and red, grape leaves can be a true friend, healing and sealing damaged capillaries and veins. This plant is a wonder for bruises, bringing down the pain, swelling, and discoloration.

I think of hyssop when there is metal or machinery involved in an injury, with a higher risk of infection, and of grape when one has banged oneself badly, though it is possible that they may be interchangeable in many situations. They are both astringent, and both mix well with witch hazel and/or yarrow. Grape leaves are more specific for helping repair damaged blood vessels, reducing varicose veins, and generally breaking up congested bruises to support healthy circulation.

Green clay, osha, plantain, and purslane. Any of these are helpful when there is an allergic swelling in response to a bite or sting. Use fresh, chewed-up purslane and plantain whenever possible; use osha root *(Ligusticum porteri)* as a tincture, and green clay in its original wet state or as a powder mixed with water. Add osha tincture to fresh plantain leaves; they work really well together on poisonous bites, and reduce inflammatory allergic reactions. Osha is one of the best antihistamine, anti-allergy helpers available to us. It is a specific for bee stings (used both externally and internally). I use it sparingly, as it is a rare plant that grows only at very high altitudes.

Fresh or dry oak leaves, twigs, and bark. All oaks, most famously white oak, are extremely tannin-rich, antibacterial, astringent medicines. They will stop bleeding and itching when applied externally. You can use the leaves or twigs of almost any oak (except poison oak, which is not really an oak but a member of the cashew family, in the same genus as poison sumac and poison /potent ivy). Use boiled or rubbed oak leaves as a poultice for cuts or bruises while hiking or camping, or make a tea from the twigs, leaves or bark to make a useful wash or soak for skin or bleeding gums (gargle with oak tea or oak-tinctured tea) and drink and apply the tea for bleeding and/or swollen hemorrhoids.

Onion. Use it mashed or roasted directly on the skin to pull out foreign objects such as splinters

Propolis. This antiseptic, resinous substance is made by bees from various saps and resins that they collect. It is a popular sore-throat remedy, and the tincture painted over a cut will act as an antiseptic band-aid.

Fresh tansy leaves *(Tanacetum vulgare).* Rub them a bit and put them into your shoes to help sore, tired, or aching feet. People who work on their feet all day have reported great success using this simple method. Fresh tansy leaves work best; they are like a time-release medicine. When you walk on them it releases more volatile oils, for ongoing foot-soothing. Unfortunately, I haven't found the oil to work nearly as well.

The following are a few sample recipes that blend several herbs together for relieving pain:

PAIN-RELIEF BLEND

3 parts St. J's wort tincture

1 part California poppy tincture

1 part skullcap tincture

This blend, taken internally in hot water, tea, or infusion offers a great combination of anti-inflammatory, anti-spasmodic, and sedating effects. Start with about 30 drops of tincture, total, in hot water, tea or infusion. You can increase the dosage as needed. (These herbs could be added into a bath, too, if you like.)

PAIN-RELIEF BATH BLEND

1 cup dried cramp bark (*Viburnum opulus* and other species)

1 cup dried St. J's wort

½ cup dried lobelia

6-inch piece of fresh ginger root

Put cramp bark leaves, twigs and/or root bark together with lobelia leaves, flowers and seedpods, St. J's wort leaves and flowers and grated ginger root in a half-gallon jar. Pour boiling water over them, filling the jar to the top. Let that stand for several hours. Pour this infusion into a nearly full bathtub. Soak for a minimum of 20 minutes—more is better—to relieve muscular or joint pain, nerve spasms, pelvic and lower-back pain.

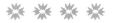

Amounts can be adjusted to suit the person and the need. Lobelia is sedative to the nervous system, muscle relaxing and deeply anti-spasmodic. This would be the bath to take after anything from a bruising car accident to running a marathon. Tinctures could be substituted for one or more of the dry herbs if necessary. For this bath blend, use about one teaspoon of tincture to equal a cup of dried herb.

PAIN-RELIEF LINIMENT
(for external use only)

**1½–2 cups fresh or 1 cup dried cramp bark leaves and twigs
(*Viburnum* species)**

1½–2 cups fresh or 1 cup dried lobelia (*Lobelia inflata*)

1 quart apple cider vinegar

Put the lobelia, cramp bark, and apple cider vinegar into a non-aluminum saucepan. Bring it to a boil, and then turn it down and simmer on the lowest possible heat for about an hour. You can use it immediately, but it will get better if you pour the liquid and herbs into a jar, and allow it to stand and infuse for weeks or even months. If possible use a lid that isn't metal; if it is, line it with unbleached parchment paper or plastic wrap to prevent corrosion.

I often use this blend externally for pulled muscles, muscle spasms and especially for pinched nerves. I first read about it in Jethro Kloss's classic herb book, *Back to Eden*. It is an old, eclectic recipe.

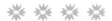

I usually bottle these mixtures and let them stand for six weeks or more—but if you don't have time to wait, don't. Let the mixture stand overnight in the saucepan (or as long as possible, even if only 10–15 minutes), then strain it and bottle it with the herbs still in it.

When you label your jar, besides writing "Lobelia/Cramp Bark Pain-Relief Liniment" and the date, also mark your bottle "for external use only." Any vinegar with lobelia in it is *not* one you want to lavish on your salads. On the other hand, cramp bark vinegar alone is safe, soothing, and delicious. So, I suggest that you make that as a simple too!

I was taking a walk one afternoon years ago when I began to get terrible menstrual cramps. I was walking by an unfamiliar tree and felt it call for my attention. I stopped and stroked the leaves, examined the bark and trunk, and quietly listened. The maple-leaved cramp bark tree *(Viburnum acerifolium)* whispered softly, "Look at my leaves. See how they spread wide open. I will help you open any tight places inside you. My leaves and twigs relieve pain."

Ever since then I have added the leaves to all my cramp "bark" medicines (teas, tinctures, liniments, and vinegars), having found that the leaves do indeed disperse and open up knots and congestion, especially in the womb, though also in other smooth and striped muscles of the body.

I use the leaves and twigs of *Viburnum acerifolium*, knowing it's easier on the small trees than to strip bark, or harvest roots for their bark. I also primarily use this species of cramp bark rather than the more generally used *Viburnum opulus* and *Viburnum prunifolium* because it's the one that is most abundant where I live. You may notice it's been hard to find written information about *V. acerifolium* until now. I worried about that for a while; even though it worked beautifully, I became concerned that I was using the "wrong" herb. Then one day I was driving Matt Wood home from a Green Nations gathering, and asked him about it. He told me that his Native American teachers told him it is the best variety of cramp bark to use! I felt affirmed, and was grateful to realize that I'd just received another gentle teaching on trusting my intuition and listening to the plants.

16

Some Additional Remedies, Recipes, and Tips

Travel Tips and Recipes

SAMPLE TRAVEL KIT

1 ounce echinacea root tincture

1 ounce St. J's wort tincture

1 ounce hawthorn berry tincture

1 ounce dandelion root tincture

1 ounce motherwort tincture

1 ounce jar plantain salve

1 ounce bottle of St. J's wort oil

2-ounce bottle lavender spray

Travel kits vary depending on the needs and concerns of the person or people traveling, the mode of travel, and where you're heading, but being able to heal bruises and cuts and prevent infection is a good place to start. One-ounce or half-ounce bottles of tinctures or other small jars and containers are usually a good size for travel kits. Consider what kinds of vulnerabilities you tend toward that you want to be prepared to take care of: Indigestion? Sore back? Sleeplessness? If there are any herbs you're currently using that you want to continue taking, you'll want to include those too.

The above sample kit contains echinacea, to be used topically and/or internally for preventing and healing infections; St. J's for muscle and nerve aches and pains, and to support good sleep through physical relaxation; hawthorn berry for joy, vitality, and good circulation. Hawthorn is helpful if you have to sit for long periods, as with plane travel. Dandelion root is great for digestive help and immune/liver/lymph strengthening. Soothing motherwort eases anxiety. You never know when you'll need her, so I always bring her along. Motherwort also relieves travel-related constipation. Lavender flower spray is refreshing, calming, mood-altering and antiseptic. Spray it on your hands to clean them. It can also be used on wounds, burns, and to repel mosquitos. Plantain salve is useful for bites, bumps, bruises, bleeding, dry skin, rashes, and more.

AIRPLANE TINCTURE COCKTAIL (STRONG VARIATION)

3 droppers St. J's (St. John's/St. Joan's wort) tincture

3 droppers hawthorn berry tincture

2 droppers echinacea tincture

1 dropper California poppy tincture

1 dropper cramp bark tincture

1 dropper elder flower tincture

1 dropper mullein leaf and/or flower tincture

These quantities make a little more than 2 teaspoons, to be taken in a cup or mug of boiled water (a high dose, but still a smaller volume of alcohol than an average dose of cough syrup). Smaller doses of the same blend can be used too. If you know you want a blend this strong, you could pre-mix one small bottle of it for traveling.

This strong blend is effective for relieving fear of flying, and for simply easing mental and physical tension on very long flights. I'm not afraid of flying and I rarely put so many herbs together, but I used it to good effect when I flew from New York to New Zealand. I carried one-ounce bottles of each tincture, and made my mix as I went along.

I first made this strong blend for a woman who was terrified of flying but had agreed to fly on a very, very long flight for a family vacation. She was concerned about everything—the flying itself, her circulation, not being able to breathe from the recycled air, getting sick from the experience, and arriving hurting all over from sitting for so long. It worked like a charm.

This blend is mentally and physically calming and tranquilizing. It prevents aches, stiffness, and infection while helping overall circulation, and supporting the sinuses, bronchia and lungs. The elder flower helps your ears with the pressure changes, and if you like to sleep on planes this blend can help you do that.

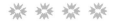

AIRPLANE TINCTURE COCKTAIL (LIGHTER VARIATION)

2 droppers St. J's (St. John's/St. Joan's wort) tincture

2 droppers hawthorn berry tincture

2 droppers echinacea tincture

1 dropper elderflower tincture

3 drops California poppy tincture

Similar to Strong Variation, above, but for use when a less strong effect is needed.

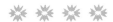

MILD FEAR OF FLYING REMEDY

Motherwort tincture

Take 10–50 drops in water as needed. And if you're not fearful, you'll still benefit from feeling more relaxed.

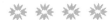

SIMPLE FLYING TIPS

Drink lots of water on the plane, especially on long trips. You'll arrive in much better shape if you do.

If your ears get painful upon takeoff and landing, take 25–30 drops of elder blossom tincture in boiled or at least hot water, as close as you can to takeoff, and then again just before you land.

If you have serious sinus or ear issues, with a history of inflammation and infections, take elderflower infusion or tincture 2–3 times a day for a week before you fly, and during the flight as described above. It can make the difference between a miserable travel experience and a perfectly comfortable one. Elder is safe for babies too; the change in pressure can be painful for tender, young ears.

Other Useful Remedies

Tension Headaches

TENSION HEADACHE TINCTURE BLEND

1 dropper St. J's (St. John's/St. Joan's wort) tincture

5 drops skullcap tincture

I start with about 25 drops of St. J's tincture, and 5–7 drops of skullcap. You can increase or decrease these amounts gradually to find out what dosage works best for you.

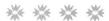

This blend is quite relaxing and helpful for relieving pain, whether you are traveling or at home; and if you're prone to tension headaches this mixture can be good to keep on hand. The St. J's tends to the physical part of the tension headache, relaxing the neck and jaw muscles and shoulders, while skullcap nurtures a sense of calm as its pain-relieving properties go to work on the headache.

In the case of St. J's, I sometimes take and give very large doses for pain, especially for things like a pinched nerve or sciatica; but with skullcap, less is usually more effective, and too high a dose can make a person jittery. If that happens to you, cut down your dosage. On the other hand, some students have told me they use high doses, up to 2 dropperfuls of skullcap, to achieve a sedative effect. Everyone is different. It's important to listen to your body, and pay attention to what you feel when you take herbs. Both of these herbs are mainstays in my herbal cabinet, and St. J's is always in my travel kit, usually as both a tincture and as infused oil for external application.

Tinctures are reasonably light and easy to take with you when traveling, to help with the muscular tension that traveling puts on the body, and to help you sleep if you have trouble sleeping away from home (or at home, for that matter). I suggest keeping different tinctures in separate bottles so that you can adjust dosages according to your needs, since needs vary in different situations.

Potent (Poison) Ivy

First, when you realize you've touched this powerful plant teacher, thank it for what it does to protect the land. Send it your respect. It is doing an important job. I believe that potent ivy is also a spiritual ally. This plant is not only a guardian of land, it teaches any willing individual to be your own guardian, to be aware of your physical space and what's around you. That is important medicine.

Some people who never used to be susceptible to the irritating oils this plant exudes are getting rashes these days. The plant seems to be getting stronger, and also growing more extensively. Where I used to only see it in disturbed soil, I now see it growing deep in the woods. I have read that it is a carbon sink, so as the carbon increases in our atmosphere, more and stronger potent ivy grows to help absorb the excess carbon.

If the oils have gotten into your bloodstream, which is a miserable situation, I suggest that you work with an herbalist to get help healing from the inside out too. (Or get medical help if needed.) Some herbal possibilities for internal healing include: oat straw infusions and baths, plantain tincture or infusion, burdock infusion or tincture, osha root tincture, and dandelion root infusions and tinctures.

MY FAVORITE POTENT IVY REMEDIES

Wash the area with cold water or, better yet, with cold water and soap as soon as possible.

Use undiluted red spruce tincture directly on the area of contact, and onto the rash when it first appears. Use caution, however, applying alcohol (in the tincture) if the rash is in "full bloom" and very raw. Try it on a small area; if it feels ok, continue applying. If it burns, don't.

For a full-blown blistery rash, use fresh burdock leaves that have been pounded and steeped for about five minutes in boiled water and allowed to cool. Apply them whole if possible over the affected areas. Don't reuse the leaves. If you only have dried leaves, cover them with boiling water, steep for about 10 minutes and apply them when they've cooled.

Fresh plantain leaves chewed up and applied are good, too, and many people swear they're the best, but I've found the other remedies sometimes help more quickly.

Use fresh, broken-open jewelweed (or jewelweed tea as the next best thing) topically after exposure to prevent an outbreak. It is almost always found growing near potent ivy. I also make a strong (triple) infusion of jewelweed (changing the herbs in the pot three times to make it ever more potent) and then freeze the infusion in ice-cube trays. I transfer those cubes to a freezer bag and label it to have on hand for anyone who might need it.

ITCH TIPS

Red spruce tincture is effective on itchy mosquito bites as well as potent ivy rash.

White pine and black birch tinctures work well, too, on both itchy bites and potent ivy rash, both preventatively and curatively.

If your skin is itching unbearably from bites or a rash, an application of fresh, wet clay is very soothing. Wash it when it hardens so it doesn't pull on your skin too much when your skin is already irritated. Reapply as needed.

Wasp or Bee Stings

The very best sting remedy is fresh yarrow leaf or flower, either rubbed open with your hands or chewed up, and then applied. This will relieve the pain quickly.

Another great pain-relieving remedy is freshly applied purslane. Mash the above-ground parts of the plant and hold them in place or bind them over the area with a piece of soft flannel. This works very well for allergic swellings from bites, too.

Plantain leaf is another effective remedy for a painful sting, cooling the area quickly.

If a stinger is embedded and needs to be drawn out, chewed up plantain leaf, moistened clay powder, or fresh clay all work well and will pull it out.

Treating a Tick Bite

According to the latest information from the Centers for Disease Control, it is thought that a tick has to be embedded for thirty-six to forty-eight hours before it can transmit an infection such as Lyme disease, but much is still unknown. Even if you don't think you were infected, it is wise to take echinacea and yarrow internally for a week or two after a bite to nourish your immunity. Even the bites of non-disease carrying ticks are challenging, usually causing swelling, pain, and/or itching.

Use sharp, pointy tweezers to make sure the entire tick is removed. If the tick didn't come out whole, don't leave even the tiniest piece of it in your skin. Clean the sharp tweezers or a needle with rubbing alcohol, and get it out. If you need help removing it, get help.

Put yarrow or echinacea tincture into a wad of chewed-up fresh plantain leaves, and apply it to the site of the bite. You can put a bandage over this to hold it in place. Change the poultice frequently, continuing until all signs of redness and swelling from the tick bite are gone.

Some Ideas about Healing

As Marshall McLuhan famously stated, "If I hadn't believed it, I wouldn't have seen it." And it's true. Our beliefs are powerful; they can support or block healing. This includes the beliefs of the healing practitioners we choose to guide and help us, whether they follow a conventional medical path or a traditional herbal one, or any other.

Extraordinary healings can and do happen every day. Sometimes they are instantaneous. What do you imagine is possible in the realm of healing yourself or another? Consider this question carefully, because reality follows your thoughts, emotions and imagination. Or, as author and astrologer Caroline Casey says, "Imagination lays the tracks for the reality train."

A woman in one of my classes healed her decades-old endometriosis following a profound realization. She changed her mind, and her body followed suit immediately.

As Albert Einstein said, "Reality is merely an illusion, albeit a very persistent one."

I saw another woman slowly heal her extensive endometriosis by changing her diet, doing daily poultices with ginger root and, just as importantly, altering her reality by realizing she was worthy of her own love and receiving love from others. She came to realize this was true even though her mother rarely showed her that she loved her, so this woman had felt unworthy of love for most of her life.

She has had no return of the endometriosis in over fifteen years, and has since had two healthy children that she wasn't supposed to be able to conceive naturally, much less give birth to—yet she did.

If someone is bleeding, I don't engage them in a philosophical discussion about the meaning and potential gift of the wound; I give them the herbs they need to stop the bleeding. But there is insight to be gained from coming through physical challenges, and wisdom waiting to be harvested.

If you ask for insight and the message you receive from "spirit" is negating and judgmental, such as, "You're so stupid—what did you expect?"—or if the answer sounds as if you are being punished for something, as in, "You knew you shouldn't have done that, so this is what you get!"—I assure you this answer is not from spirit. It is from old voices you carry around in your psyche. True communication from Spirit is always oriented toward your evolution, and is affirming even when it's fiercely discerning and asks you to confront something about yourself that makes you uncomfortable.

One of my spiritual teachers had medically diagnosed broken bones in her foot heal two days after she broke them. It amazed her as much as anyone. Upon reflection, she realized that she had truly understood and accepted the teaching, so her best guess was that she no longer needed her broken foot to be a mirror and teacher for her. Powerful medicine!

I once experienced a taste of how this can happen, not with a broken bone but by a deep realization in the core of my being. I felt it land in my body and permanently change a physical condition in less than ten seconds.

In *The Biology of Belief: Unleashing the Power of Consciousness, Matter and Miracles* by Dr. Bruce Lipton, surgeon Bruce Moseley says, "All good surgeons know there is no placebo effect in surgery." He did a study of people with severe, debilitating knee pain to determine which aspects of his surgeries were the most helpful. It included one group of patients that received elaborately faked knee surgery, and he was stunned when the outcomes of the fake surgeries and real surgeries were the same!

The placebo patients didn't find out for two years that they had benefitted from fake surgery. There were numerous cases, such as a man who had been walking with a cane, and after "surgery" he was playing basketball with his grandchildren. Upon learning the truth, he said, "I know that your mind can do miracles."

Dr. Moseley said, "My skill as a surgeon had no benefit for these patients. The entire benefit of surgery for osteoarthritis was the placebo effect."

Did you know that when a person receives a transplanted kidney, lung, heart, or other organ, some aspects of the donor's personal quirks, preferences, and even talents often show up in the personality of the organ recipient? The National Center for Biotechnology Information (NCBI) published the following report from a study of heart- and lung-transplant recipients: "Parallels included changes in food, music, art, sexual, recreational, and career preferences, as well as specific instances of perceptions of names and sensory experiences related to the donors (e.g., one donor was killed by a gunshot to the face; the recipient had dreams of seeing hot flashes of light in his face)."

· · · · ● · · · ·

A few more ideas on healing for you as you deepen your acquaintance with healing herbs:

- Every cell in your body is conscious.
- Bodies are innocent, and believe everything you tell them if you believe what you are saying/thinking.
- You can't lie to your body.
- Bodies are wise, and they always tell the truth, often inconveniently, uncomfortably, even painfully.
- Look for truth and wisdom in what goes "wrong" in the body. It speaks truths for us that we may be unaware of, or simply uncomfortable, unwilling, or unable to express.
- Your body loves you so much that it is willing to get hurt or sick in order to help you grow, evolve, and become fully alive.
- It is impossible to separate body from soul while you are living.

- Healing wounds, as well as ancestral wounds and (past-life, this-life or other-life) traumas, brings healing to you, your ancestors, and future generations. There is not really such a thing as past, present, and future. There is only now.
- Any true kindness you extend toward yourself brings more kindness into the world. That kindness extends out into the environment at a creative level, and helps compassion and thoughtfulness to grow in people.
- Compassion is more helpful than judgment in helping you to adopt new practices or release harmful habits. Whenever you can bring friendliness rather than forcefulness into your approach to healing yourself, it will help you more.
- Illness and "accidents" happen for you rather than to you. And anything that happens for you also happens for the larger world around you.
- If you look for the love letter in everything that happens, you will stand a better chance of seeing the love that is everywhere.
- Nothing is a distraction from your life, or keeping you from your life. It is all your life, moment-to-moment.
- Bodies are innately designed and oriented to heal themselves.
- Healing is as natural as breathing.
- Healing is a spiraling process, not a linear event.
- Healing sometimes means to heal into death.
- Herbs are healers. They know who they are, and what their purpose is. When you take plants into yourself as food or medicine, they can help you become who you came here to be, and to live your purpose.
- Herbs work really well. You do have to actually take them, however.
- When you look into the meaning of healing—tending to spiritual healing as well as physical—the healing goes deeper. You not only heal your body, you heal your life. When the illness alone is taken care of, the body often has to find another way to get your attention.
- Bodies are real, and they are ultimately symbolic of everything that is happening within your psyche and how you experience your relationship to the world around you.

- Without a connection to nature, including your own wild nature, a certain sense of loneliness, alienation and isolation is inevitable. This disconnection leads to the creation of our worst health problems, personally and socially. Yet what can feel so deep and irreparable is oddly simple to fix; regular walks in the woods or in a city park are a good start. Get your feet on the Earth. Move your body. Plant a garden. Drink herb teas. Grow and gather your own herbal medicine. These and other simple practices will lead you home. Remember, whatever you are seeking is also seeking you. As we the people come home to ourselves, together we can and will create a healthy world.

- Remember to try the simple things, for they often work well.

- Herbs often work surprisingly quickly.

- When the basic physical makeup of a plant has been chemically altered in a lab, it is not quite an herb anymore. Now it's an herbal product, and more prone to cause unexpected side effects.

- Self-care is not self-absorption. It is about looking out for yourself as you would for any beloved. Self-love is the greatest healing force there is.

- Condemnation and judgment are long hard roads, which will eventually lead you to acceptance; so why not choose the kinder road sooner—or even right away? No matter how long you've lived in self-judgment, the opportunity to choose self-acceptance comes around again, every instant. It is never too late to love.

- Bodies always speak to us in the language of love.

Abundant Green Blessings to you!

RESOURCES

HERBALISTS/EDUCATORS

The following list includes people whose books, blog posts, and teachings have added to my herbal education, but who may not be listed in the bibliography or notes. It wouldn't be possible to list all of the people to whom I'm indebted, so this list is by no means all-inclusive.

7Song, Northeast School for Botanical Studies, PO Box 6626, Ithaca, NY 14851, 607-539-7172, www.7Song.com. 7Song is a gifted, down-to-earth herbalist and amazing botanist whose generous online writings are clear and educational, and whose nature photography is so beautiful it makes me long to use a real camera myself one day.

Ryan Drum, PhD, PO Box 25, Waldron, WA 98297-0025, www. Ryandrum.com. Ryan is living the wild herbal life, close to the land and sea on Waldron Island, and teaches both at home and on the road. Ryan has posted a substantial number of informative articles on his website, and I've learned much of what I know about seaweed from him. He is also an expert on thyroid health.

Kiva Rose Hardin, PO Box 688, Reserve, NM 87830, www.animacenter.org. Kiva Rose has been an informative, inspirational catalyst within the herbal community, especially through her prolific blog writing filled with clear, generous and plant-intuitive writings. She and her partner, Jesse Wolf Hardin, publish a voluminous online magazine, to which I often contribute, called www.PlantHealerMagazine.com. It is gorgeous, and offers a lifetime of herbal education in each issue, as well as art and entertainment. Highly recommended!

Jim McDonald, www.herbcraft.org. Jim is an herbalist from the Great Lakes region. He is the genuine article, devoted to hands-on herbalism, and always finds ways to make challenging concepts come to life with clarity and humor. His site is also an herbal education in itself, listing his own writings, a plethora of other herbalists' articles, and a variety of resources.

ADDITIONAL HERBAL SCHOOLS AND CENTERS

I can also wholeheartedly recommend the following:

Anima Lifeways and Herbal School (see Kiva Rose, above, for contact info). Kiva Rose, Jesse Wolf Hardin, and Loba offer an array of deep, Earth-based programs in "Nature Awareness, Healing, and Rewilding Skills." Check out this beautifully illustrated site for multitudinous offerings through their books, blogs, photos, and much more. Among their fine publications is an invaluable resource book describing many of the herbal conferences offered around the country, called *The Plant Healer Conferences Guide*, which includes their own annual HerbFolk Gathering. It is available for free download at http://bearmedicineherbals.com/herbal-conferences-guide-and-directory.html.

The ArborVitae School of Traditional Herbalism, www.Arbor VitaeNY.com. is rooted in the holistic practice of herbal medicine and exists to provide quality education and training for the clinical, community, and family herbalist.

Third Root, www.ThirdRoot.org. This community health center is a worker-owned cooperative of holistic healthcare practitioners, providing accessible classes and treatments to the Brooklyn community, including herbal medicine classes and programs.

Sage Mountain Herbal Retreat Center and UpS Botanical Sanctuary, PO Box 420, E. Barre, VT 05649, 802-479-9825, www.sagemountain. com. Rosemary is a beautiful teacher, and has inspired thousands of people to love herbs and herbal medicine. She was the original founder of the California School of Herbal Studies, and has also continued to create and nourish the growth of herbal communities through conferences such as the **New England Women's Herbal Conference and the International Herb Symposium.** (See *The Plant Healer Conferences Guide* mentioned above under Anima Lifeways and Herbal School.) Additionally, Rosemary helped found NEHA (see below) and United Plant Savers, a vital plant conservation and educational organization that I encourage readers to support (see below).

Vermont Center for Integrative Herbalism, 252 Main Street, Montpelier, VT 05602, 802-224-7100, www.vtherbcenter.org/. This herbal school provides "extensive clinical training opportunities in herbal medicine, rooted in deep connection with the plants and place." It also has a sliding-scale community clinic. Herbal clinics that serve the community and provide a place for herbal students to learn have been popping up regionally over the past ten years. Cofounder Guido Masé's blog, www.aradicle.blogspot.com, is always interesting, and his new book, *The Wild Medicine Solution*, is excellent; I recommend it highly.

Wise Woman Center, PO Box 64, Woodstock, NY 12498, 845-246-8081, www.SusunWeed.com. Susun Weed is an herbal elder and the author of many books. She is devoted to women's health and spirituality, and is committed to keeping herbal medicine accessible because, as she often says, "herbal medicine is the people's medicine."

HERB COMPANIES

The following companies were created by herbalists who would also be included in my list of highly recommended teachers.

Avena Botanicals, 219 Mill St. Rockport, Maine 04856, www.avena-botanicals.com. Deb Soule's company offers the highest-quality dried herbs, many of which are hand-harvested from her beautiful herb gardens, and much more (including rose blossom glycerite). Her classes and books, and even her herbal catalog, are inspiring as well as informative.

Healing Spirits Herb Farm and Education Center, 61247 State Route 415, Avoca, NY 14809, 607-566-2701, www.healingspiritsherbfarm.com. Herbalists Andrea and Matthias Reisen have been dedicated to growing medicinal herbs for many years and their joy and passion shows in the quality of the herbal medicines they offer for sale.

Herb Haven, www.herbhaven.com. Herbalist Suki Roth offers workshops and apprenticeships out of her deep love and connection with nature. She has a product line of lovingly handmade tea blends and tinctures, including hawthorn blossom glycerite (not easy to find).

Herb Hill, 71 Ferris Lane, Poughkeepsie, NY 12601, 815-485-2563, www.gretchengould.com. Gretchen Gould focuses on topical applications of herbs, and her herbal-salve company provides many unique formulations that are tried-and-true.

Herbalist and Alchemist, 51 South Wandling Ave., Washington, NJ 07882, 908-689-9020, www.Herbalist-Alchemist.com. David Winston's herbal tincture company makes Grief Relief™ as well as many other finely crafted herbal tinctures.

Island Herbs. See Ryan Drum, above, for contact information. I've been buying various seaweeds from Ryan for nearly thirty years, and they are consistently of the best possible quality and taste.

Jean's Greens Herbal Tea Works & Herbal Essentials, 1545 Columbia Turnpike, Schodack, NY 12033, 518-479-0471, www.jeansgreens.org. Holly Applegate continues in the fine tradition of Jean Argus, offering quality herbs and herbalist supplies at reasonable costs, and shipping out with amazing efficiency.

Maine Sea Coast Vegetables, 3 George's Pond Road, Franklin, ME 04634, 207-565-2907, www.seaveg.com. This company specializes in sustainably harvested seaweeds from the North Atlantic Ocean. Founder and primary harvester Larch Hansen's connection to Earth and sea are profound. The stories and photos in his blog are inspirational.

Phoenix Botanicals, www.etsy.com/shop/PhoenixBotanicals. Herbalist Irina Adams creates perfume alive with story and scent, and wildcrafted herbal balms and remedies. She says, "The beauty and healing power of plants renews our connection to the Earth." I love her creations.

Sunstone Farm and Learning Center, www.sunstoneherbs.com/. Jen Prosser is a fabulous herbalist and teacher offering workshops, consultations, and a fine line of herbal tinctures and oils. She lives close to the Earth, and teaches a variety of homesteading skills to foster sustainable living.

Woodland Essence, 392 Teacup Street, Cold Brook, NY 13324, 315-845-1515, www.woodlandessence.com. Kate Gilday is an exceptional herbal teacher and practitioner, and her family-owned company offers medicinal mushrooms, a Fu Zhang herb blend, a delightful rose glycerite, and much more, lovingly and respectfully harvested from the forest.

Zack Woods Herb Farm, 278 Mead Road, Hyde Park, VT 05655, 802-888-7278, www.zackwoodsherbs.com. Jeff and Melanie Carpenter are conscious stewards of their land, and offer gorgeous fresh and dried herbs that sparkle with spirit.

HERBAL ORGANIZATIONS

These are just a sample of a few international, national, and regional organizations, to get you started.

American Botanical Council, www.Herbalgram.org. Founded in 1988, the American Botanical Council is a leading international non-profit organization addressing research and educational issues regarding herbs and medicinal plants.

Herbalists Without Borders, www.Herbalistswithoutborders.weebly. com. This international organization of plant people "creates educational, clinical, advocacy and grassroots model projects to fill the gaps in health care social justice internationally," fueled by a vision of affordable botanical and natural medicine for all.

North Country Herbalist Guild (NCHG), PO Box 4186, St. Paul, MN 55104, www.nchg.org. This is another active local guild that educates, creates community, brings in guest teachers to expand horizons, and actively inspires the kind of local community organizing we need to create everywhere.

Northeast Herbal Association (NEHA), PO Box 5480, Syracuse, NY 13220-5480, www.Northeastherbal.org. I am a longtime member of this lovely grassroots organization. It has a fantastic journal, an annual educational retreat, and a strong focus on creating a vibrant network of community herbalists. All who love herbs and herbal medicine are welcome.

United Plant Savers (the herbal UpS), www.UnitedPlantSavers.org. I am a member of this organization "committed to raising public awareness of the plight of our wild medicinal plants and to protecting these plants through organic cultivation, sustainable agricultural practices, and the replanting of native medicinal species back into their natural habitats." The commercialization of for-big-profit herbal medicine, as well as habitat destruction and loss, has led to the decline of native medicinal plants. UpS offers grants for starting botanical sanctuaries and native-plant gardens. (I started a medicinal plant garden on a piece of trashed public land with the help of a small UpS grant, and it is now a thriving educational medicinal-plant garden for the community.)

WEBSITES AND BLOGS

There are so many informative, well-researched and generous websites that herbalists and others have created to educate people that it is downright impossible to do justice to them all. Here is a small selection of valuable sites—and, as you know, one site leads to another. Please don't forget, as you surf and read and satisfy your mind with information, that going outside and sitting and working with the plants is the ultimate resource. I will always be adding more information and links to my own website too.

www.RobinRoseBennett.com My site features articles, links, an occasional blog, videos, information about my classes, and much more. Also see the links on my site for various online herbal discussion groups, as they are invaluable. Enjoy!

www.Acupuncturebrooklyn.com Well-grounded, meticulously researched, and prolific herbal and health information written by herbalist/acupuncturist Karen Vaughan.

www.NourishingRoot.com Emily Cavelier is an herbalist, chef, and nutrition consultant focused on helping individuals find a deeper level of nourishment and peace of mind through diet and local plants.

www.Chestnutherbs.com Herbalist Juliet Blankespoor's herbal medicine school offers in-depth programs near Asheville, North Carolina in her outdoor "classrooms." Her blog Castanea at www.blog.chestnutherbs .com is brilliant and beautiful.

www.Clearpathherbals.com Herbalist Chris Marano's writings and teaching programs are top-notch. He also offers healing consultations and meticulously hand-crafted herbal tinctures.

www.DoctorDexter.com Margaret Dexter, ND, is an herbalist, naturopathic physician, and all-around wise woman who has a practice in Hawaii and sells her line of organic herbal essentials worldwide. I would trust her with my life—and in fact, I have.

www.drjodynoe.com Jody Noé, MS, ND practices naturopathic medicine and teaches Cherokee medicine. She is a treasure.

www.HerbalConstituents.com is herbalist Lisa Ganora's stunning website on herbal chemistry. Lisa is also the director of the Colorado School of Clinical Herbalism (www.clinicalherbalism.com) in Boulder,

Colorado, and the author of *Herbal Constituents: Foundations of Phytochemistry*.

www.HerbalDale.com Clinical herbalist and registered nurse Dale Bellisfield is a gifted practitioner who is unflinching in addressing even the most challenging of health issues. She is the one other former apprentice (along with Dr. Dexter, above) whom I have trusted with my life when I was very ill.

www.Henriettesherbal.com Finnish herbalist and author Henriette Kress has an extensive herbal website replete with information from many sources and archives of herbal discussion groups and a wonderful blog, and, and, and—check it out!

www.Paulbergner.com Renowned herbalist Paul Bergner is now an elder in the herbal world, and the author of countless articles and many fine books. He teaches widely and is the director of the NAIMH (North American Institute for Medical Herbalism).

Phyllisdlight.com Herbal Studies and the Appalachian Center for Natural Health. Phyllis is a teacher whose herbalism is strongly rooted in the land that she grew up on and where she still lives, yet she travels widely and teaches with passion and skill.

www.radianthealthforlife.com. Bonnie Rogers is a talented herbalist and health coach who uses food and herbs in her practice of helping individuals to be healthy, happy, and radiant.

www.Umm.edu The University of Maryland Medical Center's website often features good articles about herbs, like this one about hawthorn: http://umm.edu/health/medical/altmed/herb/hawthorn

Here is a tiny sampling of my favorite artful, informative, and thought-provoking herbal blogs.

www.GreenManRamblings.com Herbalist, activist, witch, and exquisite writer Sean Donahue writes of plants, nature and healing. In a 2010 post he wrote, "My work as an herbalist is the work of connecting people with plants that can help them find physical, emotional, and spiritual balance. Any resemblance to work intended to diagnose or treat medical conditions is purely incidental."

www.katetemplewest.com/ by herbalist, playwright, educator, and aphrodisiac connoisseur Kate Temple-West.

www.methowvalleyherbs.com Rosalee de la Forêt, who also writes for www.HerbMentor.com, a fabulous online educational program, is not only a marvelous herbalist but a "stitcher of the herbal community," to quote 7Song. Besides her own fine work and two blogs, Rosalee compiled a "master list" of herbal blogs, which can be found at her site.

www.Plantjourneys.blogspot.com Second-generation herbalist, mother, and nature-lover Ananda Wilson's beautiful writing and spirit consistently inspire, and her writing always touches my heart. She offers handcrafted creams and perfumes and also works with Darcy Blue, another inspired blogger and wildcrafter whose blog can be found at www.gaiasgifts.blogspot.com.

http://thesagehoney.wordpress.com/ by poet, herbalist, writer, educator, and mama Mariahadessa Ekere Tallie.

ODDS AND ENDS

A few more resources for you:

Essential oils: Floracopeia makes high quality essential oils and devotes resources to community and environmental restoration projects (www.floracopeia.com).

The George Mateljan Foundation, www.whfoods.com, is a not-for-profit foundation that has published a book called *The World's Healthiest Foods,* and sends out weekly newsletters to subscribers with detailed nutritional information and helpful recipes. These are especially great for people who are trying to change their diet on their own and need some good, clear guidance.

The Herbal Highway, Karyn Sanders's long-running herbal radio show on Pacifica Radio (KPFA), is terrific. Listen up! Karyn also runs the **Blue Otter School of Herbal Medicine** (www.BlueOtterSchool.com).

Herb presses: I got a great little herb press here: https://blitz.goldrush .com/mathrespresses/order.htm.

Honey Gardens, Inc., Ferrisburgh, Vermont, www.honeygardens.com, 802-877-6766.

Jar lids: Tattlers is the only BPA-free brand I've found. I would be happy to learn of any other good options so that we can all support companies with more consciousness and conscientiousness regarding our health and the health of our planet. It may turn out, of course, that there are other chemicals in these lids to be concerned about, but for now these are the best I know of, and I've been slowly but surely replacing all my canning-jar lids with them.

Kapok silk: A company called Carolina Morning sells kapok silk by the pound at www.zafu.net/buckwheat.html.

Phytoremediation and mycoremediation: Here are two sites to visit www.cluin.org/download/citizens/a_citizens_guide_to_phytore mediation.pdf and http://fungiforthepeople.org/mushroom-info /myco-remediation. For hands-on training, see www.earthactivisttraining .org.

Rice rolling papers: The ones I like are called Club Papers, S.D. Modiano, and they can be found in fine smoke shops or online. I'm sure there are other brands, too. Some people prefer clear cellulose papers (or pipes). They can be found in the same establishments or on a great variety of websites.

NOTES

INTRODUCTION

1. There is a fantastic write-up on herbs that Matt has found indispensable in his herbal practice at www.matthewwoodherbs.com. See Bibliography for books by Matthew Wood.

CHAPTER 2

1. The quote at the beginning of the chapter is from Jean Houston's Mystery School, a program that was offered for nearly thirty years. Jean is a visionary educator now teaching social artistry for change-makers around the world. Her multidimensional teachings inspire and empower her students to fulfill their spiritual potential and become active catalysts for profound cultural transformation. More information is available from the Jean Houston Foundation, PO Box 3330, Ashland, OR 97520, 541-482-4240, www.jeanhoustonfoundation.org.

CHAPTER 3

1. I met Doña Enriqueta Contreras, much-beloved Zapotec herbalist and midwife from Oaxaca, Mexico, when she offered her heartful teachings at the International Herb Symposium (see Resources, page 508). I was most fortunate to continue learning from this very special curandera in a more intimate setting at Sage Mountain, Rosemary Gladstar's home and healing center in Vermont (see Resources, page 508). See Bibliography for Mary Margaret Návar's wonderful bilingual book about Grandmother Enriqueta's life.

2. Grandmother Twylah Nitsch (also called Yehwenode, "She Whose Voice Rides the Wind") was a beautiful teacher who founded the Seneca Indian Historical Society and began sharing Seneca wisdom teachings with non-Native people despite controversy in the 1970s. Her teachings and presence resonated deeply with me when I met her in the 1980s, and she is still the guiding light of the Wolf Clan Teaching Lodge. Her books are hard to find but worth searching for, and more information can be found at www.wolfclanteachinglodge.org.

3. Caroline Myss is an internationally noted author and speaker who, upon discovering she was a medical intuitive, left publishing to fulfill

her life's purpose—helping people to awaken to the reality of energy and spirit that underlies physical manifestation, and to help provide the tools that are needed to work within this new paradigm. In the oft-repeated quote at the beginning of this chapter, Caroline is saying that the events of our lives, and especially our emotional and energetic responses to them, literally form our bodies. We can alter our biology and stimulate healing on all levels as we learn to see and reframe our life stories with deeper levels of understanding. (See www.Myss.com, or her book *Anatomy of the Spirit*.)

4. Two good articles that include studies and references regarding hibiscus' ability to lower blood pressure, and information about additional gifts that this beautiful flower can provide, can be found at www.webmd.com/vitamins-and-supplements/hibiscus-uses-and-risks and www.motherearthnews.com/natural-health/lower-blood-pressure -naturally-zmgz11zrog.aspx

CHAPTER 9

1. Herbalist Jim McDonald says he learned much about Solomon's seal from Matt Wood's writings in *The Earthwise Herbal*, and has gone on to use it extensively in his practice. He writes about it at www.herbcraft.org/solseal.html

CHAPTER 11

1. Israeli virologist Dr. Madeleine Mumcuoglu began researching elderberries in the 1970s. When research showed how effective they are against at least ten various strains of flu, she created a company to create and market Sambucol, a syrup that now is the largest-selling elderberry product worldwide.

Also see a randomized study of the efficacy and safety of oral elderberry extract in the treatment of influenza A- and B-virus infections: Z. Zakay-Rones, E. Thom, T. Wollan, J. Wadstein. Department of Virology, Hebrew University-Hadassah Medical School, Jerusalem, Israel. Int Med Res. 2004, Mar-Apr; 32(2): 132-40. Since that original research, additional scientific studies in Israel and elsewhere have shown elderberry to be markedly effective against avian flu, and its ability to increase cytokine production to strengthen the immune system has also been studied and cited.

2. The song "Big Yellow Taxi" was written and recorded by Joni Mitchell in 1970.

CHAPTER 12

1. This information can be found on the American Cancer Society website at: www.cancer.org/treatment/treatmentsandsideeffects /complementaryandalternativemedicine/herbsvitaminsandminerals /white-birch

CHAPTER 13

1. Aviva Romm, MD, home-birth midwife, fabulous herbal educator, and author of numerous valuable herbal medicine books for women and healthcare practitioners. This information was contained in blog posts at http://avivaromm.com/blog on May 22 and June 11, 2013.

2. Rosita Arvigo is a superb herbalist whose books and classes I highly recommend. She travels frequently, often to the United States. You can find out more about her work, including Mayan uterine massage, from The Arvigo Institute, LLC, Box 189, Antrim, NH 03440, 603-588-2571, https://arvigotherapy.com/

CHAPTER 14

1. This study on using honey for burns comes from the journal of the University Department of Surgery, University Teaching Hospital, Calabar, Nigeria. *Br J Surg*, July 1988; 75(7): 679-81.

2. This 2007 study is written up at the Penn State College of Medicine, Archives of Pediatrics and Adolescent Medicine, researchers led by Ian Paul, MD, MSc.

CHAPTER 17

1. "Changes in Heart Transplant Recipients That Parallel the Personalities of Their Donors" by Dr. Paul Pearsall, Gary E. R. Schwartz, and Linda G. S. Russek was published in *The Journal of Near-Death Studies*, Volume 20, Issue 3, pp. 19–206, 2002. It is also available at www.ncbi.nlm.nih.gov/pubmed/10882878

BIBLIOGRAPHY

THE FOLLOWING WORKS WERE CONSULTED in the writing of this book and/or are recommended for further reading. Please consider the authors I referenced here (many of whom currently teach classes, run schools, guide plant walks, and/or offer consultations) as invaluable resources.

Baggaley, Ann, ed. *Human Body: An Illustrated Guide to the Human Body and How It Works.* London and New York: Dorling Kindersley (DK) Books, 2001.

Bennett, Robin Rose. *Healing Magic: A Green Witch Guidebook to Conscious Living,* 2nd ed. Bearfort Mountain, NJ: Gaia Rose Publishing, 2004.

———. "Wild Carrot: A Plant for Conscious, Natural Contraception." http://robinrosebennett.com/articles/wild-carrot-daucus-carota-a-plant-for-conscious-natural-contraception/

Bethel, May. *The Healing Power of Natural Foods.* Hollywood: Wilshire Book Company, 1978.

Binder, Dr. Hendryk (Walking Night Bear) and Stan Padilla. *Song of the Seven Herbs.* Nevada City, CA: Gold Circle Productions, 1983.

Brill, Steve (Wildman) with Evelyn Dean. *Identifying and Harvesting Edible and Medicinal Plants in Wild (and Not So Wild) Places.* NY: Hearst Books, 1994.

Buchman, Dian Dincin. *Herbal Medicine: The Natural Way to Get Well and Stay Well.* NY: Gramercy Publishing, 1980.

Buhner, Stephen Harrod. *The Secret Teachings of Plants: The Intelligence of the Heart in the Direct Perception of Nature.* Rochester, VT: Bear & Company, 2004.

Casey, Caroline W. *Making the Gods Work for You: The Astrological Language of the Psyche.* Harmony Books, 1997.

Edwards, Gail Faith. *Opening Our Wild Hearts to the Healing Plants.* Woodstock, NY: Ash Tree Publishing, 2000.

Elpel, Thomas J. *Botany in a Day: The Patterns Method of Plant Identification,* 6th ed. Hops Press, 2013.

Elson, Lawrence M. and Wynn Kapit. *The Anatomy Coloring Book,* 2nd ed. HarperCollins, 1993.

The Federation of Feminist Women's Health Centers. *How to Stay Out of the Gynecologist's Office*, 3rd ed. Culver City, CA: Women to Women Publications, 1986.

Foster, Steven and James A. Duke. *Eastern/Central Medicinal Plants*. The Peterson Field Guide Series. Houghton Mifflin, 1990.

Gladstar, Rosemary. *Herbal Healing for Women: Simple Home Remedies for Women of All Ages*. Simon and Schuster, 1993.

Goodman, Anthony, MD, FAS. *Understanding the Human Body: An Introduction to Anatomy and Physiology*. Chantilly, WV: The Great Courses, 2004.

Green, James. *The Male Herbal: Health Care for Men & Boys*. Freedom, CA: The Crossing Press, 1991.

Grieve, Maud. *A Modern Herbal, Volumes I & II*. NY: Dover, 1931. Also available online at www.botanical.com.

Hobbs, Christopher, LAc. *Medicinal Mushrooms: An Exploration of Tradition, Healing, & Culture*. Santa Cruz, CA: Botanica Press, 1995.

Hoffmann, David. *The Herb User's Guide*. Rochester, VT: Thorsons Publishing Group, 1987.

Hutchens, Alma. *Indian Herbology of North America: The Definitive Guide to Native Medicinal Plants and Their Uses*. Boston and London: Shambala, 1991.

Jarvis, D. C., MD. *Folk Medicine: A Doctor's Guide to Good Health*. London: Pan Books Limited, 1961.

Kress, Henriette. *Practical Herbs*. Helsinki: Yrtit ja yrttiterapia, 2011.

Levy, Juliette de Bairacli. *Common Herbs for Natural Health*. Woodstock, NY: Ash Tree Publishing, 1997.

Lipton, Dr. Bruce H. *The Biology of Belief: Unleashing the Power of Consciousness, Matter and Miracles*. Hay House, 2008.

Mairesse, Michelle. *Health Secrets of Medicinal Herbs*. New York: Arco Publishing, 1981.

Masé, Guido. *The Wild Medicine Solution*. Rochester, VT: Inner Traditions, 2013.

McIntyre, Anne. *Ayurveda for Women*. www.AnneMcIntyre.com

Moore, Michael. *Medicine Plants of the Pacific West*. Museum of New Mexico, 2011.

Myss, Caroline. *Anatomy of the Spirit*. Harmony, 1997.

Návar, Mary Margaret, *Zapotec Woman of the Clouds: The Life of Enriqueta Contreras Contreras*. Austin, TX: Zapotec Press, 2010.

Nissim, Rina. *Natural Healing in Gynecology: A Manual for Women*. Pandora Press, 1986.

Robertson, Diane. *Jamaican Herbs: Nutritional & Medicinal Values*. Self-published, dist. by DeSola Pinto Associates, Montego Bay, Jamaica, West Indies, 1982.

Skenderi, Gazmend. *Herbal Vade Mecum: 800 Herbs, Spices, Essential Oils, Lipids, Etc., Constituents, Properties, Uses, and Caution*. Rutherford, NJ: Herbacy Press, 2004.

Smith, Ed. *Therapeutic Herb Manual: A Guide to the Safe and Effective Use of Liquid Herbal Extracts*. Williams, OR: Ed Smith, 2004.

Somé, Malidoma Patrice. *Ritual: Power, Healing, and Community*. NY: Penguin Compass, 1997.

Thomas, Lalitha. *10 Essential Herbs*. One World Press, 2011.

Tierra, Michael, LAc, OMD. *The Way of Herbs*. Pocket Books, 1998.

Treban, Maria. *Health Through God's Pharmacy: Advice and Proven Cures with Medicinal Herbs*. Steyr, Austria: Ennsthaler Verlag, 2007.

Wardwell, Joyce. *The Herbal Home Remedy Book*. North Adams, MA: Storey Publishing, 1998.

Weed, Susun. *Healing Wise*. Woodstock, NY: Ash Tree Publishing, 1989.

———. *Breast Cancer, Breast Health!* Woodstock, NY: Ash Tree Publishing, 1996.

Winston, David. *Herbal Therapeutics: Specific Indications for Herbs and Herbal Formulas*. Broadway, NJ: Herbal Therapeutics Research Library, 2003.

——— and Steven Maimes. *Adaptogens: Herbs for Strength, Stamina, and Stress Relief*. Rochester, VT: Healing Arts Press, 2007.

Wood, Matthew. *The Book of Herbal Wisdom: Using Plants as Medicines*. Berkeley, CA: North Atlantic Books, 1997.

INDEX

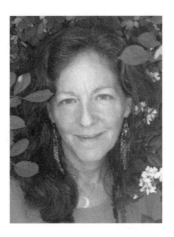

ABOUT THE AUTHOR

ROBIN ROSE BENNETT IS A COMPASSIONATE, empowering herbalist and spiritual teacher. The focus of her healing work is to share the generosity of the earth and the magic, mystery, and beauty of the web of life. Since 1986 she has taught at schools, clinics, progressive and holistic organizations, herbal conferences, and has guest lectured at Albert Einstein College of Medicine, St John's Hospital, Montefiore Teaching Hospital, Beth Israel's Nursing program, and Brown University Medical School. She is a faculty member of the Arbor Vitae School of Traditional Herbal Medicine and the New York Open Center and author of two meditation CDs. Bennett has a private consultation practice in New Jersey, and an herbalist-in-residence teaching practice at a family medical practice in Bronx, New York, offering consultations on a sliding scale. She is a long-time member of United Plant Savers and the Northeast Herbal Association. Bennett writes regularly for *Plant Healer* magazine and is proud to be a founding member, medicinal garden cocreator, and on the board of directors of SustainableWestMilford.org. Hundreds of apprentices have graduated from her three-year, in-depth apprenticeship programs over the past twenty-five years and thousands of students have benefitted from her regular classes as well as free classes that she regularly offers in her town as a community service. The author lives in Hewitt, New Jersey.